Diagnosis and Treatment of Pancreatic Cancer

Diagnosis and Treatment of Pancreatic Cancer

Edited by Russell Princeton

hayle
medical

New York

Hayle Medical,
750 Third Avenue, 9th Floor,
New York, NY 10017, USA

Visit us on the World Wide Web at:
www.haylemedical.com

ISBN: 978-1-63241-689-6

Cataloging-in-Publication Data

Diagnosis and treatment of pancreatic cancer / edited by Russell Princeton.
    p. cm.
Includes bibliographical references and index.
ISBN 978-1-63241-689-6
1. Pancreas--Cancer. 2. Pancreas--Cancer--Diagnosis. 3. Pancreas--Cancer--Treatment.
I. Princeton, Russell.
RC280.P25 D53 2019
616.994 37--dc23

Table of Contents

Preface.. IX

Chapter 1   **Deferasirox, a novel oral iron chelator, shows antiproliferative activity against pancreatic cancer in vitro and in vivo**.. 1
Hirofumi Harima, Seiji Kaino, Taro Takami, Shuhei Shinoda, Toshihiko Matsumoto, Koichi Fujisawa, Naoki Yamamoto, Takahiro Yamasaki and Isao Sakaida

Chapter 2   **γ-Tocotrienol induces apoptosis in pancreatic cancer cells by upregulation of ceramide synthesis and modulation of sphingolipid transport**........................... 11
Victoria E. Palau, Kanishka Chakraborty, Daniel Wann, Janet Lightner, Keely Hilton, Marianne Brannon, William Stone and Koyamangalath Krishnan

Chapter 3   **A non-controlled, single arm, open label, phase II study of intravenous and intratumoral administration of ParvOryx in patients with metastatic, inoperable pancreatic cancer: ParvOryx02 protocol**... 25
Jacek Hajda, Monika Lehmann, Ottheinz Krebs, Meinhard Kieser, Karsten Geletneky, Dirk Jäger, Michael Dahm, Bernard Huber, Tilman Schöning, Oliver Sedlaczek, Albrecht Stenzinger, Niels Halama, Volker Daniel, Barbara Leuchs, Assia Angelova, Jean Rommelaere, Christine E. Engeland, Christoph Springfeld and Guy Ungerechts

Chapter 4   **An elevated expression of serum exosomal microRNA-191, − 21, −451a of pancreatic neoplasm is considered to be efficient diagnostic marker**........................ 35
Takuma Goto, Mikihiro Fujiya, Hiroaki Konishi, Junpei Sasajima, Shugo Fujibayashi, Akihiro Hayashi, Tatsuya Utsumi, Hiroki Sato, Takuya Iwama, Masami Ijiri, Aki Sakatani, Kazuyuki Tanaka, Yoshiki Nomura, Nobuhiro Ueno, Shin Kashima, Kentaro Moriichi, Yusuke Mizukami, Yutaka Kohgo and Toshikatsu Okumura

Chapter 5   **Treatment of pancreatic ductal adenocarcinoma with tumor antigen specific-targeted delivery of paclitaxel loaded PLGA nanoparticles**........................ 46
Shu-ta Wu, Anthony J. Fowler, Corey B. Garmon, Adam B. Fessler, Joshua D. Ogle, Kajal R. Grover, Bailey C. Allen, Chandra D. Williams, Ru Zhou, Mahboubeh Yazdanifar, Craig A. Ogle and Pinku Mukherjee

Chapter 6   **A phase II study to evaluate LY2603618 in combination with gemcitabine in pancreatic cancer patients**.. 59
Berta Laquente, Jose Lopez-Martin, Donald Richards, Gerald Illerhaus, David Z. Chang, George Kim, Philip Stella, Dirk Richel, Cezary Szcylik, Stefano Cascinu, G. L. Frassineti, Tudor Ciuleanu, Karla Hurt, Scott Hynes, Ji Lin, Aimee Bence Lin, Daniel Von Hoff and Emiliano Calvo

Chapter 7   **Nanoliposomal irinotecan with fluorouracil for the treatment of advanced pancreatic cancer, a single institution experience**.. 68
Danielle C. Glassman, Randze L. Palmaira, Christina M. Covington, Avni M. Desai, Geoffrey Y. Ku, Jia Li, James J. Harding, Anna M. Varghese, Eileen M. O'Reilly and Kenneth H. Yu

Chapter 8   **The Warburg effect in human pancreatic cancer cells triggers cachexia in athymic mice carrying the cancer cells** 78
Feng Wang, Hongyi Liu, Lijuan Hu, Yunfei Liu, Yijie Duan, Rui Cui
and Wencong Tian

Chapter 9   **Trends in pancreatic adenocarcinoma incidence and mortality in the United States in the last four decades; a SEER-based study** 90
Anas M. Saad, Tarek Turk, Muneer J. Al-Husseini and Omar Abdel-Rahman

Chapter 10   **Programmed cell death ligand 1 cut-point is associated with reduced disease specific survival in resected pancreatic ductal adenocarcinoma** 101
Basile Tessier-Cloutier, Steve E. Kalloger, Mohammad Al-Kandari, Katy Milne,
Dongxia Gao, Brad H. Nelson, Daniel J. Renouf, Brandon S. Sheffield
and David F. Schaeffer

Chapter 11   **A phase-I trial of pre-operative, margin intensive, stereotactic body radiation therapy for pancreatic cancer: the 'SPARC' trial protocol** 110
Daniel L. P. Holyoake, Elizabeth Ward, Derek Grose, David McIntosh,
David Sebag-Montefiore, Ganesh Radhakrishna, Neel Patel, Michael Silva,
Somnath Mukherjee, Victoria Y. Strauss, Lang'o Odondi, Emmanouil Fokas,
Alan Melcher and Maria A. Hawkins

Chapter 12   **Cytoplasmic TRAIL-R1 is a positive prognostic marker in PDAC** 118
Jan-Paul Gundlach, Charlotte Hauser, Franka Maria Schlegel, Christine Böger,
Christian Röder, Christoph Röcken, Thomas Becker, Jan-Hendrik Egberts,
Holger Kalthoff and Anna Trauzold

Chapter 13   **Treatment recommendations within the leeway of clinical guidelines: A qualitative interview study on oncologists' clinical deliberation** 128
I. Otte, S. Salloch, A. Reinacher-Schick and J. Vollmann

Chapter 14   **Evaluation of pancreatic cancer cell migration with multiple parameters in vitro by using an optical real-time cell mobility assay device** 134
Akira Yamauchi, Masahiro Yamamura, Naoki Katase, Masumi Itadani,
Naoko Okada, Kayoko Kobiki, Masafumi Nakamura, Yoshiyuki Yamaguchi and
Futoshi Kuribayashi

Chapter 15   **A Phase I clinical trial of EUS-guided intratumoral injection of the oncolytic virus, HF10 for unresectable locally advanced pancreatic cancer** 145
Yoshiki Hirooka, Hideki Kasuya, Takuya Ishikawa, Hiroki Kawashima,
Eizaburo Ohno, Itzel B. Villalobos, Yoshinori Naoe, Toru Ichinose, Nobuto Koyama,
Maki Tanaka, Yasuhiro Kodera and Hidemi Goto

Chapter 16   **Inhibition of Six1 affects tumour invasion and the expression of cancer stem cell markers in pancreatic cancer** 154
Tristan Lerbs, Savita Bisht, Sebastian Schölch, Mathieu Pecqueux, Glen Kristiansen,
Martin Schneider, Bianca T. Hofmann, Thilo Welsch, Christoph Reissfelder,
Nuh N. Rahbari, Johannes Fritzmann, Peter Brossart, Jürgen Weitz,
Georg Feldmann and Christoph Kahlert

Chapter 17   **Loss of PDPK1 abrogates resistance to gemcitabine in label-retaining pancreatic cancer cells** 163
Dandan Li, John E. Mullinax, Taylor Aiken, Hongwu Xin, Gordon Wiegand,
Andrew Anderson, Snorri Thorgeirsson, Itzhak Avital and Udo Rudloff

Chapter 18   **A novel feedback loop between high MALAT-1 and low miR-200c-3p promotes cell migration and invasion in pancreatic ductal adenocarcinoma and is predictive of poor prognosis**.. 178
            Meng Zhuo, Cuncun Yuan, Ting Han, Jiujie Cui, Feng Jiao and Liwei Wang

Chapter 19   **Meta-analysis on resected pancreatic cancer: a comparison between adjuvant treatments and gemcitabine alone** 189
            Hua Chen, Ruizhi He, Xiuhui Shi, Min Zhou, Chunle Zhao, Hang Zhang and Renyi Qin

Permissions

List of Contributors

Index

Preface

When cells in the pancreas multiply uncontrollably and form a mass, the condition is called pancreatic cancer. When cancer arises in the part responsible for the production of digestive enzymes, it is termed as exocrine pancreatic cancer. When it arises in the hormone-producing tissue of the pancreas, it is called pancreatic neuroendocrine tumor (PanNET). The common symptoms associated with pancreatic adenocarcinoma are the occurrence of jaundice, diabetes, pain in the upper abdomen, unexplained weight loss, etc. PanNETs give rise to symptoms that are consistent either with the over-production of different active hormones or only show symptoms when it has spread to other parts of the body, depending on the type of the PanNET. Pancreatic cancer is diagnosed by a combination of blood tests, medical imaging techniques such as CT or ultrasound, and biopsies. The treatment of pancreatic cancer is based on the stage of the cancer. It can be treated through the modes of surgery, chemotherapy and radiotherapy or a combination of these. This book provides comprehensive insights into pancreatic cancer. It provides significant information of the clinical aspects of pancreatic cancer from diagnosis to treatment. It is appropriate for students seeking detailed information in this area as well as for experts.

Various studies have approached the subject by analyzing it with a single perspective, but the present book provides diverse methodologies and techniques to address this field. This book contains theories and applications needed for understanding the subject from different perspectives. The aim is to keep the readers informed about the progresses in the field; therefore, the contributions were carefully examined to compile novel researches by specialists from across the globe.

Indeed, the job of the editor is the most crucial and challenging in compiling all chapters into a single book. In the end, I would extend my sincere thanks to the chapter authors for their profound work. I am also thankful for the support provided by my family and colleagues during the compilation of this book.

Editor

Deferasirox, a novel oral iron chelator, shows antiproliferative activity against pancreatic cancer in vitro and in vivo

Hirofumi Harima[1†], Seiji Kaino[1*], Taro Takami[1†], Shuhei Shinoda[1], Toshihiko Matsumoto[1,2], Koichi Fujisawa[1], Naoki Yamamoto[1], Takahiro Yamasaki[2] and Isao Sakaida[1]

Abstract

Background: Iron is essential for cell replication, metabolism and growth. Because neoplastic cells have high iron requirements due to their rapid proliferation, iron depletion may be a novel therapeutic strategy for cancer. Deferasirox (DFX), a novel oral iron chelator, has been successful in clinical trials in iron-overload patients and has been expected to become an anticancer agent. However, no studies have investigated the effects of DFX on pancreatic cancer. This study aimed to elucidate the effects of DFX against pancreatic cancer.

Methods: The effects of DFX on cell cycle, proliferation, and apoptosis were examined in three human pancreatic cancer cell lines: BxPC-3, HPAF-II, and Panc 10.05. The effect of orally administered DFX on the growth of BxPC-3 pancreatic cancer xenografts was also examined in nude mice. Additionally, microarray analysis was performed using tumors excised from xenografts.

Results: DFX inhibited pancreatic cancer cell proliferation in a dose-dependent manner. A concentration of 10 μM DFX arrested the cell cycle in S phase, whereas 50 and 100 μM DFX induced apoptosis. In nude mice, orally administered DFX at 160 and 200 mg/kg suppressed xenograft tumor growth with no serious side effects ($n = 5$; average tumor volumes of 674 mm^3 for controls vs. 327 mm^3 for 160 mg/kg DFX, $p < 0.05$; average tumor volumes of 674 mm^3 for controls vs. 274 mm^3 for 200 mg/kg DFX, $p < 0.05$). Importantly, serum biochemistry analysis indicated that serum levels of ferritin were significantly decreased by the oral administration of 160 or 200 mg/kg DFX ($n = 5$; average serum ferritin of 18 ng/ml for controls vs. 9 ng/ml for 160 mg/kg DFX, $p < 0.05$; average serum ferritin of 18 ng/ml for controls vs. 10 ng/ml for 200 mg/kg DFX, $p < 0.05$). Gene expression analysis revealed that most genes in pancreatic adenocarcinoma signaling, especially transforming growth factor-ß1 (TGF-ß1), were downregulated by DFX.

Conclusions: DFX has potential as a therapeutic agent for pancreatic cancer. Iron depletion was essential for the antiproliferative effect of DFX in a preclinical model, and DFX acted through the suppression of TGF-ß signaling.

Keywords: Deferasirox, Iron chelator, Pancreatic cancer

Abbreviations: DFO, Deferoxamine; DFX, Deferasirox; EMT, Epithelial-mesenchymal transition; IPA, Ingenuity pathway analysis; MTS, 3-(4,5-dimethylthiazol-2-yl)-5-(3-carboxymethoxyphenyl)-2-(4-sulfophenyl)-2H-tetrazolium, inner salt; PBS, Phosphate-buffered saline; PI, Propidium iodide; TGF- ß, Transforming growth factor-ß

* Correspondence: kaino@yamaguchi-u.ac.jp
†Equal contributors
[1]Department of Gastroenterology and Hepatology, Yamaguchi University Graduate School of Medicine, 1-1-1 Minami-Kogushi, Ube, Yamaguchi 755-8505, Japan
Full list of author information is available at the end of the article

Background

Pancreatic cancer is the fifth leading cause of cancer-related deaths, and the number of cases has been increasing in Japan [1]. It is the fifth and fourth leading cause of cancer-related deaths in Europe and in North America, respectively [2]. Pancreatic cancer is associated with the worst prognosis among solid tumors [3]; the 5-year survival rate of pancreatic cancer, including resectable cases, is not more than 10 % [4]. Surgical resection is the only potential curative therapy, but many patients with pancreatic cancer are not candidates for surgical resection at the time of diagnosis. For patients with unresectable pancreatic cancer, chemotherapy is recommended as the current standard care [5]. During the last two decades, gemcitabine has been the standard chemotherapy for pancreatic cancer. Recently, new combination chemotherapies have been developed, such as regimens combining fluorouracil, irinotecan, oxaliplatin, and leucovorin (FOLFIRINOX) or albumin-bound paclitaxel with gemcitabine [6, 7]. However, while combination chemotherapies have shown therapeutic advantages over single-agent gemcitabine, they also have a high incidence of side effects. In addition, more than half of pancreatic cancer patients are diagnosed at an age of 65 years or older [4]. Therefore, a new chemotherapeutic strategy for pancreatic cancer is required for these patients with refractory chemotherapy due to side effects and/or advanced age.

Iron is essential for cell replication, metabolism and growth [8]. Because neoplastic cells have high iron requirements due to their rapid proliferation, iron depletion could be a novel therapeutic strategy for cancer [9]. Although iron chelators, which are commonly used for treating iron-overload disease, are not classified as anticancer drugs; they exert antiproliferative effects in several cancers [10–12]. We have reported that deferoxamine (DFO), a standard iron chelator, can prevent the development of liver preneoplastic lesions in rats [13]. We also performed a pilot study using DFO in advanced hepatocellular carcinoma patients and reported the efficacy of this iron chelator [14]. Considering the mechanism of action of iron chelators as anticancer agents, as well as other cancers, iron chelators are thought to be effective pancreatic cancer treatments. Kovacevic et al. reported that thiosemicarbazone iron chelators inhibited pancreatic cancer growth in vitro and in vivo [15]. Therefore, iron chelators represent a potential therapeutic strategy for pancreatic cancer. However, most iron chelators, including DFO and thiosemicarbazones, cannot be administered orally, thus limiting their clinical application.

Recently, deferasirox (DFX), a newly developed oral iron chelator, was successful in clinical trials in iron-overload disease patients and has been implemented as an alternative to DFO [16]. A number of in vitro and in vivo studies have demonstrated that DFX has powerful antiproliferative effects [17]. To our knowledge, there have been no studies investigating the effects of DFX against pancreatic cancer. Therefore, this study aimed to evaluate the antiproliferative activity of DFX against pancreatic cancer in vitro and in vivo.

Methods

Cell culture

The pancreatic cancer cell lines BxPC-3, HPAF-II, and Panc 10.05 were obtained from the American Type Culture Collection (Manassas, VA, USA). BxPC-3 and Panc 10.05 cells are epithelial cell lines that were derived from pancreatic adenocarcinomas. The HPAF-II cell line consists of epithelial cells derived from ascites that originated from pancreatic adenocarcinomas.

BxPC-3 cells were grown in RPMI-1640 (Life Technologies, Carlsbad, CA, USA) with 10 % (v/v) fetal calf serum. HPAF-II cells were grown in Eagle's medium (Life Technologies) with 10 % (v/v) fetal calf serum. Panc 10.05 cells were grown in RPMI-1640 (Life Technologies) containing 10 units/ml of human recombinant insulin, and 15 % (v/v) fetal calf serum. All media were supplemented with 50 μg/ml gentamicin. All cells were incubated at 37 °C in a humidified atmosphere containing 5 % CO_2.

Reagents

The oral iron chelator DFX was obtained from Novartis (Basel, Switzerland). For in vitro studies, DFX was dissolved in dimethyl sulfoxide at a stock concentration of 100 mM and was used at the concentrations indicated in the results and figures by dilution in culture media containing 10 % fetal calf serum. For in vivo studies, DFX was dissolved in sodium chloride solution (0.9 % w/v; Chemix Inc., Shinyokohama Kohoku-ku, Yokohama, Japan).

Cell proliferation

Cellular proliferation was examined using the 3-(4,5-dimethylthiazol-2-yl)-5-(3-carboxymethoxyphenyl)-2-(4-sulfophenyl)-2H-tetrazolium, inner salt (MTS) assay. Cell suspensions (2,000 cells/100 μl) were added to each well in a 96-multiwell culture plate (BD Bioscience, San Jose, CA, USA) and incubated at 37 °C for 24 h. The indicated concentrations of DFX were then added to each well, and the cells were incubated for a further 72 h. At the end of the culture period, 10 μl of MTS solution (Promega, Madison, WI, USA) was added to each 100 μl of culture media and incubated for 2 h. Absorbance at 490 nm was measured with a multimode reader (Infinite 200 PRO, Tecan Trading, AG, Switzerland), and the results are expressed as the percentage viable with respect to the untreated control.

Cell cycle analysis

Each pancreatic cancer cell line was seeded into 100-mm dishes and cultured with phosphate-buffered saline (PBS) as a vehicle control or DFX at 10, 50, or 100 μM for 72 h. After incubation, the cells were fixed with 70 % ethanol and stored overnight at -20 °C. The cells were washed and then stained with a solution containing 0.1 % Triton® X-100 (Promega), 0.02 mg/ml propidium iodide (PI; Sigma-Aldrich, St. Louis, MO, USA), and 0.2 mg/ml RNase A (Qiagen, Hilden, Germany) in the dark at 37 °C for 15 min. After staining, the cells were subjected to cellular DNA content examination by a flow cytometer (Gallios, Beckman Coulter, Fullerton, CA, USA). The data were analyzed by Multicycle for Windows software (Beckman Coulter).

Apoptosis analysis by flow cytometry

For the apoptosis analysis, the cells were cultured as described above. After harvesting, apoptosis was evaluated with an apoptosis detection kit (Annexin V Apoptosis Detection Kit APC, eBioscience, San Diego, CA, USA) according to the manufacturer's instructions. After staining, the cells were examined using a flow cytometer (Gallios, Beckman Coulter). The data were analyzed by FlowJo software (Tree star, Ashland, OR, USA).

Apoptosis analysis with the luminescence assay

Cell suspensions (2,000 cells/100 μl) were added to each well of a 96-multiwell culture plate (BD Bioscience) and were incubated at 37 °C for 24 h. PBS as a vehicle control or the indicated concentrations of DFX were then added to each well, and the cells were further incubated for 48 h. Immediately after the incubation, caspase activity was measured using the caspase 3/7 assay kit (Caspase-Glo 3/7 kit, Promega) according to the manufacturer's instructions.

Tumor xenografts in nude mice and deferasirox administration

Animal care was performed in accordance with the animal ethics requirements at Yamaguchi University School of Medicine, and the experimental protocol was approved (approval ID 21-035). Twenty female BALB/c (nu/nu) mice were purchased from Nippon SLC (Shizuoka, Japan) and were housed in sterile conditions. Experiments commenced when the mice were 8–10 weeks of age. Tumor cells (BxPC-3) in culture were harvested and resuspended in a 1:1 ratio of RPMI-1640 and Matrigel (BD Bioscience). Viable cells (5×10^6 cells) were injected subcutaneously into the backs of the mice. After engraftment, tumor size was measured using Vernier calipers every 2 days, and tumor volume was calculated as follows: tumor volume (mm^3) = (the longest diameter) (mm) $\times$ (the shortest diameter) (mm)/2. When tumor volumes reached 150 mm^3, oral treatment began (day 0). Each group of mice ($n = 5$) received DFX suspended in saline, which was administered by oral gavage every second day, with three treatments per week, over 21 days at concentrations of 120, 160, or 200 mg/kg. The control mice were treated with the vehicle alone. At the end of the experiment, the mice were sacrificed, and the tumors were excised and processed for immunohistochemistry and genetic analyses. A total of 20 blood samples were collected simultaneously during tumor removal. Serum levels of ferritin were measured using the enzyme-linked immunoassay method (Mouse Ferritin ELISA kit, Kamiya Biochemical Company, Seattle, WA, USA). Serum biochemistry with the exception of ferritin was analyzed by YAMAGUCHI Laboratory Co., Ltd. (Ube, Japan).

Immunohistochemistry

The removed tumors were fixed in 4 % paraformaldehyde (Muto-kagaku, Tokyo, Japan), sectioned, and embedded in paraffin. Immunohistochemistry was performed as previously described on the paraffin sections with antibody specific to ferritin-H (Anti-Ferritin Heavy Chain antibody, AbCam, Cambridge, MA, USA) [18]. The slides were scored according to the intensity of the immunoreactivity and the percentage of epithelial cells stained [19].

The detection of gene expression alternation in resected tumors induced by deferasirox administration

Total RNA isolation

A total of six tumors were genetically analyzed. Of these, three tumors were removed from vehicle-treated mice, and the other three tumors were removed from DFX 200 mg/kg-treated mice. According to the manufacturer's instructions, total RNA was isolated from the removal tumors using TRIzol Reagent (Invitrogen Corp., CA, USA) and purified using the SV Total RNA Isolation System (Promega). RNA samples were quantified using a NanoDrop ND-1000 spectrophotometer (Thermo Fisher Scientific Inc., Wilmington, DE, USA), and RNA quality was checked using an Experion automated electrophoresis station (Bio-Rad Laboratories Inc., Hercules, CA, USA).

Gene expression microarrays

The cRNA was amplified, labeled, and hybridized to a 60K Agilent 60-mer oligomicroarray according to the manufacturer's instructions. All hybridized microarray slides were scanned by an Agilent scanner. Relative hybridization intensities and background hybridization values were calculated using Agilent Feature Extraction Software (9.5.1.1).

Data analysis and filter criteria

The raw signal intensities of all samples were $\log_2$-transformed and normalized with a quantile algorithm from the 'preprocessCore' library package [20] on Bioconductor software [21]. We selected the probes, excluding the control probes, where the detection p-values of all samples were less than 0.05, and used them to identify differentially expressed genes. To determine significant enrichment canonical pathways, we used the tools and data provide by the Ingenuity Pathway Analysis (IPA) (Ingenuity Systems, INC. http://www.ingenuity.com). The results are the comparisons of tumors removed from vehicle-treated mice vs. the tumors removed from DFX 200 mg/kg-treated mice.

Statistical analyses

All obtained data are calculated and expressed as the mean ± SD. In the in vitro experiments, the differences were analyzed statistically using 1-way ANOVA, followed by Dannett's test. In the in vivo experiments, the differences were analyzed statistically using the Kruskal-Wallis H test, followed by Steel's test. JMP 9 statistical software (SAS Institute Inc., Cary, NC, USA) was used in the analysis. Values of p <0.05 were considered significant.

Results

DFX inhibited cell proliferation in pancreatic cancer cell lines

To examine the antiproliferative activity of DFX against pancreatic cancer in vitro, the pancreatic cancer cell lines BxPC-3, HPAF-II, and Panc 10.05 were incubated with either vehicle control (PBS) or the indicated concentrations of DFX for 72 h; then, the cell survival rates were measured using the MTS assay. The cell survival rates are shown in Fig. 1. Incubation of all three cell lines with DFX inhibited cellular proliferation in a dose-dependent manner. DFX had the same level of

antiproliferative activity in all three cell lines. As indicated in Table 1, the IC_{50} values for the BxPC-3, HPAF-II, and Panc 10.05 pancreatic cancer cell lines were 7.3 ± 1.0, 5.6 ± 1.0, and 6.1 ± 0.2 μM, respectively. There were no significant differences in the IC_{50} values of each pancreatic cancer cell line.

DFX arrested the cell cycle at the S phase in pancreatic cancer cell lines

To explore the mechanism of the antiproliferative activity of DFX, the pancreatic cancer cell lines BxPC-3, HPAF-II, and Panc 10.0 were incubated with either the vehicle control (PBS) or 10, 50, or 100 μM concentrations of DFX for 72 h, and the cell cycle was examined with flow cytometry using PI staining. The analyzed results are shown in Fig. 2a, and the percentage of S phase cells are highlighted in pink. The percentage of S phase cells for each concentration of DFX is shown in Fig. 2b. In all three cell lines, the percentage of S phase cells incubated with 10 μM concentration of DFX was increased. These results demonstrated that 10 μM DFX arrested the cell cycle of pancreatic cancer cells in S phase.

DFX induced apoptosis in pancreatic cancer cell lines

To further characterize the mechanisms of the antiproliferative activity of DFX, the pancreatic cancer cell lines BxPC-3, HPAF-II, and Panc 10.0 were incubated with either the vehicle control (PBS) or concentrations of 10, 50, or 100 μM of DFX for 72 h, and apoptosis was examined by flow cytometry using PI and Annexin V staining. The results are shown in Fig. 3a. The amount of live cells was defined as the number of cells negative for both Annexin V and PI. The amount of cells in early apoptosis was defined as cells positive for Annexin V only, whereas late apoptosis was defined as cells positive for both Annexin V and PI. The amount of necrotic cells was defined as the cells negative for Annexin V but

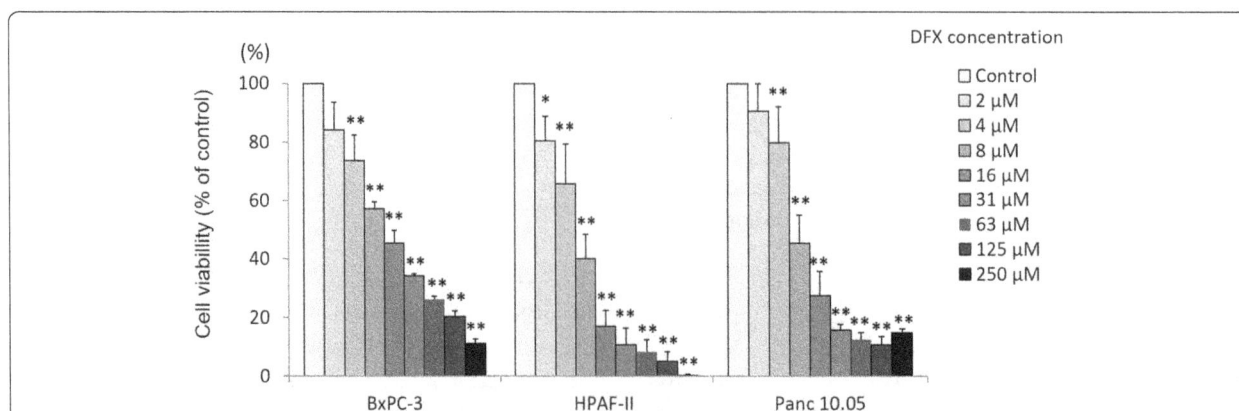

Fig. 1 DFX inhibited the proliferation of pancreatic cancer cell lines. Cell proliferation was measured using the MTS assay after cells were treated with DFX 72 h. The viability of BxPC-3, HPAF-II, and Panc 10.05 cells incubated with DFX decreased in a dose-dependent manner. The data are presented as the mean ± SD ($n = 3$–5). *p <0.05, **p <0.01 vs. control

Table 1 IC_{50} values of DFX in three pancreatic cancer cell lines after a 72-h incubation

	BxPC-3	HPAF-II	Panc 10.05
IC_{50} (μM)	7.3 ± 1.0	5.6 ± 1.0	6.1 ± 0.2

positive for PI. The percentages of live, apoptotic, and necrotic cells are shown in Fig. 3b. Incubation with 50 or 100 μM DFX significantly decreased the number of live cells compared with control cells in all three cell lines. Moreover, incubation with 50 or 100 μM DFX typically increased the number of cells in late apoptosis in all three cell lines. Apoptosis was also examined by measuring the caspase 3/7 activity with a luminescence assay. The analyzed results are shown in Fig. 4. In all three cell lines, the caspase 3/7 activities were significantly higher in cells incubated with 100 μM of DFX compared with control cells. These results demonstrated that 50 and 100 μM DFX induced apoptosis in pancreatic cancer cells.

DFX inhibited the growth of human pancreatic cancer xenografts

Next, the antiproliferative activity of DFX against pancreatic cancer was assessed in vivo using BxPC-3 pancreatic cancer xenografts in BALB/c nude mice. As DFX is given to patients orally, we administered DFX as a saline suspension given orally in accordance with previous studies [22, 23]. DFX administered orally at 160 and 200 mg/kg (every second day, three treatments per week for 21 days) resulted in marked inhibition of tumor growth as determined by measurements of tumor volume and tumor weight (Fig. 5a, b, and c). After 21 days of oral treatment with the vehicle control (saline solution),

the tumor xenografts reached an average volume of 674 ± 150 mm^3. In contrast, the tumor volumes were significantly reduced to 327 ± 45 and 274 ± 67 mm^3 in mice treated with 160 and 200 mg/kg DFX, respectively (Fig. 5a). At the end of the experiment, the tumors were excised and measured. The control tumors weighed 0.6 ± 0.2 g, whereas tumors treated with 160 and 200 mg/kg oral DFX weighed significantly less than the control tumors at 0.4 ± 0.04 and 0.3 ± 0.1 g, respectively (Fig. 5c). Furthermore, in the blood sample examinations, DFX administered orally at 160 and 200 mg/kg for 3 weeks significantly decreased serum levels of ferritin to 8.6 ± 1.5 and 9.8 ± 1.5 ng/ml, respectively, compared with mice that received vehicle alone (18.3 ± 1.9 ng/ml; Table 2). While DFX administered at 160 and 200 mg/kg inhibited tumor growth and decreased the serum levels of ferritin, the mice did not show body weight loss or altered serum biochemistry, with the exception of the serum levels of ferritin (Fig. 5d and Table 2). On the other hand, DFX administered at 120 mg/kg did not significantly inhibit tumor growth, compared with mice administered vehicle alone. Additionally, it is important to note that DFX administered at 120 mg/kg also failed to reduce the serum levels of ferritin in mice. These observations are consistent with immunohistochemical studies on tumor xenografts that performed semi-quantitative analyses of tumor sections. While tumors treated with 160 and 200 mg/kg oral DFX significantly reduced ferritin-H protein levels compared with tumors treated with the vehicle alone, tumors treated with 120 mg/kg oral DFX did not significantly decrease the ferritin-H protein levels compared with tumors treated with the vehicle alone (Fig. 6a and b). These data indicated that tumor growth could be suppressed when tumors were treated with a sufficient dose of DFX, which functions as an iron chelator.

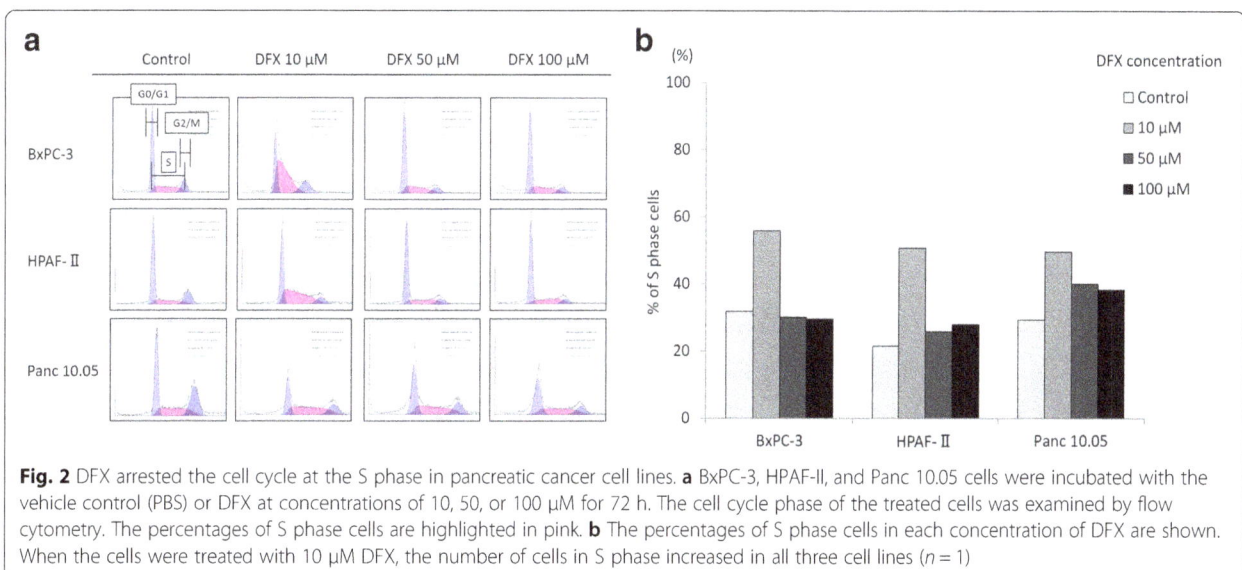

Fig. 2 DFX arrested the cell cycle at the S phase in pancreatic cancer cell lines. **a** BxPC-3, HPAF-II, and Panc 10.05 cells were incubated with the vehicle control (PBS) or DFX at concentrations of 10, 50, or 100 μM for 72 h. The cell cycle phase of the treated cells was examined by flow cytometry. The percentages of S phase cells are highlighted in pink. **b** The percentages of S phase cells in each concentration of DFX are shown. When the cells were treated with 10 μM DFX, the number of cells in S phase increased in all three cell lines ($n = 1$)

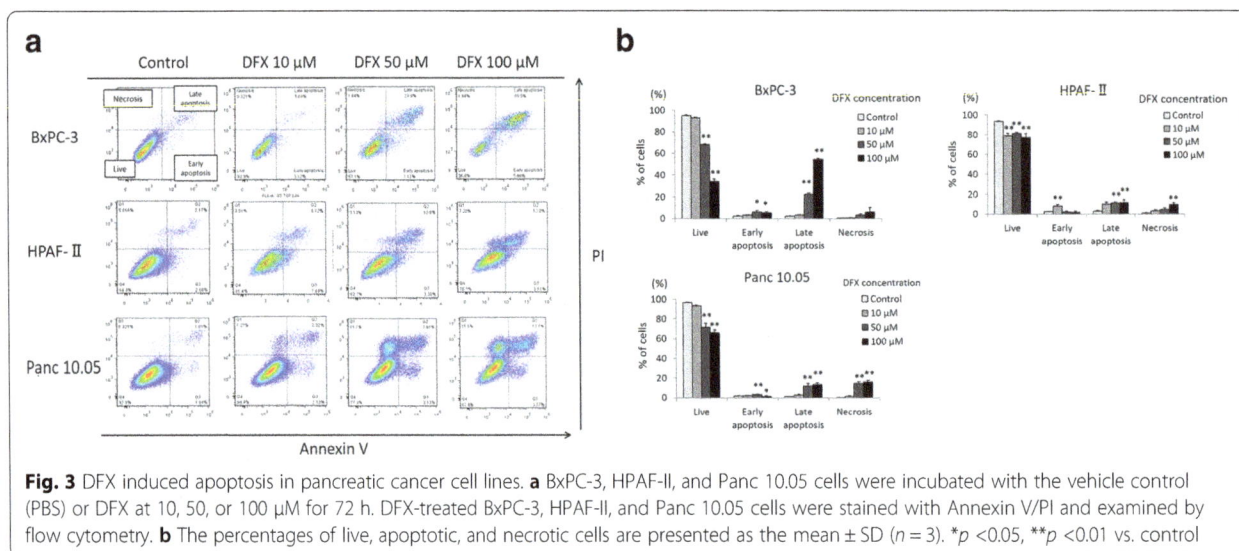

Fig. 3 DFX induced apoptosis in pancreatic cancer cell lines. **a** BxPC-3, HPAF-II, and Panc 10.05 cells were incubated with the vehicle control (PBS) or DFX at 10, 50, or 100 μM for 72 h. DFX-treated BxPC-3, HPAF-II, and Panc 10.05 cells were stained with Annexin V/PI and examined by flow cytometry. **b** The percentages of live, apoptotic, and necrotic cells are presented as the mean ± SD ($n = 3$). *p <0.05, **p <0.01 vs. control

DFX downregulated genes in the pancreatic adenocarcinoma signaling pathway

To investigate the genetic effect of DFX in pancreatic cancer, we examined gene expression alternations in the removed tumors exposed to DFX. From the results of the cancer xenograft experiments, we found that the tumors treated with 200 mg/kg oral DFX were suitable for examining gene expression alterations. Thus, three tumors were randomly chosen from the tumors treated with 200 mg/kg oral DFX, and another three tumors were randomly chosen from the control tumors. After the whole genome microarray analysis, a total of 2412 genes were recognized as differentially expressed with a significance cutoff of p <0.05. These genes were imported into the IPA, and pathway analyses were performed. The

top canonical pathways are shown in Fig. 7a. Pancreatic adenocarcinoma signaling was identified as one of the top canonical pathways. This observation indicated that DFX strongly affected xenografted pancreatic cancer genetically. A heatmap of differently expressed genes included in pancreatic adenocarcinoma signaling is shown in Fig. 7c. Genes highlighted in red indicate upregulation versus the control tumors, while green indicates downregulation in the treated tumors. According to the heatmap, most genes in the pancreatic adenocarcinoma signaling pathway were downregulated by DFX. Specifically, transforming growth factor-ß1 (TGF- ß1) was strongly inhibited. The top upstream regulators are shown in Fig. 7b; TGF- ß1 was also a top upstream regulator. These data demonstrated that the antiproliferative activities of DFX were sustained genetically.

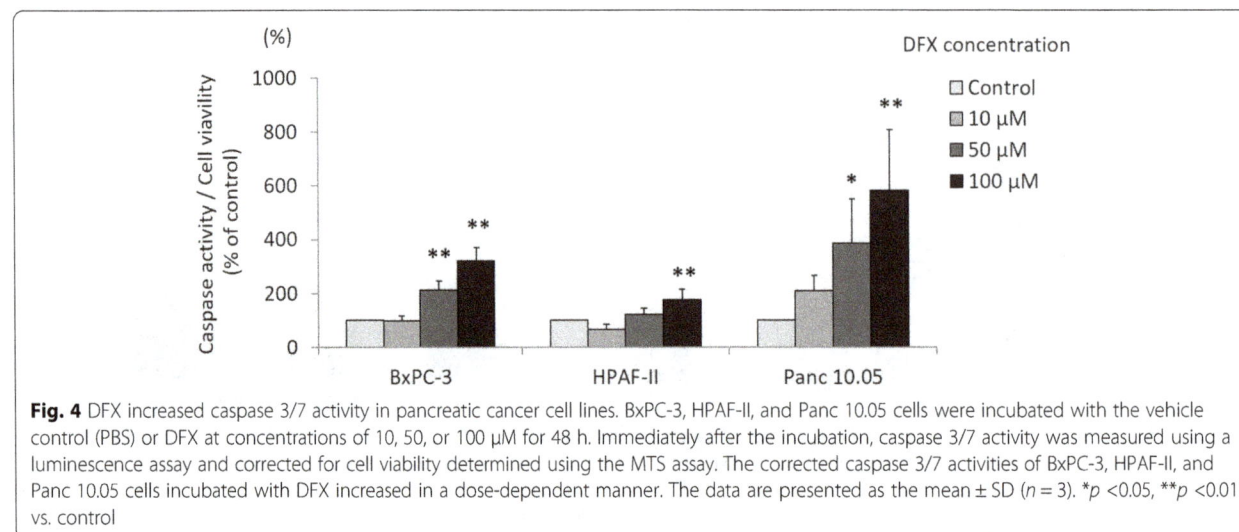

Fig. 4 DFX increased caspase 3/7 activity in pancreatic cancer cell lines. BxPC-3, HPAF-II, and Panc 10.05 cells were incubated with the vehicle control (PBS) or DFX at concentrations of 10, 50, or 100 μM for 48 h. Immediately after the incubation, caspase 3/7 activity was measured using a luminescence assay and corrected for cell viability determined using the MTS assay. The corrected caspase 3/7 activities of BxPC-3, HPAF-II, and Panc 10.05 cells incubated with DFX increased in a dose-dependent manner. The data are presented as the mean ± SD ($n = 3$). *p <0.05, **p <0.01 vs. control

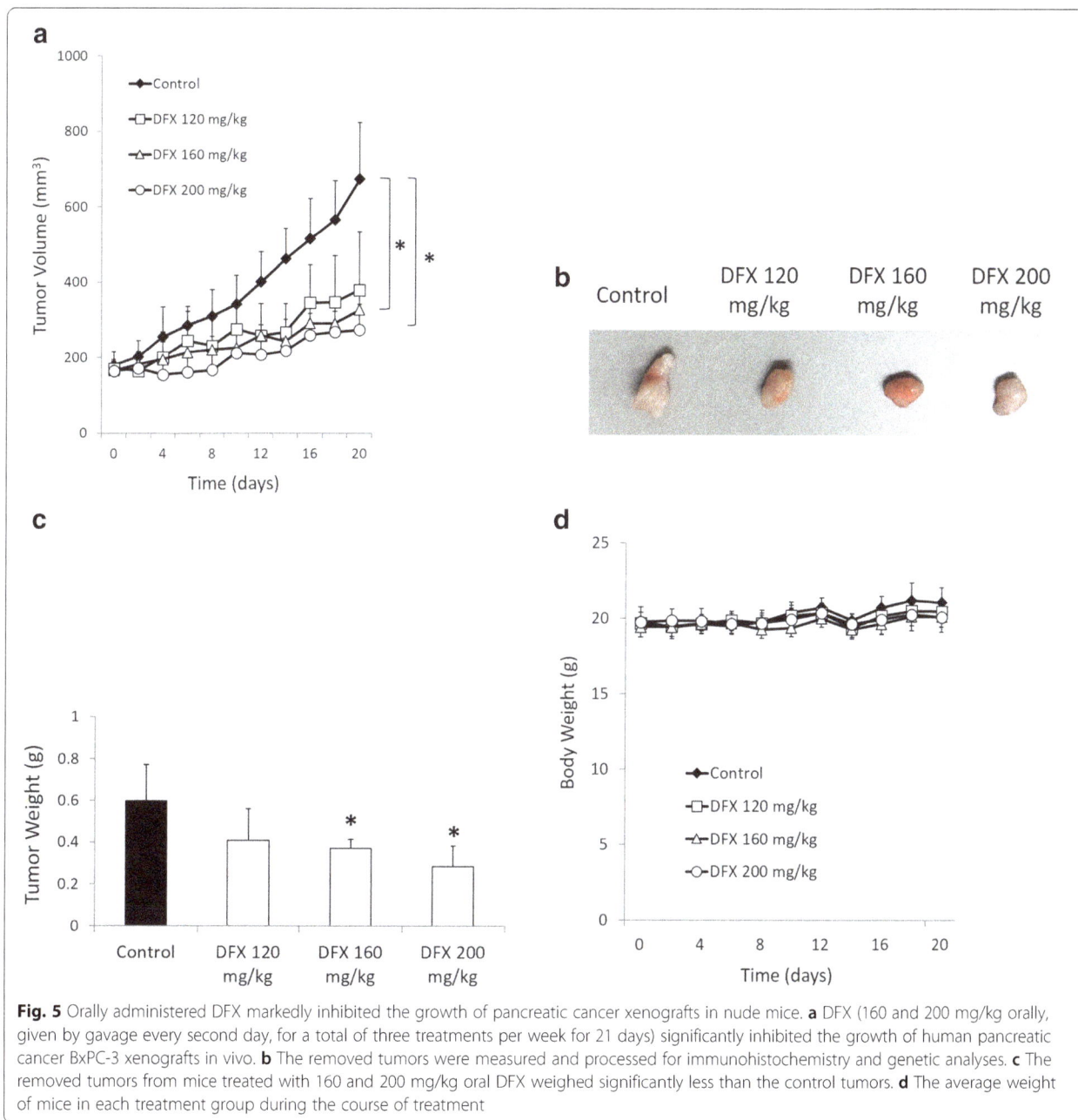

Fig. 5 Orally administered DFX markedly inhibited the growth of pancreatic cancer xenografts in nude mice. **a** DFX (160 and 200 mg/kg orally, given by gavage every second day, for a total of three treatments per week for 21 days) significantly inhibited the growth of human pancreatic cancer BxPC-3 xenografts in vivo. **b** The removed tumors were measured and processed for immunohistochemistry and genetic analyses. **c** The removed tumors from mice treated with 160 and 200 mg/kg oral DFX weighed significantly less than the control tumors. **d** The average weight of mice in each treatment group during the course of treatment

Discussion

The antiproliferative activity of iron chelators was first demonstrated on leukemia in cell cultures and clinical trials [24, 25]. Then, the antiproliferative activity of iron chelators was demonstrated in solid tumors, including pancreatic cancer tumors, and in cell culture in recent studies [15, 26, 27]. DFO was the first commercially available iron chelator to be used for the treatment of iron-overload disease [28]. DFO has also been used for studies researching the antiproliferative activity of iron chelators in cell cultures and clinical trials [13–15, 25–27]. Although DFO exhibits antiproliferative activity, this chelator has serious limitations because it is not utilized by the body if administered orally and has a short serum half-life. DFO needs to be given parenterally (either subcutaneously or intravenous infusion) for long periods, typically 8–12 h per day, which has led to poor patient compliance. On the other hand, DFX, a recently identified iron chelator, can be administered orally once daily because it is orally active and has a long half-life of 7–18 h. DFX is currently used for the treatment of iron-overload disease and is considered an alternative to DFO [16]. The antiproliferative activity of DFX has been investigated in various cancers [22, 23, 29, 30]. However, there have

Table 2 Serum indices from nude mice bearing a BxPC-3 xenograft that were treated orally by gavage with either the vehicle control or DFX (120, 160, or 200 mg/kg) every second day (three treatments per week) for 21 days

	Units	Treatment groups			
		Vehicle control	Deferasirox		
			120 mg/kg	160 mg/kg	200 mg/kg
Ferritin	ng/ml	18.3 ± 1.9	20.6 ± 2.9	8.6 ± 1.4*	9.8 ± 1.5*
Total protein	g/dl	5.0 ± 0.3	5.4 ± 0.3	5.3 ± 0.4	5.3 ± 0.3
Albumin	g/dl	3.2 ± 0.2	3.3 ± 0.1	3.4 ± 0.1	3.4 ± 0.1
Aspartate aminotransferase	U/l	89.2 ± 15.8	106.2 ± 32.6	155.2 ± 97.9	146 ± 58.9
Alanine transaminase	U/l	23.6 ± 1.9	29.2 ± 8.2	28.4 ± 9.6	28.8 ± 7.2
Lactate dehydrogenase	U/l	243.6 ± 37.9	242.6 ± 18.2	243.8 ± 23.1	243.6 ± 21.7
Blood urea nitrogen	mg/dl	560.6 ± 112.7	578.2 ± 65.5	669 ± 43.9	689.8 ± 101.9
Creatinine	mg/dl	17.6 ± 1.2	14.2 ± 2.1	14.4 ± 0.6	15.8 ± 1.3

*$p < 0.05$ vs. control

previously been no studies of the effects of DFX in pancreatic cancer; this study is the first to elucidate the antiproliferative activity of DFX against pancreatic cancer cells.

We examined the in vitro antiproliferative activity of DFX using an MTS assay in three pancreatic cancer cell lines: BxPC-3, HPAF-II, and Panc 10.05. We observed a dose-dependent antiproliferative activity of DFX in pancreatic cancer cell lines, consistent with the results of previous studies in esophageal cancer cell lines [22] or lung cancer cell lines [23]. Although a number of studies have attempted to elucidate the anti-cancer mechanisms of iron chelators, their mechanisms are not well known [12]. Especially in pancreatic cancer, there have been few studies investigating the effect of iron chelators as anticancer agents [15]. To investigate the mechanisms of the antiproliferative activity of DFX, we examined the effects of DFX on the cell cycle and apoptosis in pancreatic

cancer cell lines. We observed that 10 μM DFX inhibited pancreatic cancer cell proliferation by arresting the cell cycle in the S phase, and 50 and 100 μM DFX inhibited pancreatic cancer cell proliferation by inducing apoptosis. These anti-cancer mechanisms of DFX are consistent with those found in previous reports for most iron chelators [15, 31, 32].

We next assessed the ability of DFX to inhibit pancreatic cancer growth in vivo using a murine xenograft model. We administered DFX at doses of 120, 160, and 200 mg/kg every second day, totaling three treatments per week for 3 weeks. The doses of 160 and 200 mg/kg of DFX successfully inhibited tumor growth and decreased serum and tumor levels of ferritin. Initially, we attempted to administer DFX at doses of 20–40 mg/kg every second day, for three treatments per week for 3 weeks because a 20 mg/kg per day regimen is considered suitable

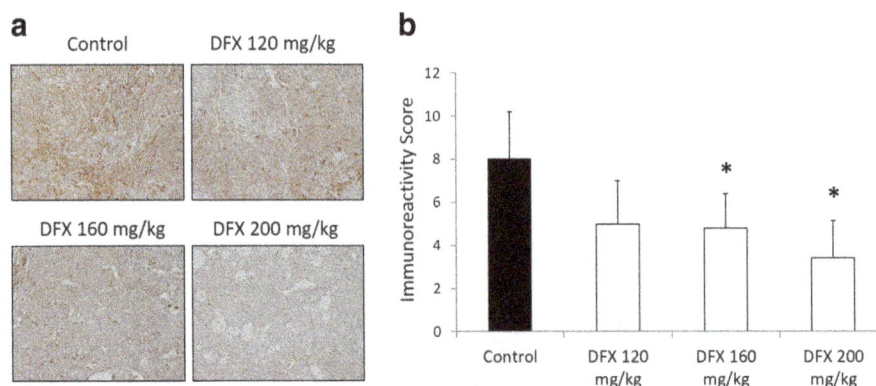

Fig. 6 Orally administered DFX reduced ferritin-H protein levels of removed tumors in immunohistochemical analyses. **a** Immunohistochemistry was performed on the removed tumors with antibody specific to ferritin-H. **b** The slides were scored for the percentage of positive cells (0 = 0–5, 1 = 6–25, 2 = 26–50, 3 = 51–75 and 4 = 76–100 %) and intensity (0 = negative, 1 = weak, 2 = moderate, 3 = strong). The immunoreactivity score was calculated as the percentage of positive cells multiplied by the score for the staining intensity. The immunoreactivity scores of removed tumors treated orally with 160 and 200 mg/kg of DFX were significantly lower than that of control tumors. The data are presented as the mean ± SD (n = 5 mice per group). For statistical analysis, each treatment was compared with the control. *$p < 0.05$, **$p < 0.01$ vs. control

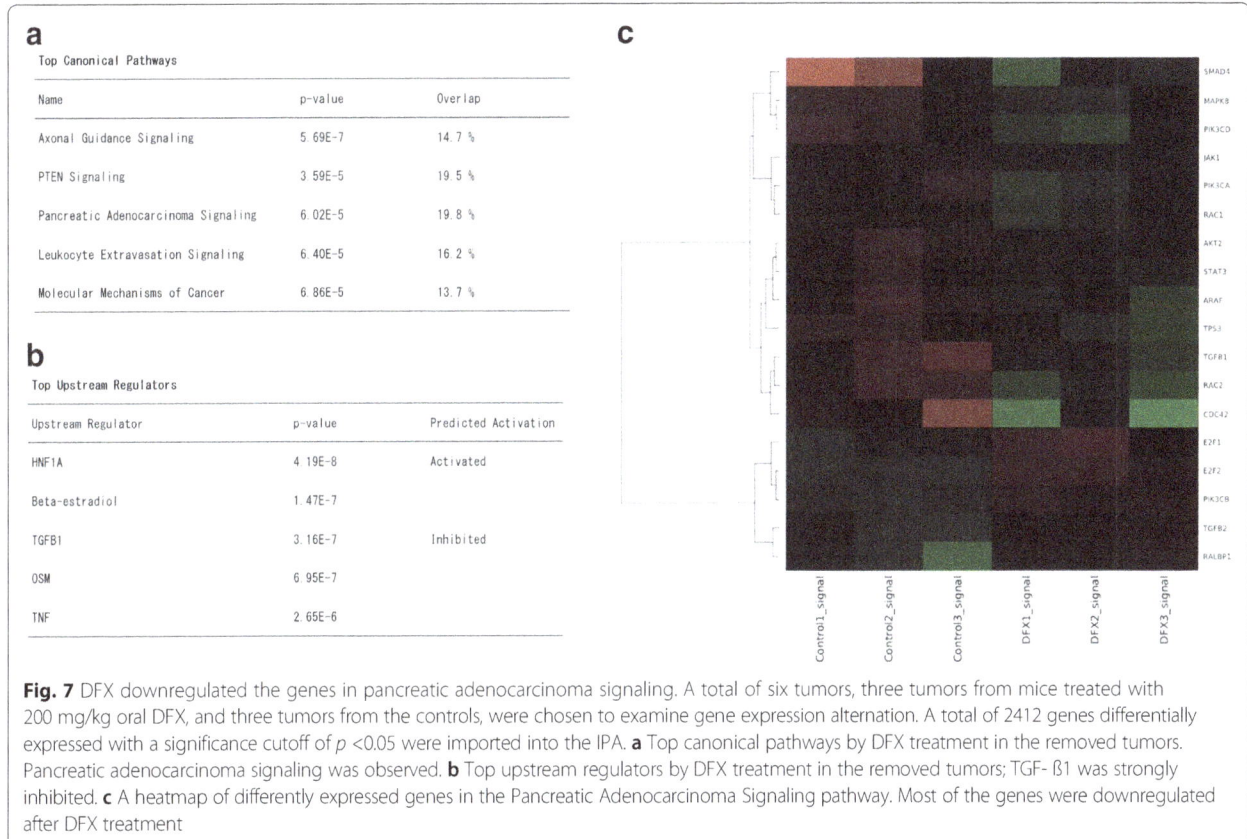

Fig. 7 DFX downregulated the genes in pancreatic adenocarcinoma signaling. A total of six tumors, three tumors from mice treated with 200 mg/kg oral DFX, and three tumors from the controls, were chosen to examine gene expression alternation. A total of 2412 genes differentially expressed with a significance cutoff of $p < 0.05$ were imported into the IPA. **a** Top canonical pathways by DFX treatment in the removed tumors. Pancreatic adenocarcinoma signaling was observed. **b** Top upstream regulators by DFX treatment in the removed tumors; TGF- ß1 was strongly inhibited. **c** A heatmap of differently expressed genes in the Pancreatic Adenocarcinoma Signaling pathway. Most of the genes were downregulated after DFX treatment

in patients with iron overload [33]. However, in nude mice, 20–40 mg/kg DFX did not inhibit tumor growth or reduce serum levels of ferritin (data not shown). In fact, even a dose of 120 mg/kg of DFX failed to significantly suppress either tumor growth or serum and tumor ferritin levels. The 3-week experiment may have been too short to assess the effects of a normal dose of DFX in this xenograft model. However, it is important to note that decreased serum and tumor levels of ferritin were observed in the mice that received 160 or 200 mg/kg doses of DFX administration, and the xenografted tumors were markedly suppressed. Furthermore, no serious effects on body weight and biological indices were observed. A previous in vivo study using DFX also demonstrated the importance of iron depletion in the xenografted tumor for cancer therapy [22]. According to our study, we believe that DFX demonstrates antiproliferative activity by decreasing serum levels of ferritin, which is reflected as iron depletion in the tumor.

To assess the genetic effects of DFX for pancreatic cancer, we conducted microarray analysis using in vivo samples. Most genes included in pancreatic adenocarcinoma signaling, especially TBF- ß1, were downregulated by DFX administration. A previous study revealed that TGF- ß overexpression is associated with early recurrence following resection and decreased survival in

patients with pancreatic cancer [34]. TGF- ß1 also plays pivotal roles in driving epithelial-mesenchymal transition (EMT) in the pathogenesis of pancreatic cancer [35, 36]. In fact, the TGF- ß signaling inhibitor displays antiproliferative activity for pancreatic cancer [37]. A recent review article also demonstrated that iron chelators can target several pathways, including the TBF- ß pathway, to subsequently inhibit cellular proliferation, EMT and metastasis [38]. This evidence, combined with the results of our microarray analysis, indicates that DFX works as anticancer agent by suppressing TGF- ß signaling.

Conclusions

We first elucidated that DFX has potential as a therapeutic agent for pancreatic cancer. We demonstrated that DFX inhibits pancreatic cancer cell growth by arresting the cell cycle and inducing apoptosis. Furthermore, DFX inhibited pancreatic cancer growth in vivo in a murine xenograft model. Genetically, TGF- ß1 plays a key role in the effect of DFX against pancreatic cancer. Because DFX is a commercially available oral iron chelator, its clinical application can be considerable. While further extensive studies are required, the DFX treatment strategy can be considered a novel effective and safe pancreatic cancer therapy in the near future.

Acknowledgments
Not applicable.

Funding
This study was supported by the Strategic Research Promotion Program from Yamaguchi University, the Translational Research Program from Yamaguchi University Hospital, and the Pancreatic Disease Research Award from the Pancreas Research Foundation of Japan.

Authors' contributions
HH and TT drafted the manuscript. SK and TY designed the study. SS, TM, KF, and NY acquired and analyzed the study data. IS approved the final manuscript. All authors read and approved the final manuscript.

Competing interests
The authors declare that they have no competing interest.

Author details
[1]Department of Gastroenterology and Hepatology, Yamaguchi University Graduate School of Medicine, 1-1-1 Minami-Kogushi, Ube, Yamaguchi 755-8505, Japan. [2]Department of Oncology and Laboratory Medicine, Yamaguchi University Graduate School of Medicine, 1-1-1 Minami-Kogushi, Ube, Yamaguchi 755-8505, Japan.

References
1. Egawa S, Toma H, Ohigashi H, Okusaka T, Nakao A, Hatori T, et al. Japan pancreatic cancer registry; 30th year anniversary: Japan Pancreas Society. Pancreas. 2012;41:985–92.
2. Ferlay J, Soerjomataram I, Dikshit R, Eser S, Mathers C, Rebelo M, et al. Cancer incidence and mortality worldwide: sources, methods and major patterns in GLOBOCAN 2012. Int J Cancer. 2015;136:E359–86.
3. Magee CJ, Ghaneh P, Neoptolemos JP. Surgical and medical therapy for pancreatic carcinoma. Best Pract Res Clin Gastroenterol. 2002;16:435–55.
4. SEER: Surveillance, Epidemiology, and End Results Program. Cancer statistics review, 1975–2012. National Cancer Institute. 2015. http://seer.cancer.gov/archive/csr/1975_2012/. Accessed 18 Nov 2015.
5. National Comprehensive Cancer Network. NCCN clinical practice guidelines in oncology, pancreatic adenocarcinoma. National Comprehensive Cancer Network. 2015. https://www.nccn.org/. Accessed 3 June 2015.
6. Conroy T, Desseigne F, Ychou M, Bouché O, Guimbaud R, Bécouarn Y, et al. FOLFIRINOX versus gemcitabine for metastatic pancreatic cancer. N Engl J Med. 2011;364:1817–25.
7. Von Hoff DD, Ramanathan RK, Borad MJ, Laheru DA, Smith LS, Wood TE, et al. Gemcitabine plus nab-paclitaxel is an active regimen in patients with advanced pancreatic cancer: a phase I/II trial. J Clin Oncol. 2011;29:4548–54.
8. Crichton R. Iron metabolism: from molecular mechanisms to clinical consequences. Hoboken: Wiley; 2009.
9. Yu Y, Wong J, Lovejoy DB, Kalinowski DS, Richardson DR. Chelators at the cancer coalface: desferrioxamine to Triapine and beyond. Clin Cancer Res. 2006;12:6876–83.
10. Kicic A, Chua AC, Baker E. Effect of iron chelators on proliferation and iron uptake in hepatoma cells. Cancer. 2001;92:3093–110.
11. Yu Y, Gutierrez E, Kovacevic Z, Saletta F, Obeidy P, Suryo Rahmanto Y, et al. Iron chelators for the treatment of cancer. Curr Med Chem. 2012;19:2689–702.
12. Torti SV, Torti FM. Iron and cancer: more ore to be mined. Nat Rev Cancer. 2013;13:342–55.
13. Sakaida I, Hironaka K, Uchida K, Okita K. Iron chelator deferoxamine reduces preneoplastic lesions in liver induced by choline-deficient L-amino acid-defined diet in rats. Dig Dis Sci. 1999;44:560–9.
14. Yamasaki T, Terai S, Sakaida I. Deferoxamine for advanced hepatocellular carcinoma. N Engl J Med. 2011;365:576–8.
15. Kovacevic Z, Chikhani S, Lovejoy DB, Richardson DR. Novel thiosemicarbazone iron chelators induce up-regulation and phosphorylation of the metastasis suppressor N-myc down-stream regulated gene 1: a new strategy for the treatment of pancreatic cancer. Mol Pharmacol. 2011;80:598–609.
16. Cappellini MD, Taher A. Deferasirox (Exjade) for the treatment of iron overload. Acta Haematol. 2009;122:165–73.
17. Bedford MR, Ford SJ, Horniblow RD, Iqbal TH, Tselepis C. Iron chelation in the treatment of cancer: a new role for deferasirox? J Clin Pharmacol. 2013;53:885–91.
18. Boult J, Roberts K, Brookes MJ, Hughes S, Bury JP, Cross SS, et al. Overexpression of cellular iron import proteins is associated with malignant progression of esophageal adenocarcinoma. Clin Cancer Res. 2008;14:379–87.
19. Di Martino E, Wild CP, Rotimi O, Darnton JS, Olliver RJ, Hardie LJ. IGFBP-3 and IGFBP-10 (CYR61) up-regulation during the development of Barrett's oesophagus and associated oesophageal adenocarcinoma: potential biomarkers of disease risk. Biomarkers. 2006;11:547–61.
20. Bolstad BM, Irizarry RA, Astrand M, Speed TP. A comparison of normalization methods for high density oligonucleotide array data based on variance and bias. BioInformatics. 2003;19:185–93.
21. Gentleman RC, Carey VJ, Bates DM, Bolstad B, Dettling M, Dudoit S, et al. Bioconductor: open software development for computational biology and bioinformatics. Genome Biol. 2004;5:R80.
22. Ford SJ, Obeidy P, Lovejoy DB, Bedford M, Nichols L, Chadwick C, et al. Deferasirox (ICL670A) effectively inhibits oesophageal cancer growth in vitro and in vivo. Br J Pharmacol. 2013;168:1316–28.
23. Lui GY, Obeidy P, Ford SJ, Tselepis C, Sharp DM, Jansson PJ, et al. The iron chelator, deferasirox, as a novel strategy for cancer treatment: oral activity against human lung tumor xenografts and molecular mechanism of action. Mol Pharmacol. 2013;83:179–90.
24. Kontoghiorghes GJ, Piga A, Hoffbrand AV. Cytotoxic and DNA-inhibitory effects of iron chelators on human leukaemic cell lines. Hematol Oncol. 1986;4:195–204.
25. Estrov Z, Tawa A, Wang XH, Dubé ID, Sulh H, Cohen A, et al. In vitro and in vivo effects of deferoxamine in neonatal acute leukemia. Blood. 1987;69:757–61.
26. Brard L, Granai CO, Swamy N. Iron chelators deferoxamine and diethylenetriamine pentaacetic acid induce apoptosis in ovarian carcinoma. Gynecol Oncol. 2006;100:116–27.
27. Hoke EM, Maylock CA, Shacter E. Desferal inhibits breast tumor growth and does not interfere with the tumoricidal activity of doxorubicin. Free Radic Biol Med. 2005;39:403–11.
28. Olivieri NF, Brittenham GM. Iron-chelating therapy and the treatment of thalassemia. Blood. 1997;89:739–61.
29. Lescoat G, Chantrel-Groussard K, Pasdeloup N, Nick H, Brissot P, Gaboriau F. Antiproliferative and apoptotic effects in rat and human hepatoma cell cultures of the orally active iron chelator ICL670 compared to CP20: a possible relationship with polyamine metabolism. Cell Prolif. 2007;40:755–67.
30. Ohyashiki JH, Kobayashi C, Hamamura R, Okabe S, Tauchi T, Ohyashiki K. The oral iron chelator deferasirox represses signaling through the mTOR in myeloid leukemia cells by enhancing expression of REDD1. Cancer Sci. 2009;100:970–7.
31. Jin H, Xu Z, Li D, Huang J. Antiproliferative activity and therapeutic implications of potassium tris(4-methyl-1-pyrazolyl) borohydride in hepatocellular carcinoma. Chem Biol Interact. 2014;213:69–76.
32. Yu Y, Kovacevic Z, Richardson DR. Tuning cell cycle regulation with an iron key. Cell Cycle. 2007;6:1982–94.
33. Nisbet-Brown E, Olivieri NF, Giardina PJ, Grady RW, Neufeld EJ, Séchaud R, et al. Effectiveness and safety of ICL670 in iron-loaded patients with thalassaemia: a randomised, double-blind, placebo-controlled, dose-escalation trial. Lancet. 2003;361:1597–602.
34. Friess H, Yamanaka Y, Büchler M, Ebert M, Beger HG, Gold LI, et al. Enhanced expression of transforming growth factor beta isoforms in pancreatic cancer correlates with decreased survival. Gastroenterol. 1993;105:1846–56.
35. Yin T, Wang C, Liu T, Zhao G, Zhou F. Implication of EMT induced by TGF-beta1 in pancreatic cancer. J Huazhong Univ Sci Technolog Med Sci. 2006;26:700–2.
36. Ellenrieder V, Hendler SF, Boeck W, Seufferlein T, Menke A, Ruhland C, et al. Transforming growth factor beta1 treatment leads to an epithelial-mesenchymal transdifferentiation of pancreatic cancer cells requiring extracellular signal-regulated kinase 2 activation. Cancer Res. 2001;61:4222–8.
37. Lou C, Zhang F, Yang M, Zhao J, Zeng W, Fang X, et al. Naringenin decreases invasiveness and metastasis by inhibiting TGF-β-induced epithelial to mesenchymal transition in pancreatic cancer cells. PLoS ONE. 2012;7:e50956.

γ-Tocotrienol induces apoptosis in pancreatic cancer cells by upregulation of ceramide synthesis and modulation of sphingolipid transport

Victoria E. Palau[1,2], Kanishka Chakraborty[1], Daniel Wann[3], Janet Lightner[1], Keely Hilton[1], Marianne Brannon[4], William Stone[4] and Koyamangalath Krishnan[1]* (iD)

Abstract

Background: Ceramide synthesis and metabolism is a promising target in cancer drug development. γ-tocotrienol (GT3), a member of the vitamin E family, orchestrates multiple effects that ensure the induction of apoptosis in both, wild-type and RAS-mutated pancreatic cancer cells. Here, we investigated whether these effects involve changes in ceramide synthesis and transport.

Methods: The effects of GT3 on the synthesis of ceramide via the *de novo* pathway, and the hydrolysis of sphingomyelin were analyzed by the expression levels of the enzymes serine palmitoyl transferase, ceramide synthase-6, and dihydroceramide desaturase, and acid sphingomyelinase in wild-type RAS BxPC3, and RAS-mutated MIA PaCa-2 and Panc 1 pancreatic cancer cells. Quantitative changes in ceramides, dihydroceramides, and sphingomyelin at the cell membrane were detected by LCMS. Modulation of ceramide transport by GT3 was studied by immunochemistry of CERT and ARV-1, and the subsequent effects at the cell membrane was analyzed via immunofluorescence of ceramide, caveolin, and DR5.

Results: GT3 favors the upregulation of ceramide by stimulating synthesis at the ER and the plasma membrane. Additionally, the conversion of newly synthesized ceramide to sphingomyelin and glucosylceramide at the Golgi is prevented by the inhibition of CERT. Modulation ARV1 and previously observed inhibition of the HMG-CoA pathway, contribute to changes in membrane structure and signaling functions, allows the clustering of DR5, effectively initiating apoptosis.

Conclusions: Our results suggest that GT3 targets ceramide synthesis and transport, and that the upregulation of ceramide and modulation of transporters CERT and ARV1 are important contributors to the apoptotic properties demonstrated by GT3 in pancreatic cancer cells.

Keywords: γ-Tocotrienol, Vitamin E, Pancreatic cancer, ARV-1, CERT, Ceramide transport, Ceramide synthesis, Ceramide distribution, Lipid transport, Membrane lipid, Free radicals

* Correspondence: krishnak@etsu.edu
[1]Division of Hematology-Oncology, Department of Internal Medicine, James H. Quillen College of Medicine, East Tennessee State University, Johnson City, TN 37614, USA
Full list of author information is available at the end of the article

Background

Pancreatic cancer is the fourth leading cause of cancer-related deaths in the United States [1]. Since available treatment options are limited, novel therapeutic agents that demonstrate the ability to inhibit signaling pathways implicated in the proliferation and survival of pancreatic cancer cells need to be evaluated for drug development. Promising agents may uncover new targets and alternate treatment strategies that have the potential to contribute to the understanding of pancreatic carcinogenesis and progression. It has been known for a long time that ceramides can inhibit cell proliferation and induce apoptosis in cancer cells via various stress stimuli such as tumor necrosis factor-α and platelet-activating factor [2, 3]. Furthermore, recent studies in the synthesis and metabolism of ceramides suggest that changes in the expression levels of these compounds may contribute to metastasis and resistance to therapy [4]. The syntheses of ceramides occur through multiple pathways that include: *de novo* synthesis from serine and palmitoyl-CoA substrates, salvage, from sphingosine [5] and from the hydrolysis of sphingomyelin by acid sphingomyelinase (ASM). The *de novo* synthesis is initiated in the cytoplasmic face of the endoplasmic reticulum by serine palmitoyl transferase (SPT), to form 3-keto-sphinganine, which is subsequently reduced to sphinganine (SA). Ceramide synthase (CerS) acetylates SA followed by desaturation by ceramide desaturase (DES) to form ceramide [6, 7]. There are six CerSs that regulate ceramide synthesis to produce a variety of compounds with di-and tri-hydroxy long-chain bases linked to fatty acids of variable length [8] and with C16 and C24 ceramides being most abundant in mammalian cells. These highly hydrophobic molecules can displace cholesterol and disrupt lipids rafts that may be associated with signaling molecules, thus affecting their function [9]. Moreover, the biophysical properties of ceramides may influence lipid reorganization in the membrane and cause destabilization, efflux and fusion. Hence, their expression levels and localization are tightly controlled.

Tocotrienols are members of the vitamin E family that unlike tocopherols possess an unsaturated isoprenoid side-chain [10]. These compounds have shown cytotoxic activity on pancreatic cancer cells via a multi-pronged mechanism. We had previously shown that γ-tocotrienol (GT3) is cytotoxic to pancreatic cancer cells, and is significantly more potent in its ability to inhibit cell viability as compared to alpha-tocopherol [11]. The ability of tocotrienols to selectively inhibit the PI3 kinase/Akt pathway, Ras/Raf/Erk signaling [11], HMG CoA reductase, and transcription factor NF-κB [12], are contributors to these properties. In pancreatic cancer, the oncogenic process is frequently driven by aberrant K-Ras. We have shown that GT3 can cause inhibition of cellular proliferation and survival in pancreatic cancer cells regardless of their K-Ras

status [11]. However, the mechanism of action is not completely understood. It has been reported that vitamin E isoforms other than tocotrienols can increase cellular ceramide and dihydroceramide levels. Alpha-TEA, a modified form of alpha tocopherol, can increase membrane ceramide levels in mammary cancer cells [13], and γ-tocopherol has a similar effect on prostate cancer cells [14]. In vivo, pharmacokinetics studies have demonstrated the bioavailabilty of tocotrienols in humans [15]. These studies led us to determine whether the observed apoptotic effects in pancreatic cancer cells dosed with GT3 involved changes in ceramide transport and levels in K-Ras mutated cells as compared to wild type. Here we show that GT3 causes an increase in the levels of certain ceramides at the plasma membrane by the upregulation of enzymes involved in both the *de novo* pathway and the hydrolysis of sphingomyelin, and the modulation of ceramide transporters regardless of K-Ras status. The apoptotic nature of these changes is confirmed by the clustering of death receptor 5 at the membrane and confirming previous observations of the mechanism of action by which GT3 inhibits cell proliferation and survival in pancreatic cancer cells.

Methods

Cell lines and culture conditions

MIA PaCa-2 (CRM-CRL-1420), BxPc3 (CRL-1687), and Panc 1 (CRL-1469) cells were obtained from the American Type Culture Collection (Manassas, VA) and were maintained as described before [11]. Human pancreatic ductal epithelial cells (HPDE-E6E7), a generous gift from Dr. Ming-Sound Tsao (Ontario Cancer Institute, Toronto, Ontario, Canada), were cultured in keratinocyte medium (Fisher Scientific, Waltham, MA) as described elsewhere [16]. For immunoblotting experiments, lentiviral transduction, LC/MS and qRT-PCR, cells were seeded on 60 mm plates at high density (~5x10^4 cells/cm^2) to obtain confluency in 2–3 days. For immunofluorescence experiments, the cells were seeded on 12mm round cover slips (Fisher Scientific) or 6-mm Transwell-Clear^{TM} filters (Corning Costar) at high density (~5x10^4 cells/cm^2) and treated at 70% confluency.

SDS PAGE and immunoblotting

Cells (70% confluent) were treated with GT3 (Cayman Chemical, Ann Arbor, MI) dissolved in ethanol, at a concentration of 40 μM or dissolution vehicle as a control and incubated for 2, 4, or 6 hours. The cells were rinsed with phosphate-buffered saline and lysed in the plate with buffer (20 mM Imidazole-HCl, pH 6.8, 100 mM KCl, 1 mM MgCl2, 10 mM EGTA, 0.2% (v/v) Triton X-100,) containing phosphatase and protease inhibitors (Sigma Aldrich, St. Louis, MO). The protein concentration of the cell lysates was determined using the Advanced protein assay reagent (Cytoskekleton, Denver, CO). Equal amounts of proteins in cell lysates were separated in 7 or 10% SDS-PAGE. The proteins were transferred to nitrocellulose membranes (Pall Life Sciences, Ann Arbor, MI). Immunoblot procedures were done according to the protocol for each antibody. Membranes were probed with primary antibodies against ASM, DEGS1, SPT, Collagen type IV alpha-3-binding protein, also known as ceramide transfer protein CERT, DDIT3 (Abcam, Cambridge, MA), ceramide synthase 6 (Abgent, San Diego, CA), ACAT-related enzyme-2 required for viability, also known as ARV1 (Santa Cruz Biotechnology, Dallas, TX), DR5 (Sigma Aldrich), and caveolin (Cell Signaling Technology, Danvers, MA).

Lentiviral transduction of ARV1 shRNA

shRNA-expressing lentiviral particles against human ARV1 (NM_022786) were obtained from Sigma Aldrich (5'CCGGGCCAGAAACCTGTAGACAAATCTCGAGA TTTGTCTACAGGTTT CTGGCTTTTTG-3') clone no. TCRN0000107011; MIA PaCa-2 cells were transduced at 70% confluency and treated with GT3 or dissolution vehicle, 48h after lentiviral transduction.

qRT-PCR for ARV-1 and ceramide enzymes

To study the levels of ARV1, quantitative RT-PCR was performed on MIA PaCa-2 cells. Total RNA was isolated using Trizol (Invitrogen) according to the manufacturer's instructions and treated with DNase I using the RNeasy Mini Kit and on-column RNase free DNase kit (Qiagen). 1.0 μg RNA was reverse-transcribed with the Super script II Kit (Invitrogen) as recommended. The ARV-1 primers used were: (GCC ACC ACC TCA GGT ATG CTT C) and (GTG CAA AGC TCA GGC CTA CAG AC).

Immunofluorescence

Cells were dosed with 40μM GT3 or ethanol as a control and processed for immunofluorescence as described before [17]. Briefly, cells were rinsed with phosphate-buffered saline and fixed with 4% p-formaldehyde. Then the cells were rinsed and permeabilized with 0.2% Triton-X100, followed by quenching with NH4Cl. Cells were then incubated with primary antibody in 1% bovine serum albumin at room temperature for one hour. Antibodies against ceramide, death receptor 5 (DR5) (Sigma) and caveolin (Cell Signaling Technology) were used as primary antibodies for immunofluorescence. Cells were then rinsed and incubated for one hour in the dark with secondary antibody conjugated to fluorescent dyes Alexa Fluor 488® and Texas Red® (Molecular Probes, Eugene, OR). DAPI stain was used to visualize nuclei. Cells were then mounted in 10% polyvinyl alcohol, 30% glycerol, 1% n-propyl gallate and SlowFade™ (Molecular Probes). Laser confocal microscopy was performed with a Zeiss LSM 710 confocal microscope (Carl Zeiss MicroImaging GmbH, Germany) in the Imaging Core, Quillen College of Medicine, East Tennessee State University. Cell

monolayers were analyzed using a 63 x oil immersion objective. The images were collected using the LSM 710 software (Carl Zeiss Micro Imaging).

Preparation of cellular samples for LC/MS

All solvents for sample extraction and LC/MS were LC/MS grade (Fisher Scientific), other reagents were purchased from Sigma-Aldrich (St. Louis, MO, USA) or Fisher Scientific. Calibration standards and internal standards were purchased from Avanti Polar Lipid, Inc. (Alabaster, AL). Crude plasma membrane isolation was carried out at 4°C. Briefly, cells were resuspended in lysis buffer (NaHCO3 1mM, NaCO3 0.011mM, CaCl2 1mM, MgCl2 1mM, pH 7.4), and incubated on ice for 20 minutes, followed by homogenization with a Dounce homogenizer. The homogenates were centrifuged at 500 g for 5 minutes; the resulting supernatant was transferred to another microcentrifuge tube, and the remaining pellet containing the nuclear fraction was discarded. An equal volume of 510mM sucrose solution was added to the supernatant, and separated by centrifugation at 20,000g for 30minutes. The supernatant was transferred to an ultracentrifuge tube, and the remaining pellet containing mitochondria, Golgi apparatus and part of the microsome was set aside. The supernatant was ultracentrifuged at 240,000 g for 2 hrs. The resulting supernatant was transferred to another tube as cytosol sample, whereas the crude plasma membrane was settled in the pellet. The pellet was washed with lysis buffer and resuspended with PBS as plasma membrane sample. Samples were frozen at -80 C for later analysis. The extraction of lipids from the plasma membrane was performed in the following manner, 1 ml of methanol containing 20μl of 2μM of each internal standard (C12 ceramides, C12 dihydroceramide, C12 sphingomyelin, C17 sphingosine, C17 sphinganine, C17 sphingosine-1-phosphate, and C17 sphinganine-1-phosphate) were added to 100μl aliquot of sample in a clean glass tube. The mixture was centrifuged at 3,000g for 10 minutes and the supernatant was transferred to a second glass tube and evaporated under a nitrogen stream. The extracted lipids were reconstituted in methanol: acetonitrile (v:v=50:50) and transferred to LC/MS autosampler vials (Waters, Milford, MA) for injection.

LC/MS

All experiments were carried out on a Waters Xevo TQ MS ACQUITY UPLC system (Waters). The system was controlled by Mass Lynx Software version 4. 1. The sample was maintained at 4°C in the autosampler and was loaded onto a Waters ACQUITY UPLC BEH Phenyl column (3 mm inner diameter × 100 mm with 1.7 μm particles), preceded by a 2.1×5 mm guard column containing the same packing. The column was maintained at 40°C throughout analysis. The UPLC flow rate was continuously 300μL/min in a binary gradient mode with the following mobile phase: initial flow conditions were 20% solvent A (H2O, containing 0.2% formic acid and 0.1% ammonium formate) and 80% solvent B (acetonitrile, containing 0.2% formic acid and 0.1% ammonium formate). Solvent B was increased linearly to 95% over a 2 min period and to 98% in the subsequent 6 min. This was followed by a reduction of solvent B to 80% starting at 8.2 min and continuing through 9 min. Ceramides of interest eluted between 4.0 and 7.5 min. Positive ESI-MS/MS mass spectrometry was performed to identify ceramide species. Different species were confirmed by comparing the retention times of experimental compounds with those of authentic standards. Concentrations of ceramides in the samples were quantified by comparing integrated peak areas for those of each ceramide against those of known amounts of purified standards. Loss during extraction was accounted for by adjusting for the recovery of the internal standard added before extraction. Positive ESI-MS/MS was performed using the parameters described under supplementary information.

Statistical analysis. Data are represented as the mean ± SE. In all cases, *n* refers to the number of independent experiments. When comparisons were done relative to the control, statistical analyses were run by Student's *t* test, *p* < 0.05 was considered significant. Statistical significance of comparisons between different treatments was assessed using ANOVA (GraphPad Prism 7, La Jolla, CA).

Results

Upregulation of ceramide via the de novo pathway and the hydrolysis of sphingomyelin by GT3 in pancreatic cancer cells regardless of their Ras status. Previous studies had shown that apoptosis is induced by GT3 in both wild type and mutated K-Ras pancreatic cancer cell lines via a mechanism that involves disruption of signaling of receptor tyrosine kinase ErbB2. To test whether changes in ceramide expression levels occur, we probed the ceramide *de novo* synthesis pathway by analyzing the expression of enzymes SPT, CERS-6, DEGS1 at 2, 4, and 6 hours after dosing with GT3, K-Ras mutated MIA PaCa-2 (Fig. 1a-f) and Panc 1 (Fig. 2a-f), and wild type BxPC3

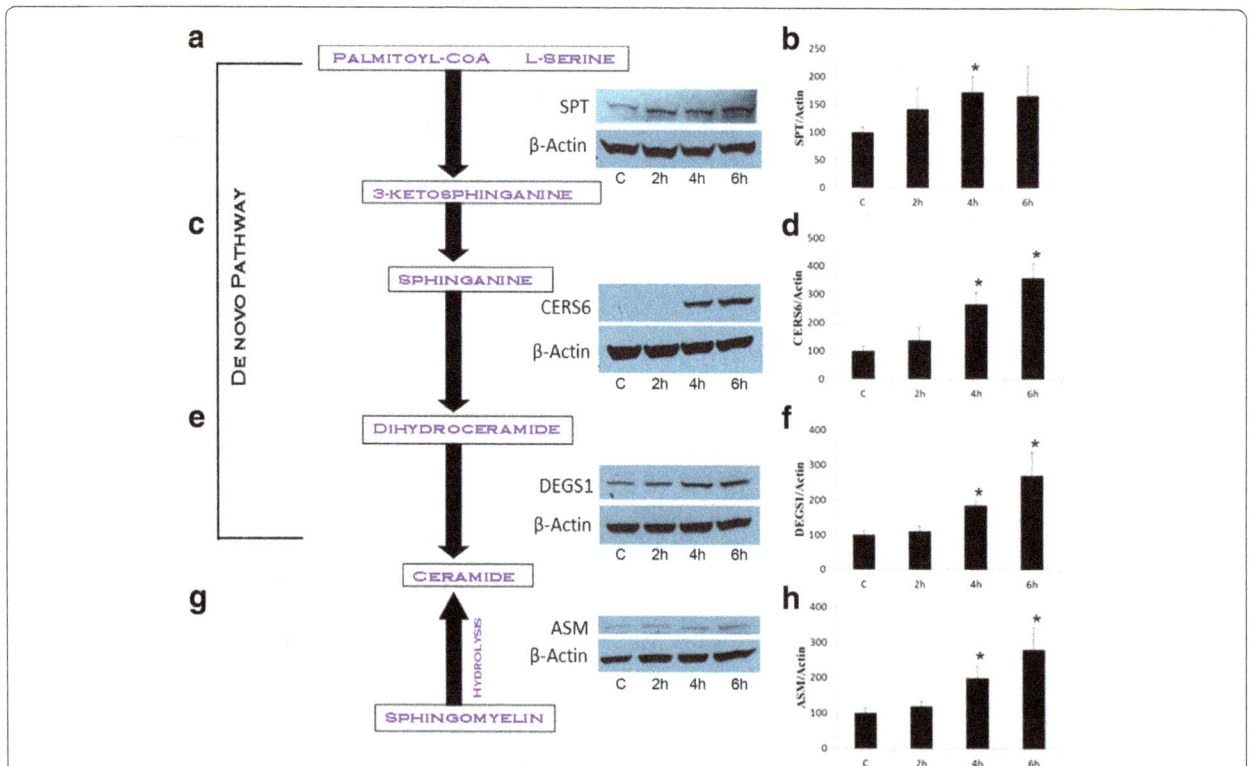

Fig. 1 *Time-dependent increase of ceramide synthesis enzymes in GT3 treated MIA-PaCa-2 cells.* Ceramide is produced via the *de novo* pathway (**a, c, e**) each step is catalyzed by the following enzymes, SPT(**b**), CER6 (**d**), and DEGS1(**f**). It is also produced by hydrolysis of sphingomyelin (**g**) by ASM (**h**). Pancreatic cancer MIA PaCa-2 cells were treated with GT3 at a concentration of 40 μM or dissolution vehicle as a control for different time periods (2, 4, 6 h). Cell lysates were analyzed by immunoblot. Membranes were incubated with antibodies against SPT(**b**), CERS6 (**d**), DEGS1(**f**), and ASM(**h**). The membranes were reprobed with actin as a loading control. All assays were conducted at least three times and blots shown are representative of the results obtained. For quantification band densities from the treatment conditions identified by the lane labels, were calculated as percentages of the value for the treated, untreated cells (100%), and shown averages ± standard deviations from three independent experiments (*p<0.05)

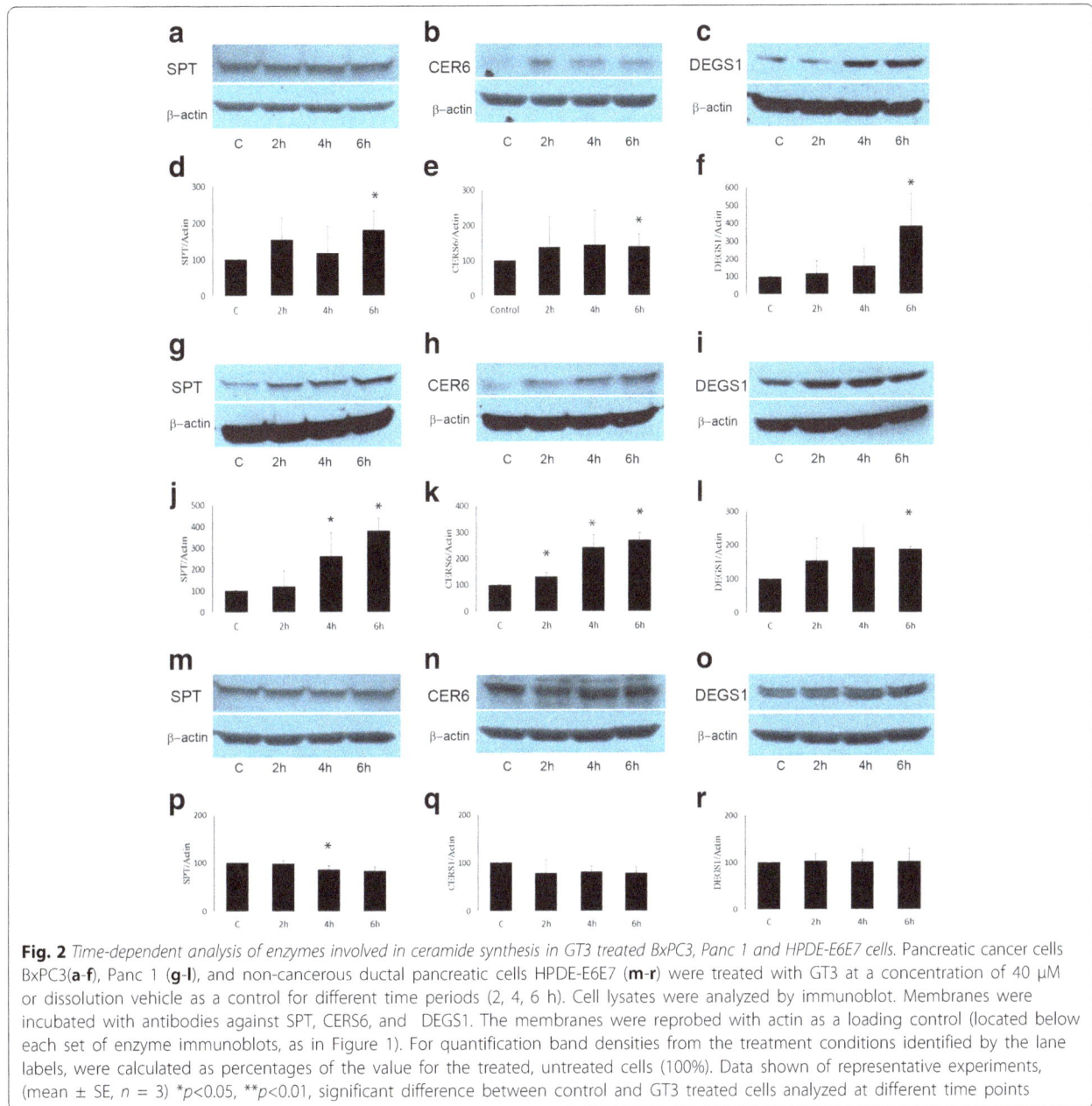

Fig. 2 *Time-dependent analysis of enzymes involved in ceramide synthesis in GT3 treated BxPC3, Panc 1 and HPDE-E6E7 cells.* Pancreatic cancer cells BxPC3(**a-f**), Panc 1 (**g-l**), and non-cancerous ductal pancreatic cells HPDE-E6E7 (**m-r**) were treated with GT3 at a concentration of 40 μM or dissolution vehicle as a control for different time periods (2, 4, 6 h). Cell lysates were analyzed by immunoblot. Membranes were incubated with antibodies against SPT, CERS6, and DEGS1. The membranes were reprobed with actin as a loading control (located below each set of enzyme immunoblots, as in Figure 1). For quantification band densities from the treatment conditions identified by the lane labels, were calculated as percentages of the value for the treated, untreated cells (100%). Data shown of representative experiments, (mean ± SE, n = 3) *p<0.05, **p<0.01, significant difference between control and GT3 treated cells analyzed at different time points

pancreatic cancer cells (Fig. 2g-l). The expression levels of all enzymes tested increased in a time-dependent manner in MIA PaCa-2, Panc 1, and BxPC3 pancreatic cancer cells. A 1.5 fold increase of SPT is apparent 2 hours after dosing MIA PaCa -2 cells with GT3 as compared to the control (Fig. 1a and b). Similarly, DEGS1 levels increase in all cell lines tested with up to 3.0 fold increase in MIA PaCa-2 cells (Fig. 1e and f). A robust increase in the CERS6 levels at 4 and 6 hours after treatment with GT3 also support the activation of this pathway (Fig. 1c and d). Many recent studies have demonstrated the central role of ASM in the apoptotic process via the formation of ceramide-enriched

membrane domains, specifically by gamma radiation [18, 19], UV light [20, 21], and chemotherapeutic agents such as cisplatin [22] and doxorubicin [23]. To determine whether GT3 activates the hydrolysis of sphingomyelin, we probed the levels of ASM. Our results indicate that GT3 may also favor the hydrolysis of sphingomyelin to produce ceramide by increasing the concentration of ASM by 3.4 fold in MIA PaCa-2 cells after treatment with GT3 (Fig. 1g and h). A similar trend on the levels of ASM was observed in Panc 1 and BxPC3 pancreatic cancer cells (results not shown). These results suggest that the activation of ceramide synthesis by GT3 is likely to increase the ceramide levels in the treated cells. Conversely, in non-cancerous human pancreatic ductal epithelial cells (HPDE-E6E7), GT3 has no significant effects on any of the enzymes tested, as compared to the control (Fig. 2m-r).

Pancreatic cancer cells MIA PaCa-2 have higher total ceramide content than non-malignant pancreatic HPDE-E6E7 epithelial cells and GT3 cause a further increase in ceramides and dihydroceramides in MIA PaCa-2 cells. Ceramide is an important regulator of cellular homeostasis, involved in signaling pathways of apoptosis, senescence, and differentiation [24]. However, its expression levels are normally low and upregulation of ceramide concentration is tightly controlled. Increased levels of ceramides are known to cause apoptosis and are also involved in oncogenesis. To test whether pancreatic cancer MIA PaCa-2 cells have higher ceramide levels than epithelial pancreatic HPDE-E6E7 cells, the total content of ceramides was analyzed by LCMS. The results obtained are in agreement with previous studies in other cancers, and show that MIA PaCa-2 cells have approximately three-fold expression levels than non-malignant (HPDE-E6E7) pancreatic cells (Fig. 3a). Further accumulation of ceramides in the cell membrane may activate their apoptotic function, and support the observations in studies that have shown inhibition of cell viability by GT3. LCMS analysis showed that GT3 cause a further increase of 72.9%±1.82 total membrane ceramides in MIA PaCa-2 cells, confirming the observations on the activation of synthesis pathways of ceramide (Fig. 3b). Dihydroceramides are present at significantly lower concentrations as compared to ceramides in both MIA PaCa-2 and HPDE-E6E7 cells. Unlike ceramides, dihydroceramide levels in the membrane are three fold higher in HPDE-E6E7 than in MIA PaCa-2 cells. These compounds show an increase of 80.5 %±1.16, and 42.97%±3.47 after treatment with GT3 of MIA PaCa-2 and HPDE-E6E7 cells, respectively (Fig. 3b).

Membrane sphingomyelin is significantly decreased in MIA PaCa-2 and HPDE-E6E7 cells treated with GT3. Besides the *de novo* pathway, ceramide synthesis can occur via the hydrolysis of sphingomyelin. In order to determine whether there is a significant change in sphingomyelin content, LCMS analysis was conducted on cell lysates of GT3 treated and untreated MIA PaCa-2 and HPDE-E6E7 cells. In untreated cells, non-malignant cells have only slightly higher levels of sphingomyelin than pancreatic cancer cells (Fig. 3c). A significant decrease in membrane sphingomyelin of 26.54%±0.071 in MIA PaCa-2, and 70. 05% ±11.17 in HPDE-E6E7 was observed after treatment with GT3, supporting our previous data on the activation of the ceramide synthesis pathway via sphingomyelin hydrolysis (Fig. 3c).

GT3 cause an increase in membrane ceramides and dihydroceramides C16, C24:1, and C24 and a decrease in sphingomyelins in MIA PaCa-2 cells Ceramides with a

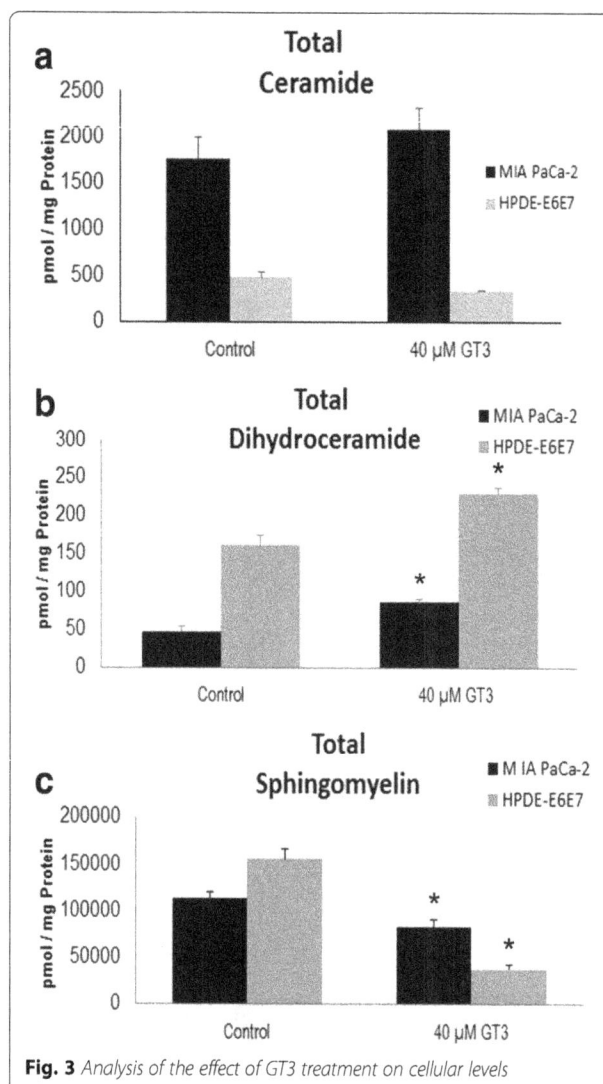

Fig. 3 *Analysis of the effect of GT3 treatment on cellular levels of ceramide,dihydroceramide, and sphingomyelin.* A. LC/MS analysis of sphingolipids present in theplasma membrane for ceramides (**a**), dihydroceramides (**b**), and sphingomyelin (**c**), in MIA Paca-2, and HPDE-E6E7 cells treated with dissolution vehicle (control) or 40 µMGT3. Results are shown as pmol of each indicated sphingolipid / mg of protein in the sample analyzed. The values shown are the averages ± standard deviations obtained from three independentexperiments. * p <0.05, significant difference between control and GT3 treated cells

different fatty acid chain length, have different cellular functions. It has been previously reported that increase in the levels of C16, C24:1 and C24 ceramides, can induce cell death in lymphoma cells after treatment with cannabinoids [25], and the specific upregulation of C16 ceramide in leukemia and colon cancer cells can cause apoptosis [26]. To test whether membrane C16, C24:1, and C24 ceramides are altered by GT3 treatment of MIA PaCa-2 and HPDE E6E7 cells, we analyzed these compounds by LC/MS. Our data show that in untreated cells, C16 is present at 2.7-fold higher levels in MIA PaCa-2 than in HPDE E6E7 cells. Similarly, C24:1, and

C24 ceramides, are also present at 7.5-fold and 3.5 fold higher levels in MIA PaCa-2 than in HPDE E6E7 cells. Treatment with GT3 produce a significant change only in C16 ceramide, with an increase of 32.36% as compared to the control (Fig. 4a). Conversely, in non-malignant HPDE-E6E7 cells, the only membrane ceramide that is observed to change significantly is also C16 with a 41.47% decrease as compared to the control (Fig. 4b). Dihydroceramides are present at significantly lower concentrations than ceramides in MIA PaCa-2 cells. However, these compounds may contribute to the total content of cellular ceramides. Our results show that GT3 cause an increase in dihydroceramides of 79.08% 87.34%, and 83.44% for C16, C24:1, and C24, respectively as compared to the control (Fig. 4c). HPDE-E6E7 cells have higher concentrations of dihydroceramides at the cellular membrane than MIA PaCa-2 cancer cells. Our results show that only C16 display a significant

increase of 59.52% (Fig. 4d). All sphingomyelins tested displayed a significant decrease in MIA PaCa-2 cells after treatment with GT3. LCMS analysis of sphingomyelin in MIA PaCa-2 cells treated with GT3 showed a significant decrease of 29. 2% (C16), 24.44 (C24:1), and 45.0% (C24). (Fig. 4e). Similarly to sphingomyelins in MIA PaCa-2 cells, GT3 cause a significant decrease in HPDE-E6E7 -E6E7 cells of 79.5% (C16), 74.8% (C24:1), and 79.3% (C24) (Fig. 4f).

Ceramide transporter CERT is downregulated and ER-localized sterol transport protein ARV1 is upregulated by GT3 in MIA PaCa-2, BxPC3, and Panc1 pancreatic cancer cells.

To determine whether the activation of the pathways of ceramide synthesis cause an effect on the expression levels of ceramide transporters, we probed ceramide transport protein CERT and ARV-1. The function of the ceramide transport protein CERT, is to transport newly

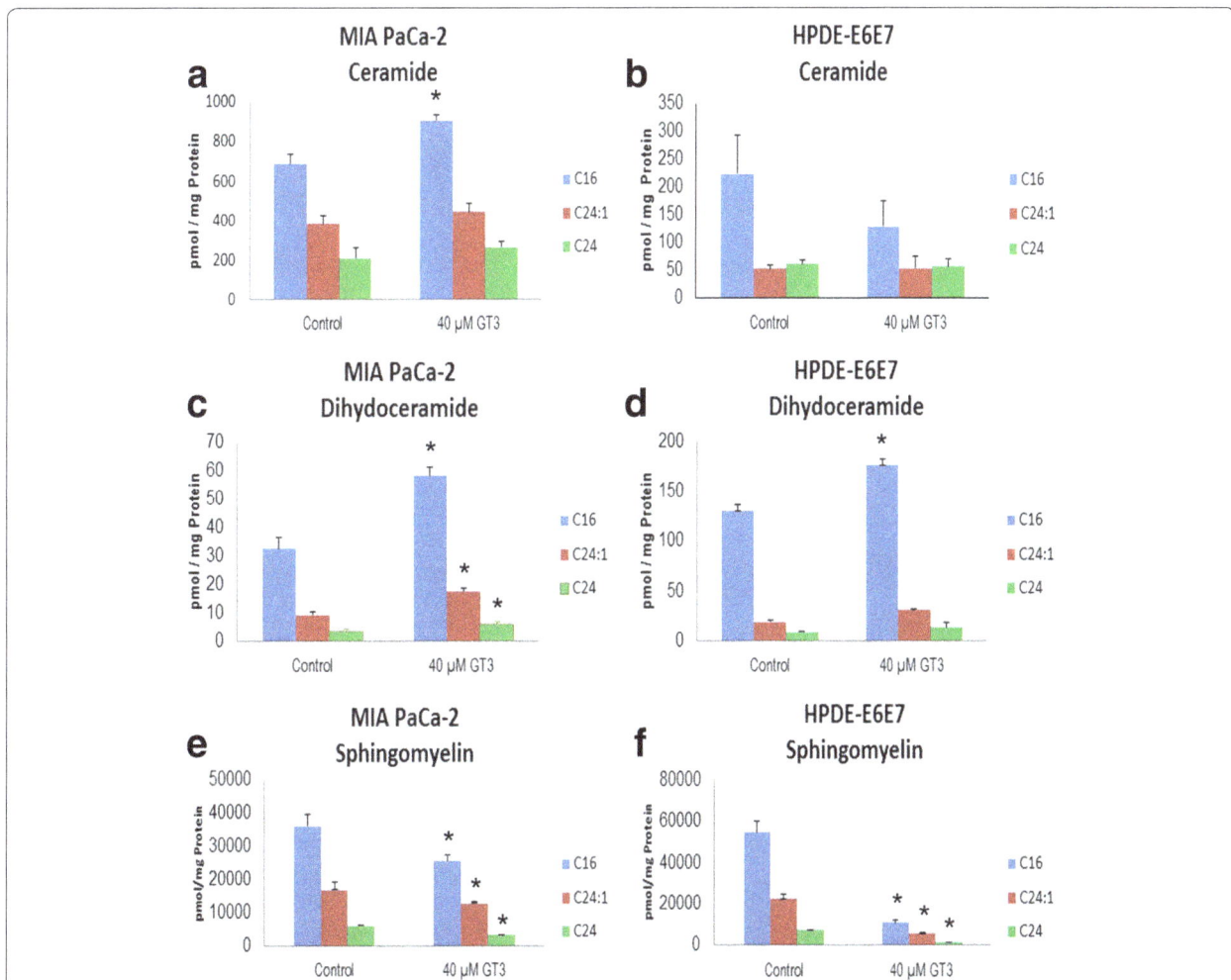

Fig. 4 *Analysis of the effect of GT3 treatment on the expression levels of ceramides C16, C24:1 and C24. A. LC/MS of C16, C24:1 and C24 ceramides in MIA PaCa-2 cells (**a**), and HPDE-E6E7(**b**) dihydroceramides (**c** and **d**), and sphingomyelin (**e** and **f**) treated with dissolution vehicle (control) or 40μM GT3. Results are shown as pmol of each indicatedsphingolipid/mg of protein in the sample analyzed. The values shown are the averages ± standard deviations obtained from three independent experiments. * p <0.05, significant differencebetween control and GT3 treated cells*

synthesized ceramide from the ER to the Golgi [27], where the latter is hydrolyzed to sphingomyelin by sphingomyelinase [28]. To determine whether treatment of MIA PaCa-2, BxPC3, and Panc 1 cancer cells with GT3 favor the transport of newly synthesized ceramide to the Golgi, the levels of CERT and its phosphorylated form were probed by immunoblot. As shown in Fig. 5a and b, there is a significant decrease of both, the activated form and total CERT levels in GT3 treated MIA PaCa-2 cells as compared to the control. We also probed ARV1, a sterol/ceramide transport protein that interacts with genes involved in GPI anchor synthesis; it has been shown that GPI assembly is required for ceramide transport from the ER [29]. As shown in Fig. 5c, d and f, ARV-1 displays a dose-dependent increase in expression levels in MIA PaCa-2, BxPC3 and Panc 1 cells treated with GT3 at 5, 10, 20, and 40µM, with ARV-1 expression levels reaching a 3-fold increase at the highest concentration tested in MIA PaCa-2 cells. A similar trend was observed in BxPC3 and Panc 1 cells, suggesting a decrease in sphingomyelin biosynthesis from newly synthesized ceramide (Fig. 5g).This trend is also evident in

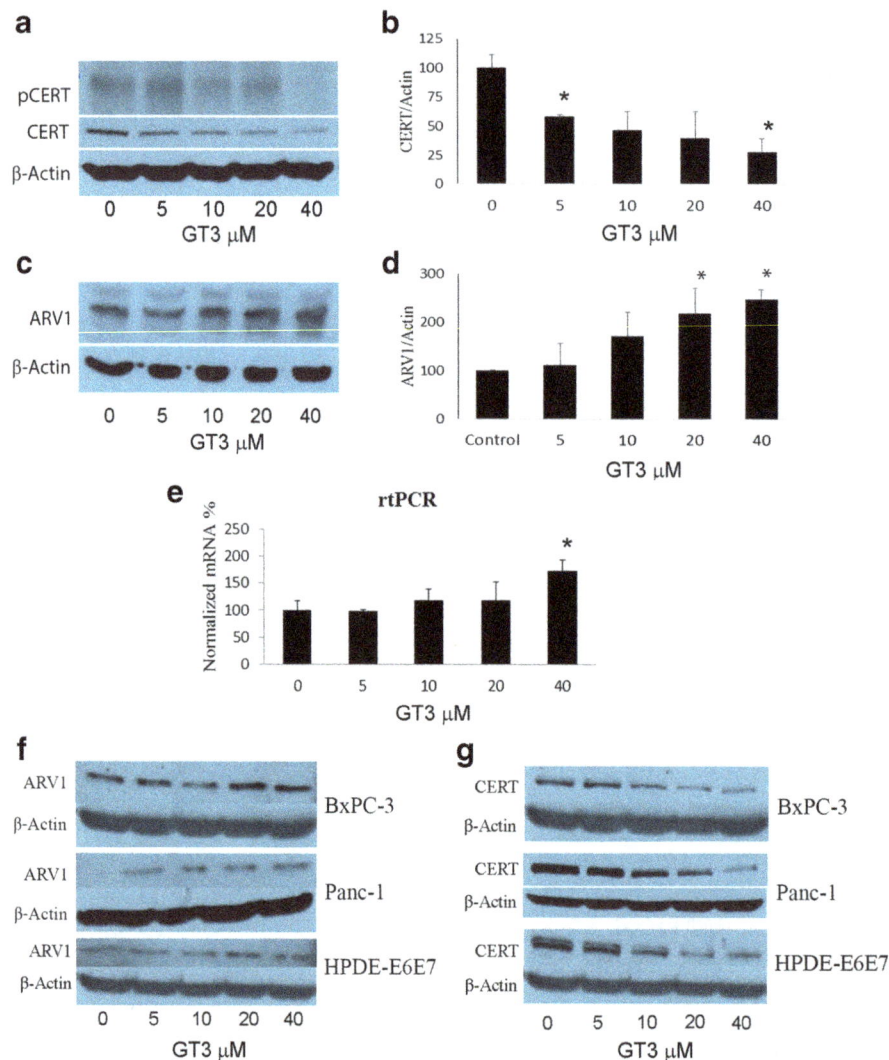

Fig. 5 *Downregulation of ceramide transporter CERT and upregulation of transport protein, ARV-1 in MIA PaCa-2, BxPC3, Panc 1 and HPDE-E6E7 cells treated with GT3.* Pancreatic cancer cells MIA PaCa-2, BxPC3, and Panc 1, as well as HPDE-E6E7cells were treated for 4 hours with increasing concentrations of GT3 over a dose range from 0-40µM and probed for CERT and its activated form (**a** and **b** for MIA PaCa-2 assays, and **g** for BxPC3, Panc1, and HPDE-E6E7), ARV-1 (**c** and **d** for MIA PaCa-2 assays and **f** for BxPC3, Panc1, and HPDE-E6E7), and analyzed by western immunoblot. The membranes were reprobed with actin as a loading control. Quantitative RT-PCR using ARV-1 primers was performed on MIA PaCa-2 cells treated with increasing concentrations of GT3 in the same manner as described above (**e**). All assays were conducted in triplicate and blots shown are representative of the results obtained. For quantification, (graphs) band densities from the treatment conditions identified by the lane labels, were calculated as percentages of the value for the treated, untreated cells (100%). Data shown of representative experiments, (mean ± SE, $n = 3$). * $p < 0.05$, significant difference between control and GT3 treated cells at different concentrations

rtPCR analysis suggesting that GT3 effect on ARV-1 may occur at the transcription level (Fig. 5e).

GT3 treatment of ARV-1 inhibited MIA PaCa-2 cells causes upregulation of the expression levels of caveolin-1. To test whether the effect of GT3 on ARV-1 occurs mainly at the messenger level, protein expression levels were analyzed by immunoblot in MIA PaCa-2 cells transduced with ARV-1 shRNA and treated with GT3. As shown in Fig. 6a and b, ARV-1 is effectively downregulated by ARV-1 shRNA (Fig. 6a and b). GT3 has no significant effect on the expression of ARV-1 (Fig. 6a and b). One of the functions of ARV-1 is to regulate sterol trafficking and plasma membrane

structure. It is also known that ceramide is present in caveolae in cancer cells. To test whether GT3 has an effect on caveolin-1, we probed the expression levels of this protein in the presence and in the absence of ARV-1 in MIA PaCa-2 cells. Data shown in Fig. 6c and d suggest that in the presence of ARV-1, there is no significant change in the expression levels of this molecule. However, substantial upregulation is observed in the absence of ARV-1 regardless of GT3 treatment. Caveolin-1 is present in caveolae and is a major component of the vesicular transport system of the trans-Golgi network [27]. To study the role of ARV-1 in the localization of ceramide and caveolin in GT3 treated cells,

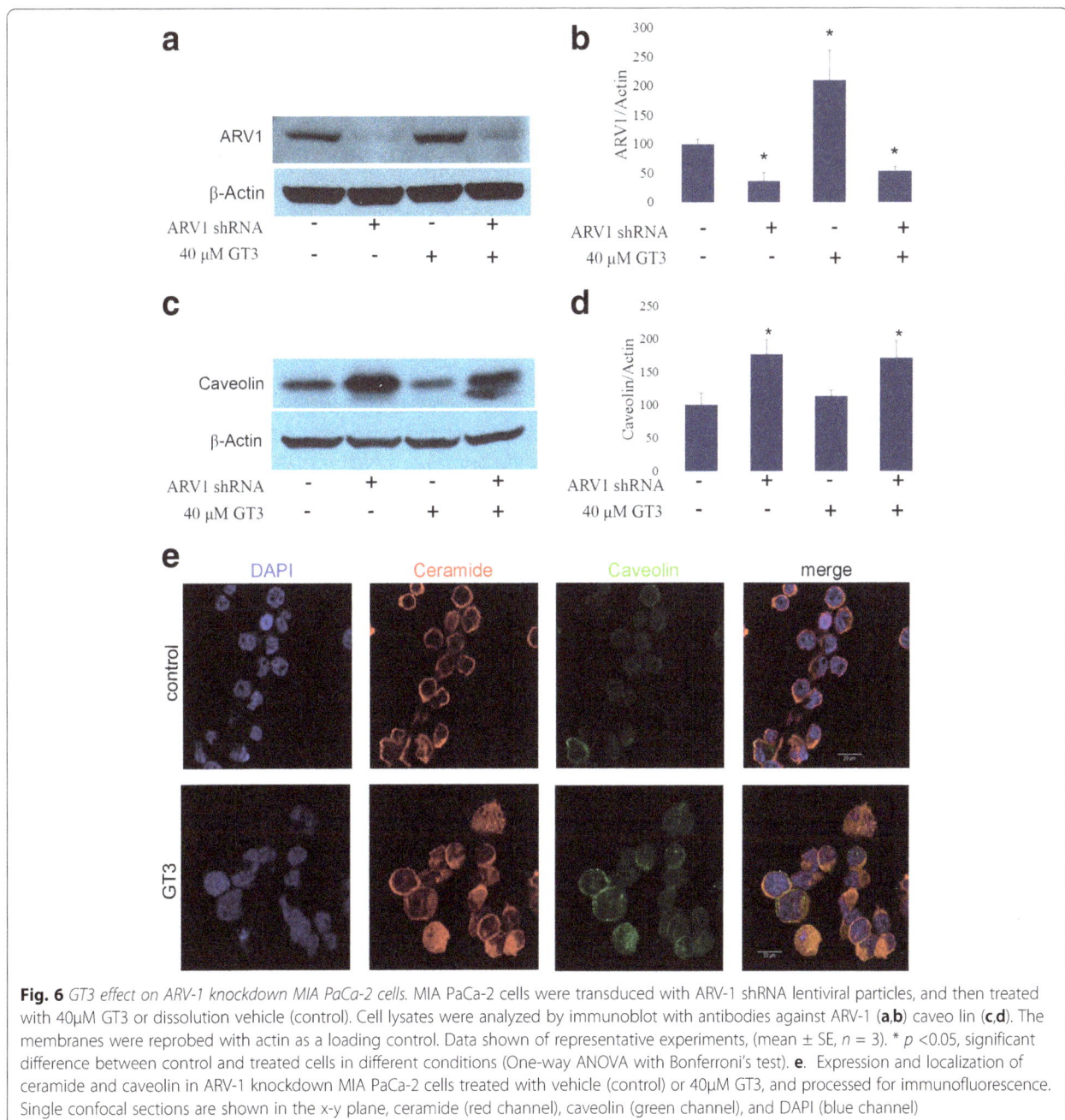

Fig. 6 *GT3 effect on ARV-1 knockdown MIA PaCa-2 cells.* MIA PaCa-2 cells were transduced with ARV-1 shRNA lentiviral particles, and then treated with 40μM GT3 or dissolution vehicle (control). Cell lysates were analyzed by immunoblot with antibodies against ARV-1 (**a,b**) caveo lin (**c,d**). The membranes were reprobed with actin as a loading control. Data shown of representative experiments, (mean ± SE, $n = 3$). * $p < 0.05$, significant difference between control and treated cells in different conditions (One-way ANOVA with Bonferroni's test). **e.** Expression and localization of ceramide and caveolin in ARV-1 knockdown MIA PaCa-2 cells treated with vehicle (control) or 40μM GT3, and processed for immunofluorescence. Single confocal sections are shown in the x-y plane, ceramide (red channel), caveolin (green channel), and DAPI (blue channel)

ARV-1 shRNA transduced cells were processed for immunofluorescence. In the absence of ARV-1, caveolin (green channel) and ceramide (red channel) are localized at the plasma membrane and intracellularly in GT3 treated cells (Fig. 6e).

Ceramide-rich caveolae favor clustering of DR5 in GT3 treated pancreatic cancer cells. It has been reported that a high presence of ceramide in caveolae in human colon cancer cells, favors apoptosis via clustering of Death Receptor 5 [28]. We have previously shown that GT3 has a potent inhibitory effect on ErbB2 phosphorylation [11]. Since ErbB2 is co-localized with caveolin [30], we probed whether the increase of membrane ceramides and the onset of apoptosis by GT3 include the clustering of DR5, by determining the presence and localization of the receptor via immunofluorescence. In untreated and treated cells, ceramide and DR5 are localized at the membrane, red and green channels respectively, Fig. 7a xy and xz planes. Intensity correlation analysis of 14 fields, each with an average of 12.5 cells, showed no significant change with a percentage of colocalization of 74.6% in untreated cells (Fig. 7b) and 73.8% in treated cells (Fig. 7d). However, there was a substantial increase in fluorescence intensity on treated cells, of 3-fold for DR5, and 1.5-fold for ceramide (Fig. 7e) as compared to the control (Fig. 7c). To confirm these observations, analysis of mean intensities of the red and green channels was conducted in these cells (Fig. 8a) GT3 treated cells showed a significant increase in intensities of both channels as compared to untreated cells (Fig. 8b). These results suggest that the activation of apoptosis by GT3 in pancreatic cancer cells may include the participation of DR5 and an increase of ceramide expression levels at the cell membrane suggesting the presence of ceramide micro domains that have been described previously [31].

Discussion

Our previous work indicated that GT3 has potent antiproliferative activity in both k-Ras wild type and k-Ras mutated pancreatic cancer cells, but not on noncancerous pancreatic duct epithelial HPDE-E6E7 cells. The mechanism of action included inhibitory effects on transcription factor NF-κB [12], ErbB2, and the PI3K, MAPK, and HMG CoA reductase pathways, as well as induction of apoptotic signaling through Foxo3 and GSK-3β [11]. However, the coordination of these multi-pronged effects is not completely understood. The results presented in this study suggest that the modulation of expression and localization of ceramide is a relevant factor contributing to the previously observed effects on cell signaling pathways and cell survival. The increase of expression of ASM, responsible for the production of ceramide from sphingomyelin, lends support to this notion. ASM localizes in sphingolipid and cholesterol-enriched membrane domains [32], and the ceramide molecules thus generated, freely associate with each other forming strongly stabilized [33] ceramide-enriched membrane domains [25] by the selective displacement of cholesterol [9]. These changes in membrane composition alter the relatively rapid lateral diffusion characteristic of cholesterol-rich liquid-ordered state [26], and cause destabilization in the structure and function of membrane domains where ErbB2 and other signaling molecules are known to be localized. We had previously shown that cholesterol depletion result in the loss of ErbB2 activation and subsequent inhibition of the ERK pathway [17] It has also been shown that ceramide can cause apoptosis via inactivation of the Ras-Raf/MEK pathway [34]. Thus the exclusion of cholesterol from the plasma membrane, and the downregulation of cholesterol synthesis through inhibition of the HMG CoA reductase pathway by GT3, are likely contributors to the profound changes at the cell membrane imposed by the upregulation of ceramide synthesis. Furthermore, ASM activity also leads to cholesterol displacement from the plasma membrane [35–38] supporting a shift in membrane composition and structure, and subsequently altering signaling function. The resulting ceramide-enriched membrane domains [31], may then favor the presence and clustering of death receptors [28, 39], in agreement with our observation of DR5 localization and clustering at the plasma membrane. These events are required for the formation of death-inducing signaling complexes [40, 41] and are indicative of the activation of the extrinsic apoptotic (JNK) pathway [42], which lend support to our previous results on the upregulation and activation of c-JUN and caspase 8 by GT3 [11]. The role of ceramide in the activation of the JNK pathway and initiation of apoptosis has been demonstrated in several studies [43, 44]. Additionally, DR5 is a component of the TRAIL apoptotic signaling, important for its selective toxicity towards tumor cells [45] and its relation to resistance and sensitization to chemotherapy agents [46]. Our results suggest that GT3 cytotoxic effects carried out via various signaling molecules, are facilitated by the upregulation of expression levels of enzymes involved in the synthesis of ceramide and the subsequent shift in cellular membrane composition and function. However, this set of finely orchestrated events that may obviate the aberrant survival mechanisms present in pancreatic cancer cells, would not be functional without the upregulation of ARV-1 [47] and downregulation of CERT. ARV-1 is involved in sterol transport [48] as well as sphingolipid [49] and glycosylphosphatidyl- inositol [29] biosynthesis. Thus suggesting that GT3 may exert an effect on multiple targets related to control of transcription and molecular synthesis, as well as lipid trafficking and distribution. Loss of membrane cholesterol stimulate sphingolipid transport via CERT [36], and changes in membrane composition by the increase in ceramide

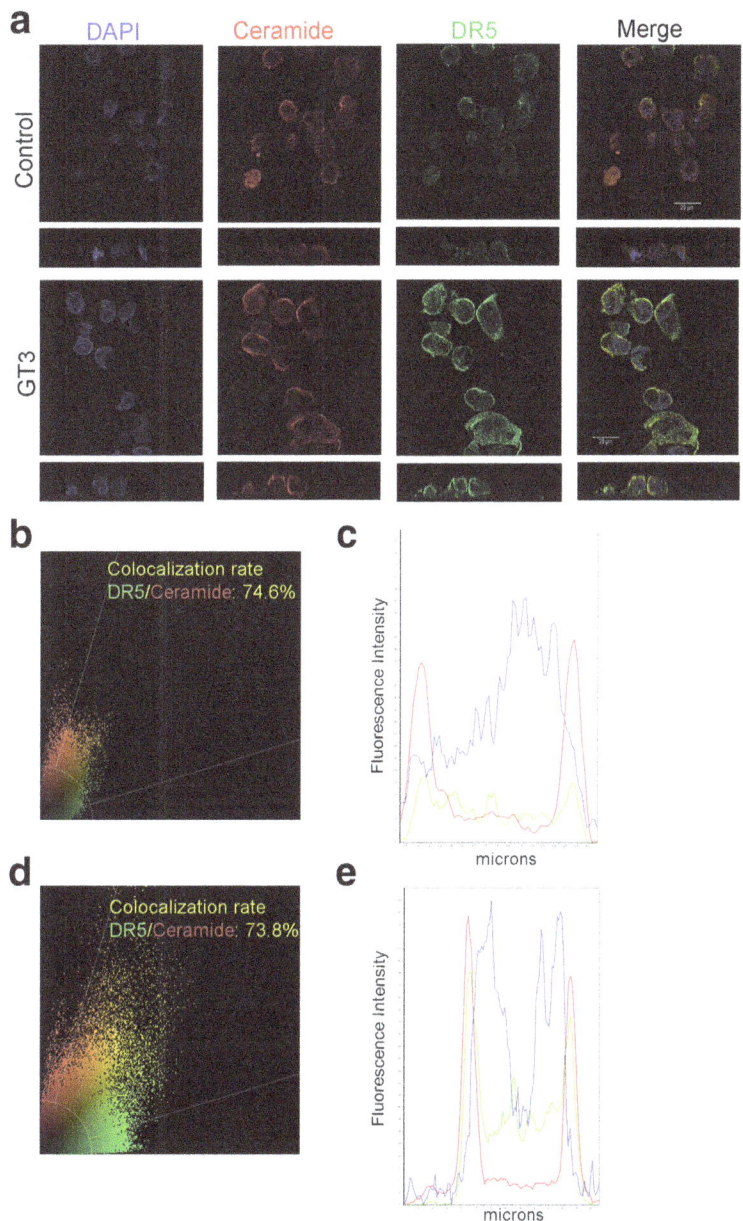

Fig. 7 *Colocalization analysis of ceramide and DR5 after GT3 treatment in MIA PaCa-2 cells.* MIA PaCa-2 cells were treated with dissolution vehicle (**a** top panels) or 40μM GT3 (**a** bottom panels), fixed, and processed for immunofluorescence. Single confocal sections shown in the x–y plane, and 3D reconstructions of the confocal stack in the x–z plane perpendicular to the monolayer, apical side up, show localization of DR5 (green channel), ceramide (red channel), and nuclei using DAPI (blue channel). Intensity correlation analysis of 14 fields, each with an average of 12.5 cells from at least three independent experiments, using the Leica Software were run for control cells (**b**) and (**c**) and treated cells (**d**) and were plotted for both sets of cell populations. The values shown are the averages ± standard deviations obtained from at least three independent experiments. Images are representative of fields analyzed. Graphs illustrating the quantification of relative fluorescence for control cells (**c**) and treated cells (**e**) show the merge for ceramide and DR5 channels. Images shown are representative of the fields observed

content, cause displacement of cholesterol [9]. However, GT3 effectively downregulates CERT, thus causing inhibition of sphingomyelin synthesis in the Golgi from ceramide by diminishing the transport of newly produced ceramide from the ER [50, 51]. Additionally, upregulation of sterol transporter ARV-1, and ceramide synthesis enzymes cause redistribution and upregulation of ceramide

at the cellular membrane strongly promoting a profound change in membrane composition and function. Thus, GT3 displays remarkable efficacy in inhibiting the survival mechanisms present in pancreatic cancer cells by its direct involvement in multiple pro-apoptotic events. Specifically, the inhibition of the MAPK and PI 3K/AKT pathways affecting proliferation and survival, the activation of GSK3β

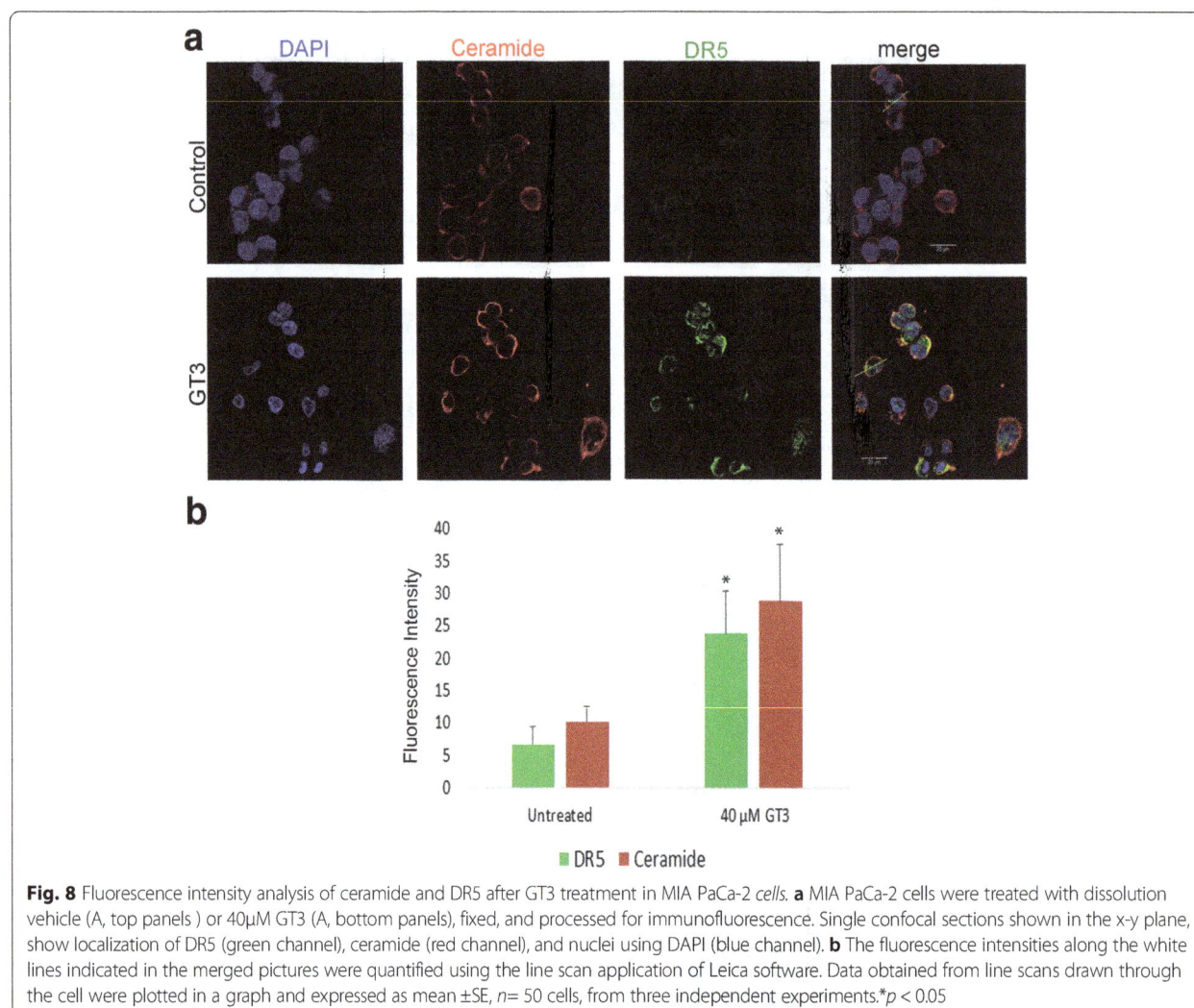

Fig. 8 Fluorescence intensity analysis of ceramide and DR5 after GT3 treatment in MIA PaCa-2 *cells*. **a** MIA PaCa-2 cells were treated with dissolution vehicle (A, top panels) or 40μM GT3 (A, bottom panels), fixed, and processed for immunofluorescence. Single confocal sections shown in the x-y plane, show localization of DR5 (green channel), ceramide (red channel), and nuclei using DAPI (blue channel). **b** The fluorescence intensities along the white lines indicated in the merged pictures were quantified using the line scan application of Leica software. Data obtained from line scans drawn through the cell were plotted in a graph and expressed as mean ±SE, n= 50 cells, from three independent experiments.*$p < 0.05$

and Foxo3 translocation to the nucleus causing G1-phase cell cycle arrest, and activation of the JNK apoptotic pathway via upregulation of and clustering of DR5 at the cell membrane, with subsequent phosphorylation of c-JUN and activation of caspases (10). Additionally, the increase of synthesis of ceramides, specifically, C:16 ceramide a pro-apoptotic molecule. Since most of the newly synthesized ceramides in the ER are used in the Golgi for the synthesis of sphingomyelin and glycosphingolipids [52], the inhibition of CERT [50] causes accumulation of ceramides at the ER, favoring cellular stress and apoptosis. Previous studies have shown increased cytotoxic effects by upregulation of ceramide synthesis in cancer cells.

However, tumor cells treated with drugs that target one or two of the pathways, are likely to fail. Eight approaches to raise ceramide levels have been identified, and many studies suggest that a multiple approach is best to attain a successful intervention [53]. This study has shown that GT3 effectively addresses four of these: stimulation of ceramide synthesis by the *de novo* pathway and sphingomyelin

hydrolysis, inhibition of glycoceramide and sphingomyelin synthesis from ceramide. The latter is due to the inhibition of CERT and results in the downregulation of the MDR1 [54] suggesting the involvement of ceramide with the multidrug resistance pathway. The mechanism of action of several current chemotherapeutic agents include the upregulation of cellular levels of ceramide. Treatment with daunorubicin activate the *de novo* ceramide synthesis pathway [55], and may like cisplatin, stimulate sphingomyelin hydrolysis (32, 33).

Conclusion

Ceramide is a recognized target in oncotherapy. However, in order to obviate the effects of abnormal signaling pathways that result in various mechanisms of resistance in cancer cells, it has been determined that activation of several pathways conducive to raising ceramide levels is necessary for successful activation of apoptosis. The concerted effects on ceramide synthesis, localization and transport by GT3 and its effects on membrane receptors may provide important insight into the targeted pathways necessary to lead pancreatic cancer cells to initiate the apoptotic process and guide the design and development of new therapies for the treatment of pancreatic cancer.

Abbreviations
ARV-1: ACAT-related enzyme-2 required for viability; ASM: acid sphingomyelinase; CERS6: Ceramide synthase 6; CERT: Collagen type IV alpha-3-binding protein, also known as ceramide transfer protein; DEGS1: Delta(4)-desaturase sphingolipid 1; DR5: Death receptor 5; GT3: γ-tocotrienol; SPT: Serine palmitoyl transferase

Acknowledgements
Dr. Hongfeng Jiang at the Biomarkers Core Laboratory, The Irving Institute for Clinical and Translational Research, Columbia University for his help with the acquisition of the LC/MS data. Ms. Rhesa Dykes from the Molecular Biology Core facility at East Tennessee State University, Quillen College of Medicine for her PCR work. Dr. Scott Olenych at the David H. Murdock Research Institute (Kannapolis, NC) for assistance in the use of their Zeiss confocal microscope.

Funding
This work was supported in part by endowment funds from the Dishner Chair of Excellence in Medicine to Dr. K. Krishnan, the National Institutes of Health grant C06RR0306551, as well as by the National Center for Advancing Translational Sciences, National Institutes of Health, through Grant Number UL1 TR000040. The content is solely the responsibility of the authors and does not necessarily represent the official views of the NIH.

Authors' contributions
VEP: Conception, design, data acquisition and analysis, drafting and revising of the manuscript. KC: Conception, design, data acquisition and analysis, drafting and revising of the manuscript. DW: Design, data analysis, drafting and revising of the manuscript. JL: Data acquisition and analysis, drafting of the figures and revising the manuscript. KH: Enzyme data acquisition and analysis, drafting of the figures and revising the manuscript. MB: Design, data acquisition and analysis, and revising of the manuscript.
WS: Design, data analysis, drafting and revising of the manuscript. KK: Design, data acquisition and analysis, drafting and revising of the manuscript, funding. All authors have read and approved the manuscript.

Competing interests
The authors declare that they have no competing interests.

Author details
[1]Division of Hematology-Oncology, Department of Internal Medicine, James H. Quillen College of Medicine, East Tennessee State University, Johnson City, TN 37614, USA. [2]Department of Pharmaceutical Sciences, Gatton College of Pharmacy, East Tennessee State University, Johnson City, TN 37614, USA. [3]Department of Internal Medicine, Beth Israel Deaconess Medical Center, Harvard Medical School, Boston, MA 02215, USA. [4]Department of Pediatrics, James H. Quillen College of Medicine, East Tennessee State University, Johnson City, TN 37614, USA.

References
1. Jemal A, Bray F, Center MM, Ferlay J, Ward E, Forman D. Global cancer statistics. *CA Cancer J Clin*. 2011;61(2):69–90.
2. Bose R, Verheij M, Haimovitz-Friedman A, Scotto K, Fuks Z, Kolesnick R. Ceramide synthase mediates daunorubicin-induced apoptosis: an alternative mechanism for generating death signals. *Cell*. 1995;82(3):405–14.
3. Bruno AP, Laurent G, Averbeck D, Demur C, Bonnet J, Bettaieb A, Levade T, Jaffrezou JP. Lack of ceramide generation in TF-1 human myeloid leukemic cells resistant to ionizing radiation. *Cell Death Differ*. 1998;5(2):172–82.
4. Karahatay S, Thomas K, Koybasi S, Senkal CE, Elojeimy S, Liu X, Bielawski J, Day TA, Gillespie MB, Sinha D, et al. Clinical relevance of ceramide metabolism in the pathogenesis of human head and neck squamous cell carcinoma (HNSCC): attenuation of C(18)-ceramide .0in HNSCC tumors correlates with lymphovascular invasion and nodal metastasis. *Cancer letters*. 2007;256(1):101–11.
5. Tettamanti G, Bassi R, Viani P, Riboni L. Salvage pathways in glycosphingolipid metabolism. *Biochimie*. 2003;85(3-4):423–37.
6. Mandon EC, Ehses I, Rother J, van Echten G, Sandhoff K. Subcellular localization and membrane topology of serine palmitoyltransferase, 3-dehydrosphinganine reductase, and sphinganine N-acyltransferase in mouse liver. *J Biol Chem*. 1992;267(16):11144–8.
7. Shimeno H, Soeda S, Sakamoto M, Kouchi T, Kowakame T, Kihara T. Partial purification and characterization of sphingosine N-acyltransferase (ceramide synthase) from bovine liver mitochondrion-rich fraction. *Lipids*. 1998;33(6):601–5.
8. Mizutani Y, Kihara A, Igarashi Y. Mammalian Lass6 and its related family members regulate synthesis of specific ceramides. *Biochem J*. 2005;390(Pt 1):263–71.
9. Megha LE. Ceramide selectively displaces cholesterol from ordered lipid domains (rafts): implications for lipid raft structure and function. *J Biol Chem*. 2004;279(11):9997–10004.
10. Brigelius-Flohe R, Traber MG. Vitamin E: function and metabolism. *FASEB J*. 1999;13(10):1145–55.
11. Shin-Kang S, Ramsauer VP, Lightner J, Chakraborty K, Stone W, Campbell S, Reddy SA, Krishnan K. Tocotrienols inhibit AKT and ERK activation and suppress pancreatic cancer cell proliferation by suppressing the ErbB2 pathway. *Free Radic Biol Med*. 2011;51(6):1164–74.
12. Ahn KS, Sethi G, Krishnan K, Aggarwal BB. Gamma-tocotrienol inhibits nuclear factor-kappaB signaling pathway through inhibition of receptor-interacting protein and TAK1 leading to suppression of antiapoptotic gene products and potentiation of apoptosis. *J Biol Chem*. 2007;282(1):809–20.
13. Li J, Yu W, Tiwary R, Park SK, Xiong A, Sanders BG, Kline K. alpha-TEA-induced death receptor dependent apoptosis involves activation of acid sphingomyelinase and elevated ceramide-enriched cell surface membranes. *Cancer Cell Int*. 2010;10:40.
14. Jiang Q, Wong J, Fyrst H, Saba JD, Ames BN. gamma-Tocopherol or combinations of vitamin E forms induce cell death in human prostate cancer cells by interrupting sphingolipid synthesis. *Proc Natl Acad Sci U S A*. 2004;101(51):17825–30.
15. Yap SP, Yuen KH, Wong JW. Pharmacokinetics and bioavailability of alpha-, gamma- and delta-tocotrienols under different food status. *J Pharm Pharmacol*. 2001;53(1):67–71.
16. Ouyang H, Mou L, Luk C, Liu N, Karaskova J, Squire J, Tsao MS. Immortal human pancreatic duct epithelial cell lines with near normal genotype and phenotype. *Am J Pathol*. 2000;157(5):1623–31.
17. Pfister AB, Wood RC, Salas PJ, Zea DL, Ramsauer VP. Early response to ErbB2 over-expression in polarized Caco-2 cells involves partial segregation from ErbB3 by relocalization to the apical surface and initiation of survival signaling. *J Cell Biochem*. 2010;111(3):643–52.
18. Paris F, Fuks Z, Kang A, Capodieci P, Juan G, Ehleiter D, Haimovitz-Friedman A, Cordon-Cardo C, Kolesnick R. Endothelial apoptosis as the primary lesion initiating intestinal radiation damage in mice. *Science*. 2001;293(5528):293–7.
19. Santana P, Pena LA, Haimovitz-Friedman A, Martin S, Green D, McLoughlin M, Cordon-Cardo C, Schuchman EH, Fuks Z, Kolesnick R. Acid sphingomyelinase-deficient human lymphoblasts and mice are defective in radiation-induced apoptosis. *Cell*. 1996;86(2):189–99.
20. Charruyer A, Grazide S, Bezombes C, Muller S, Laurent G, Jaffrezou JP. UV-C light induces raft-associated acid sphingomyelinase and JNK activation and translocation independently on a nuclear signal. *J Biol Chem*. 2005;280(19): 19196–204.
21. Zhang Y, Mattjus P, Schmid PC, Dong Z, Zhong S, Ma WY, Brown RE, Bode AM, Schmid HH, Dong Z. Involvement of the acid sphingomyelinase pathway in uva-induced apoptosis. *J Biol Chem*. 2001;276(15):11775–82.

22. Lacour S, Hammann A, Grazide S, Lagadic-Gossmann D, Athias A, Sergent O, Laurent G, Gambert P, Solary E, Dimanche-Boitrel MT. Cisplatin-induced CD95 redistribution into membrane lipid rafts of HT29 human colon cancer cells. *Cancer Res.* 2004;64(10):3593–8.

23. Morita Y, Perez GI, Paris F, Miranda SR, Ehleiter D, Haimovitz-Friedman A, Fuks Z, Xie Z, Reed JC, Schuchman EH, et al. Oocyte apoptosis is suppressed by disruption of the acid sphingomyelinase gene or by sphingosine-1-phosphate therapy. *Nat Med.* 2000;6(10):1109–14.

24. Jarvis WD, Grant S, Kolesnick RN. Ceramide and the induction of apoptosis. *Clin Cancer Res.* 1996;2(1):1–6.

25. Holopainen JM, Subramanian M, Kinnunen PK. Sphingomyelinase induces lipid microdomain formation in a fluid phosphatidylcholine/sphingomyelin membrane. *Biochemistry.* 1998;37(50):17562–70.

26. Almeida PF, Vaz WL, Thompson TE. Lateral diffusion in the liquid phases of dimyristoylphosphatidylcholine/cholesterol lipid bilayers: a free volume analysis. *Biochemistry.* 1992;31(29):6739–47.

27. Kurzchalia TV, Dupree P, Parton RG, Kellner R, Virta H, Lehnert M, Simons K. VIP21, a 21-kD membrane protein is an integral component of trans-Golgi-network-derived transport vesicles. *The Journal of cell biology.* 1992;118(5):1003–14.

28. Martin S, Phillips DC, Szekely-Szucs K, Elghazi L, Desmots F, Houghton JA. Cyclooxygenase-2 inhibition sensitizes human colon carcinoma cells to TRAIL-induced apoptosis through clustering of DR5 and concentrating death-inducing signaling complex components into ceramide-enriched caveolae. *Cancer Res.* 2005;65(24):11447–58.

29. Kajiwara K, Watanabe R, Pichler H, Ihara K, Murakami S, Riezman H, Funato K. Yeast ARV1 is required for efficient delivery of an early GPI intermediate to the first mannosyltransferase during GPI assembly and controls lipid flow from the endoplasmic reticulum. *Mol Biol Cell.* 2008;19(5):2069–82.

30. Nagy P, Claus J, Jovin TM, Arndt-Jovin DJ. Distribution of resting and ligand-bound ErbB1 and ErbB2 receptor tyrosine kinases in living cells using number and brightness analysis. *Proc Natl Acad Sci U S A.* 2010;107(38):16524–9.

31. Kilkus J, Goswami R, Testai FD, Dawson G. Ceramide in rafts (detergent-insoluble fraction) mediates cell death in neurotumor cell lines. *J Neurosci Res.* 2003;72(1):65–75.

32. Grassme H, Jekle A, Riehle A, Schwarz H, Berger J, Sandhoff K, Kolesnick R, Gulbins E. CD95 signaling via ceramide-rich membrane rafts. *J Biol Chem.* 2001;276(23):20589–96.

33. Xu X, Bittman R, Duportail G, Heissler D, Vilcheze C, London E. Effect of the structure of natural sterols and sphingolipids on the formation of ordered sphingolipid/sterol domains (rafts). Comparison of cholesterol to plant, fungal, and disease-associated sterols and comparison of sphingomyelin, cerebrosides, and ceramide. *J Biol Chem.* 2001;276(36):33540–6.

34. Basu S, Bayoumy S, Zhang Y, Lozano J, Kolesnick R. BAD enables ceramide to signal apoptosis via Ras and Raf-1. *J Biol Chem.* 1998;273(46):30419–26.

35. Chatterjee S. Neutral sphingomyelinase action stimulates signal transduction of tumor necrosis factor-alpha in the synthesis of cholesteryl esters in human fibroblasts. *J Biol Chem.* 1994;269(2):879–82.

36. Ridgway ND, Lagace TA, Cook HW, Byers DM. Differential effects of sphingomyelin hydrolysis and cholesterol transport on oxysterol-binding protein phosphorylation and Golgi localization. *J Biol Chem.* 1998;273(47):31621–8.

37. Ridgway ND. Interactions between metabolism and intracellular distribution of cholesterol and sphingomyelin. *Biochim Biophys Acta.* 2000;1484(2-3):129–41.

38. Slotte JP, Lundberg B, Bjorkerud S. Intracellular transport and esterification of exchangeable cholesterol in cultured human lung fibroblasts. *Biochim Biophys Acta.* 1984;793(3):423–8.

39. Stancevic B, Kolesnick R. Ceramide-rich platforms in transmembrane signaling. *FEBS letters.* 2010;584(9):1728–40.

40. Dumitru CA, Gulbins E. TRAIL activates acid sphingomyelinase via a redox mechanism and releases ceramide to trigger apoptosis. *Oncogene.* 2006;25(41):5612–25.

41. Miyaji M, Jin ZX, Yamaoka S, Amakawa R, Fukuhara S, Sato SB, Kobayashi T, Domae N, Mimori T, Bloom ET, et al. Role of membrane sphingomyelin and

ceramide in platform formation for Fas-mediated apoptosis. *J Exp Med.* 2005;202(2):249–59.

42. Min Y, Shi J, Zhang Y, Liu S, Liu Y, Zheng D. Death receptor 5-recruited raft components contributes to the sensitivity of Jurkat leukemia cell lines to TRAIL-induced cell death. *IUBMB Life.* 2009;61(3):261–7.

43. Verheij M, Bose R, Lin XH, Yao B, Jarvis WD, Grant S, Birrer MJ, Szabo E, Zon LI, Kyriakis JM, et al. Requirement for ceramide-initiated SAPK/JNK signalling in stress-induced apoptosis. *Nature.* 1996;380(6569):75–9.

44. Tepper AD, Ruurs P, Wiedmer T, Sims PJ, Borst J, van Blitterswijk WJ. Sphingomyelin hydrolysis to ceramide during the execution phase of apoptosis results from phospholipid scrambling and alters cell-surface morphology. *The Journal of cell biology.* 2000;150(1):155–64.

45. Ashkenazi A. Targeting death and decoy receptors of the tumour-necrosis factor superfamily. *Nat Rev Cancer.* 2002;2(6):420–30.

46. Marks P, Rifkind RA, Richon VM, Breslow R, Miller T, Kelly WK. Histone deacetylases and cancer: causes and therapies. *Nat Rev Cancer.* 2001;1(3):194–202.

47. Beh CT, Rine J. A role for yeast oxysterol-binding protein homologs in endocytosis and in the maintenance of intracellular sterol-lipid distribution. *J Cell Sci.* 2004;117(Pt 14):2983–96.

48. Tinkelenberg AH, Liu Y, Alcantara F, Khan S, Guo Z, Bard M, Sturley SL. Mutations in yeast ARV1 alter intracellular sterol distribution and are complemented by human ARV1. *J Biol Chem.* 2000;275(52):40667–70.

49. Swain E, Stukey J, McDonough V, Germann M, Liu Y, Sturley SL, Nickels JT Jr. Yeast cells lacking the ARV1 gene harbor defects in sphingolipid metabolism. Complementation by human ARV1. *J Biol Chem.* 2002;277(39):36152–60.

50. Hanada K, Kumagai K, Yasuda S, Miura Y, Kawano M, Fukasawa M, Nishijima M. Molecular machinery for non-vesicular trafficking of ceramide. *Nature.* 2003;426(6968):803–9.

51. Perry RJ, Ridgway ND. Oxysterol-binding protein and vesicle-associated membrane protein-associated protein are required for sterol-dependent activation of the ceramide transport protein. *Mol Biol Cell.* 2006;17(6):2604–16.

52. Tafesse FG, Ternes P, Holthuis JC. The multigenic sphingomyelin synthase family. *J Biol Chem.* 2006;281(40):29421–5.

53. Radin NS. Killing tumours by ceramide-induced apoptosis: a critique of available drugs. *Biochem J.* 2003;371(Pt 2):243–56.

54. Gouaze-Andersson V, Yu JY, Kreitenberg AJ, Bielawska A, Giuliano AE, Cabot MC. Ceramide and glucosylceramide upregulate expression of the multidrug resistance gene MDR1 in cancer cells. *Biochim Biophys Acta.* 2007;1771(12):1407–17.

55. Jaffrezou JP, Levade T, Bettaieb A, Andrieu N, Bezombes C, Maestre N, Vermeersch S, Rousse A, Laurent G. Daunorubicin-induced apoptosis: triggering of ceramide generation through sphingomyelin hydrolysis. *EMBO J.* 1996;15(10):2417–24.

A non-controlled, single arm, open label, phase II study of intravenous and intratumoral administration of ParvOryx in patients with metastatic, inoperable pancreatic cancer: ParvOryx02 protocol

Jacek Hajda[1*] ⓘ, Monika Lehmann[1], Ottheinz Krebs[2], Meinhard Kieser[3], Karsten Geletneky[4], Dirk Jäger[5], Michael Dahm[2], Bernard Huber[2], Tilman Schöning[6], Oliver Sedlaczek[7], Albrecht Stenzinger[8], Niels Halama[9], Volker Daniel[10], Barbara Leuchs[11], Assia Angelova[11], Jean Rommelaere[11], Christine E. Engeland[5], Christoph Springfeld[5†] and Guy Ungerechts[5†]

Abstract

Background: Metastatic pancreatic cancer has a dismal prognosis, with a mean six-month progression-free survival of approximately 50% and a median survival of about 11 months. Despite intensive research, only slight improvements of clinical outcome could be achieved over the last decades. Hence, new and innovative therapeutic strategies are urgently required. ParvOryx is a drug product containing native parvovirus H-1 (H-1PV). Since H-1PV was shown to exert pronounced anti-neoplastic effects in pre-clinical models of pancreatic cancer, the drug appears to be a promising candidate for treatment of this malignancy.

Methods: ParvOryx02 is a non-controlled, single arm, open label, dose-escalating, single center trial. In total seven patients with pancreatic cancer showing at least one hepatic metastasis are to be treated with escalating doses of ParvOryx according to the following schedule: i) 40% of the total dose infused intravenously in equal fractions on four consecutive days, ii) 60% of the total dose injected on a single occasion directly into the hepatic metastasis at varying intervals after intravenous infusions. The main eligibility criteria are: age ≥ 18 years, disease progression despite first-line chemotherapy, and at least one hepatic metastasis. Since it is the second trial within the drug development program, the study primarily explores safety and tolerability after further dose escalation of ParvOryx. The secondary objectives are related to the evaluation of certain aspects of anti-tumor activity and clinical efficacy of the drug.

(Continued on next page)

* Correspondence: Jacek.Hajda@med.uni-heidelberg.de
†Equal contributors
[1]Coordination Centre for Clinical Trials, University Hospital Heidelberg,
Marsilius-Arkaden, Tower West, Im Neuenheimer Feld 130.3, 69120
Heidelberg, Germany
Full list of author information is available at the end of the article

(Continued from previous page)

Discussion: This trial strongly contributes to the clinical development program of ParvOryx. The individual hazards for patients included in the current study and the environmental risks are addressed and counteracted adequately. Besides information on safety and tolerability of the treatment after further dose escalation, thorough evaluations of pharmacokinetics and intratumoral spread as well as proof-of-concept (PoC) in pancreatic cancer will be gained in the course of the trial.

Keywords: H-1 parvovirus, Parvovirus, Oncolytic virotherapy, Pancreatic cancer, Pancreatic ductal adenocarcinoma, PDAC, Clinical protocol

Background

According to epidemiological estimations for 40 European countries the overall incidence of pancreatic cancer in the year 2012 amounted to approximately 10.5 cases per 100,000 inhabitants [1]. The figures for mortality were only slightly lower with 10.1 cases per 100,000, indicating the limited treatment options for this disease [1, 2]. Unlike in other neoplasms, the apparent mortality from pancreatic cancer has increased gradually in the past decades and was approximately 20 to 30% higher in 2014 than in 1970. This is probably due to an improvement of diagnostic procedures with a parallel increase in the number of properly documented disease cases. Nevertheless, pancreatic cancer is the only major cancer showing nearly no improvement of therapeutic outcome over the last decades [1–3].

Currently, there are no modalities for early diagnosis or screening for pancreatic cancer so that the disease is typically discovered only at advanced stages. Based on the analysis of the US National Cancer Database (NCDB) performed by the American Joint Committee on Cancer (AJCC) for the period between 1992 and 1998, the following relative distribution of disease stages at the time of the initial diagnosis can be assumed: stage I 9.8, stage II 21.9, stage III: 13.0, and stage IV 55.2%. The corresponding 5-year survival rates are: 25.3, 11.6, 2.7, and 0.7%, respectively [4]. The locally advanced (stage III) and metastatic disease (stage IV) are primarily not eligible for surgical intervention and therefore associated with poor prognosis. The current standard of care for these tumor stages relies upon different chemotherapeutic regimens.

Based on the results of a randomized, controlled clinical trial comparing the therapeutic efficacy of a combination of oxaliplatin, leucovorin, irinotecan, and 5-FU (FOLFIRINOX) to monotherapy with gemcitabine, FOLFIRINOX has been established as the first-line therapy in patients with inoperable pancreatic cancer who are in good physical condition([5]). Another phase III randomized, controlled clinical trial including 861 patients compared the clinical outcome

after treatment with a combination of nab-paclitaxel and gemcitabine to gemcitabine alone [6]. As the drug combination showed significant increase in overall survival with acceptable toxicity, it was approved for the first-line treatment of inoperable disease by the US Food and Drug Administration (FDA) [7]. However, neither FOLFIRINOX nor the combination of nab-paclitaxel and gemcitabine bring about any relevant advantage in terms of long-term clinical outcome [5, 6].

Trial rationale/justification

As briefly outlined above, despite intense efforts to improve treatment, the prognosis for pancreatic cancer patients is still disappointing. Therefore, all agents showing antitumor effects with an acceptable safety profile should undergo rapid clinical development to assess their therapeutic potential.

ParvOryx is a drug that contains parvovirus H-1 (H-1PV) as active substance. H-1PV is a small, single-stranded rodent DNA virus. The natural host is rat, but like other related parvoviruses, H-1PV is able to infect and replicate in cells of various other species including humans. Parvoviruses exert cytopathic effects mainly in neoplastic cells: they preferentially kill in-vitro-transformed and tumor-derived human and rodent cell lines, with limited-to-no cytocidal action in non-transformed cells [8]. Moreover, these viruses have been shown to have oncosuppressive properties, inhibiting the formation of spontaneous as well as chemically or virally induced tumors in laboratory animals [8, 9]. Furthermore, implants of tumor cells, including human neoplastic cells, were shown to be targets for parvoviral anti-cancer activity (oncolysis) in recipient animals [8–12]. Parvoviral cytotoxicity seems to be attributed to the viral nonstructural protein NS-1 [13].

H-1PV showed efficacy in preclinical, in-vitro models of pancreatic cancer. All investigated human pancreatic cancer cell lines, both of primary tumor and of metastatic origin, were susceptible to the stand-alone treatment with H-1PV, although to a varying extent [14, 15]. Synergistic increase of efficacy could be achieved by combination with valproic acid (VPA), a histone deacetylase inhibitor (HDACI) [14]. Moreover, based on the results from investigations on cellular pathways affected by H-1PV as well as by gemcitabine, synergistic effects of concomitant treatment with both agents can be anticipated [15]. Consecutive preclinical in-vivo investigations in animal models of pancreatic cancer carried out in mice and rats showed promising effects of H-1PV in the dose range between 1E09 and 2.5E09 plaque forming units (pfu). The anti-tumor effects were dose-dependent and the viral proteins were selectively expressed in the tumor as opposed to normal tissues. H-1PV virotherapy in an orthotopic pancreatic carcinoma model led to a significant delay in tumor growth and prolongation of survival, with 20% of the treated animals remaining disease-free for 16 weeks [15]. Importantly, in some cases, complete remission of pre-existing tumors was observed. Moreover, inoculation of the primary tumor with H-1PV at early stages of tumor development resulted in almost 50% suppression of distant metastases involving the visceral lymph nodes of the upper abdominal cavity and liver [15]. Also in animal models, the co-administration of VPA increased the potency of H-1PV, allowing a dose reduction by one power of ten down to 2.5E08 pfu without loss of efficacy [14].

Based on the findings described above, ParvOryx can reasonably be assumed to show efficacy against pancreatic cancer in humans. Ideally, the drug would not only be directly cytotoxic to the neoplastic cells but also induce anti-cancer vaccination by destruction of cancer cells and activation of the adaptive immune system. Based on the preclinical investigations synergistic effects with gemcitabine, a drug commonly used for treatment of pancreatic cancer, can be assumed. Thus, there is a strong rationale for treating patients suffering from pancreatic cancer with a combination regimen of ParvOryx and gemcitabine.

Design and methods
Aim
The trial aims at investigation of safety and tolerability, virus distribution and shedding as well as at evaluation of anti-tumor activity and clinical efficacy after multiple intravenous and a single intrametastatic administration of ParvOryx to patients suffering from pancreatic cancer.

Objectives
Primary objectives
The primary objectives of the trial are related to the safety and tolerability of the Investigational Medicinal Product (IMP):

- Safety and tolerability assessed on the basis of physical examinations, chosen laboratory parameters, 12-lead electrocardiogram (ECGs), adverse events (AEs), and serious adverse events (SAEs),
- Assessment of humoral immune response to H-1PV after intravenous infusions and intrametastatic injection (detection of anti-drug-antibodies (ADA)),
- Investigation of the kinetics of H-1PV genomes in blood following intravenous and intrametastatic administration of the IMP by means of quantitative real-time polymerase chain reaction (qPCR),
- Investigation of virus shedding in faeces, urine, and saliva following intravenous and intrametastatic administration of the IMP.

Secondary objectives
The secondary objectives of the study are related to the anti-tumor activity and clinical efficacy of the IMP:

- Investigation of anti-tumor effects of ParvOryx by means of the following histo-immuno-pathological findings: i) extent of metastatis necrosis, proliferation rate and other pathological characteristics, ii) density of tumor-infiltrating immune cells,
- Quantity of cytokines and chemokines in tumor tissue,
- Investigation of viral replication in the tumor tissue by means of NS-1 detection in the tumor material,
- Investigation of the cellular immune response against viral proteins and tumor antigens by means of enzyme-linked immunospot assay (ELISPOT) and fluorescence-activated cell sorting (FACS),
- Progression-free survival (PFS) up to 6 months after the first administration of the IMP (determined by RECIST criteria),
- Morphological changes of the liver metastasis assessed by ultrasonography,
- Overall survival (OS) up to 6 months after the first administration of the IMP,
- Course of the tumor marker carbohydrate antigen 19-9 (CA 19-9) up to 6 months after the first administration of the IMP.

Design
ParvOryx02 is a non-controlled, single arm, open label, dose-escalating, single center trial.

Due to an exploratory approach with regard to safety and tolerability of the IMP, no positive control is used. In face of the small size of the trial population and the intensity of collecting the biological samples, including multiple liver biopsies, no negative control (placebo) was implemented.

In a foregoing, first-in-man trial, referred to as ParvOryx01, comprehensive information on safety and tolerability of the IMP up to the total dose of 5E09 pfu administered by systemic (intravenous) as well as by local (intratumoral and intracerebral) route was obtained. Since the current trial includes further dose escalation up to the total dose of 1E10 pfu, a sequential design, including intervals of at least 28 days between treatments of consecutive subjects, is employed.

Due to the complex handling and administration of the IMP this trial is being performed in a single center with a sound experience in clinical research as well as in clinical management of patients with pancreatic cancer.

Eligibility

Histologically confirmed pancreatic ductal adenocarcinoma with at least one hepatic metastasis is a prerequisite for inclusion in this trial. Moreover, patients have to fulfill the following main inclusion criteria: i) at least 18 years of age, ii) disease progression despite first-line therapy, iii) ECOG performance scale 0 or 1, iv) adequate main organ function, including normal thyroid function, v) negative beta-HCG-test and willingness to abide by the rules of adequate contraception.

Main criteria for exclusion of patients are: i) eligibility for surgery, ii) symptomatic cerebral, pulmonary, osseous metastases and/or peritoneal carcinomatosis, (iii) liver cirrhosis, previous splenectomy and/or severe respiratory impairment, (iv) chemo- and/or radiotherapy within 2 and 6 weeks prior to trial inclusion, respectively, (v) known allergy to iodinated contrast media, (vi) presumed contact to pregnant women and/or infants within 2 months after the first administration of the IMP.

Sample size

As no confirmatory hypothesis tests are performed in this trial, the choice of sample size was not based on formal sample size calculation but on the following pragmatic considerations. The trial aims at evaluating safety and

tolerability as well as proof-of-concept (PoC) regarding efficacy of ParvOryx in the treatment of pancreatic cancer. The number of seven subjects is assumed to be adequate to gain information on safety and tolerability of ParvOryx at the scheduled dose levels as required for continuation of the clinical drug development. Moreover, since PoC is mainly related to pathological and immunological parameters, the size of the trial population seems to be sufficient.

Course of the trial

A schematic overview of the trial is given in Fig. 1. For each individual subject, the trial consists of three phases, i.e. screening, treatment (including observation until study Day 28) and follow-up phase between study Day 28 and 6 months:

- *Screening*
  Screening of patients, aiming at assessment of their eligibility for the trial and collection of the baseline parameters, must be carried out within 2 weeks prior to the study inclusion. Potentially eligible patients are provided with comprehensive written and verbal information. Procedures that are carried out during the screening include:
  Written informed consent, demography and medical history, concomitant medication, physical examination, vital signs and 12-lead ECG, clinical chemistry, hematology and coagulation, CA19-9, ELISPOT and FACS, H-1PV-specific antibodies, serology of human immunodeficiency virus (HIV), hepatitis B virus (HBV) and hepatitis C virus (HCV), pregnancy test, thoracic computed tomography (CT) and abdominal magnetic resonance imaging (MRI), abdominal ultrasonography.
  At the end of the screening phase the inclusion and exclusion criteria will be reviewed and the final

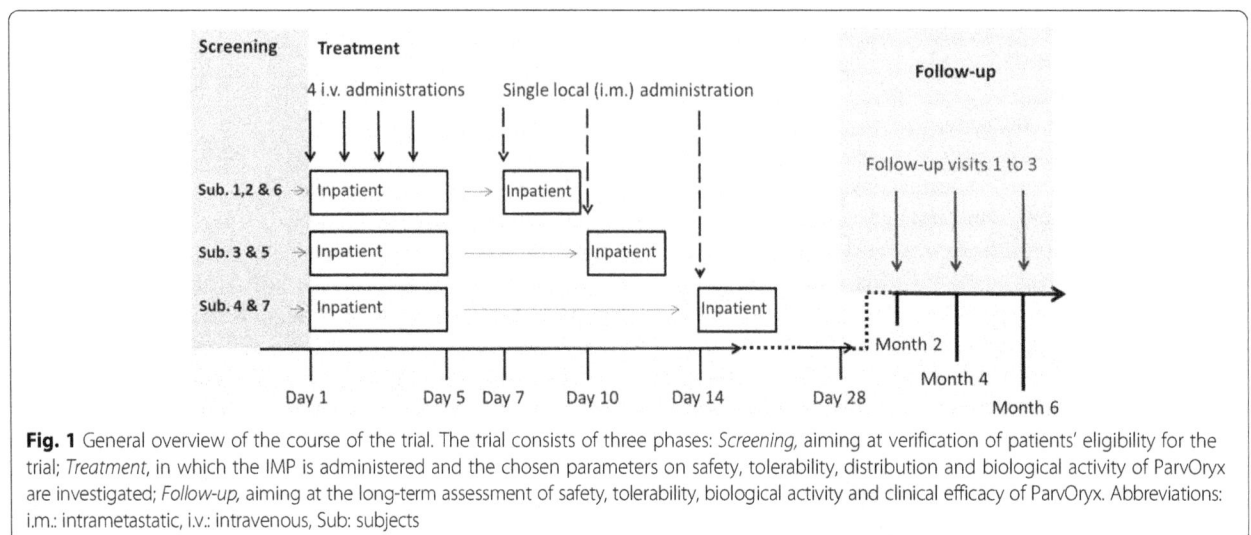

Fig. 1 General overview of the course of the trial. The trial consists of three phases: *Screening*, aiming at verification of patients' eligibility for the trial; *Treatment*, in which the IMP is administered and the chosen parameters on safety, tolerability, distribution and biological activity of ParvOryx are investigated; *Follow-up*, aiming at the long-term assessment of safety, tolerability, biological activity and clinical efficacy of ParvOryx. Abbreviations: i.m.: intrametastatic, i.v.: intravenous, Sub: subjects

judgment on the subject's eligibility will be made. If eligible, the subject will enter the treatment phase and receive the study-specific intervention.

- *Treatment (main intervention)*
  The IMP in this trial is ParvOryx, i.e. a GMP-grade preparation of H-1PV. The administration of the IMP is carried out as follows: i) 40% of the total dose, divided into four equal fractions (10% of the total dose each) infused intravenously (i.v.) over 2 h on four consecutive days, ii) 60% of the total dose injected on a single occasion directly into the hepatic metastasis under ultrasound guidance. The timing of intrametastatic injection differs between the trial subjects. The injection is to be performed either 6 or 9 or 13 days after the first i.v. administration of the IMP (see Fig. 1). The total doses of ParvOryx are: 1E09 pfu in the first subject, 5E09 pfu in three further subjects and 1E10 pfu in the last three subjects (see Table 1). The dose escalation and maintenance at the given dose level is only allowed if ParvOryx proved safe and well-tolerated in the previously treated subjects.

The different time points for the intrametastatic injection were chosen to explore the most appropriate schedule for boosting the anticipated anti-tumor immune reaction. Furthermore, the tissue samples taken in parallel to the intrametastatic treatment will allow for assessment of pharmacokinetics and pharmacodynamics at the respective time points.

There are two chemotherapeutics defined as non-investigational medicinal products (NIMP) in this trial: i) Gemcitabine, administered at the dose of 1000 mg/m^2 of body surface area (BSA) on days 1, 8 and 15 of each 28-day cycle. The administration (cycle 1, day 1) is to be commenced 27 days after the first intravenous administration of ParvOryx, ii) Nab-paclitaxel, administered at the dose

of 125 mg/m^2 of BSA, given on days 1, 8 and 15 of each 28-day cycle, immediately prior to gemcitabine. Nab-paclitaxel is to be introduced only in case of disease progression despite previous treatment with ParvOryx and gemcitabine. Nab-paclitaxel has emerged as a second-line treatment option in PDAC after FOLFIRINOX failure [16]. Mechanistically, preclinical data suggest that nab-paclitaxel increases gemcitabine levels by decreasing intratumoral cytidine deaminase activity [17]. In absence of preclinical data of combining ParvOryx, gemcitabine and nab-paclitaxel, a triple therapy was not feasible within this trial. Nevertheless, this treatment option should be made available to patients with disease progression.

Although the primary objective of this trial refers to the safety and tolerability of ParvOryx, the investigations related to the local anti-tumor activity and to the pharmacokinetics (PK) of H-1PV genomes are of substantial importance. In order to detect possible time-dependent differences, study days appointed for biopsies and PK sampling differ interindividually (see Fig. 2). Likewise, the thorough blood PK evaluations (PK profiles) are scheduled for different study days, i.e. they are performed either on the last day of i.v. administration (3 subjects) or on the day of intrametastatic administration (the remaining four subjects) of ParvOryx. In either case the timing of blood collection is as follows: The first sample is taken prior to the dosing of the IMP, the second sample up to 10 min after the end of the administration procedure, i.e. either at the end-of-infusion or after intrametastatic injection is completed; further samples are obtained 0.5, 1, 2, 4, 7 and 22 h thereafter. Three biopsies per subject are to be collected: i) prior to the overall first administration of the IMP, ii) 6, 9, or 13 days after the first i.v. administration of ParvOryx, directly prior to the intrametastatic administration, iii) either

Table 1 Dosing of ParvOryx in the current trial

Total dose	Study Time	Individual dose and route of administration	Duration
Dose level 1 (1 subject)			
1E09 pfu	Day 1–4	1E08 pfu, intravenous infusion	2 h
	Day 7	6E08 pfu, intrametastatic injection	As slowly as feasible
Dose level 2 (3 subjects)			
5E09 pfu	Day 1–4	5E08 pfu, intravenous infusion	2 h
	Day 7 or 10 or 14	3E09 pfu, intrametastatic injection	As slowly as feasible
Dose level 3 (3 subjects)			
1E10 pfu	Day 1–4	1E09 pfu, intravenous infusion	2 h
	Day 7 or 10 or 14	6E09 pfu, intrametastatic injection	As slowly as feasible

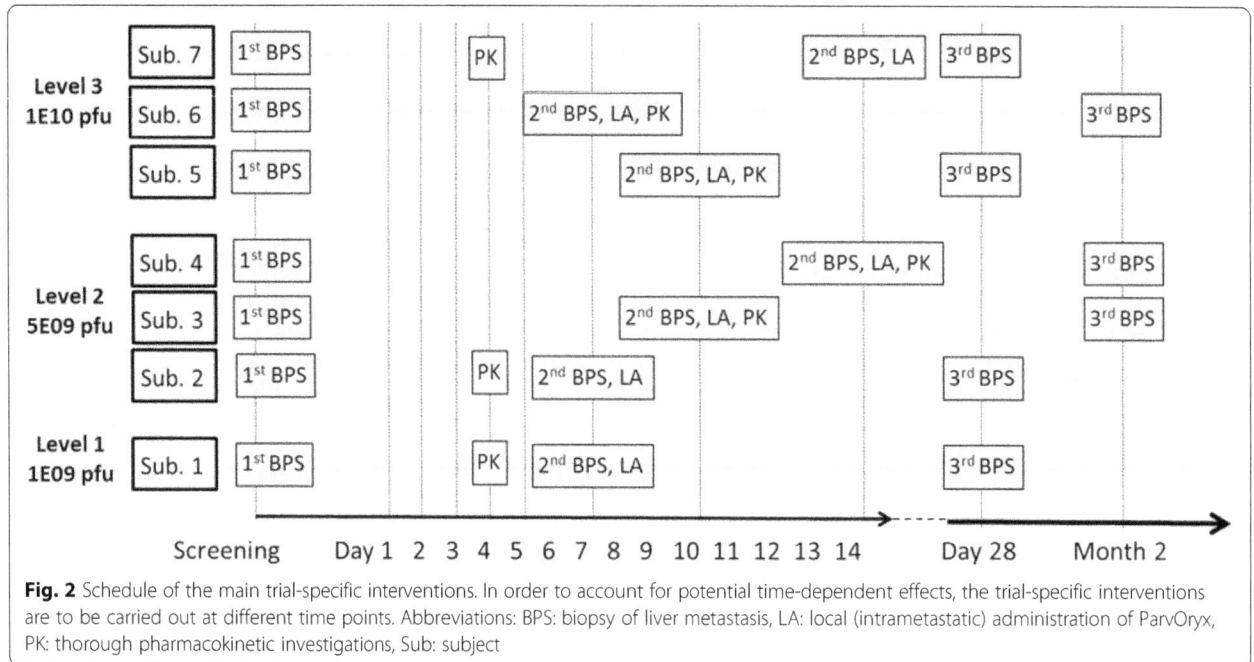

Fig. 2 Schedule of the main trial-specific interventions. In order to account for potential time-dependent effects, the trial-specific interventions are to be carried out at different time points. Abbreviations: BPS: biopsy of liver metastasis, LA: local (intrametastatic) administration of ParvOryx, PK: thorough pharmacokinetic investigations, Sub: subject

one or 2 months after the first i.v. administration of ParvOryx. Since cycle 1 of gemcitabine begins on day 27, effects of chemotherapy will be accounted for when interpreting biopsies taken 2 months after i.v. ParvOryx.

- *Follow-up*
  During the follow-up phase, which extends up to 6 months after the first administration of the IMP, delayed and/or long-term effects of ParvOryx are evaluated. If no complications occur, the subjects are to attend the study visits at months 2, 4 and 6. At each visit safety, tolerability and clinical efficacy will be assessed by the parameters described above.

- *Trial schedule and duration*
  ParvOryx02 is the overall second clinical trial with the IMP ParvOryx. In this trial further dose escalation is planned. Since the starting dose level equals to the concluding dose level of the previous trial (ParvOryx01), a sequential escalation design is used. The subsequent patient may only receive the first dose of ParvOryx if the treatment proved safe and well-tolerated in the previous subject, i.e. if none of the following pre-defined events occurred up to 27 days after the first i.v. administration: i) elevation of alanine aminotransferase (ALAT), aspartate aminotransferase (ASAT), alkaline phosphatase (AP), bilirubin or c-reactive protein (CRP) > 3 times the baseline ii) neutrophil count <1.0 × 1E09/L or >12E09/L, iii) hemoglobin <7.5 g/L, iv) platelet count <5E10/L, v) INR > 2.5, aPTT >50 s., vi)

occurrence of neurological symptoms with no other explanation than the administration of the IMP, vii) occurrence of thromboembolic event(s), vii) serious adverse events (SAE(s)) classified as at least 'possibly' related to the IMP viii) deteriorations in medical monitoring parameters (laboratory values, ECG, etc.), classified as at least 'possibly' related to the IMP and requiring countermeasures to avert conditions fulfilling at least one of the 'seriousness'-criteria, ix) medical necessity to interrupt or to prematurely terminate the scheduled treatment. If any of the before mentioned events occur, an independent data safety monitoring board (DSMB) will be provided with all required data and consulted regarding the trial continuation and/or implementation of any modifications.

The overall duration of the clinical trial, including completion of all follow-up visits related to the efficacy of the IMP in all subjects, is scheduled to last approximately 12 months.

Specific hygienic measures

ParvOryx contains the active, replication-competent virus. Therefore, environmental safety has to be considered as an important factor in the context of administering ParvOryx.

Based on the findings from the previous clinical trial, the risk of virus transmission from study patients to other persons is very low even after the planned dose escalation, if the general hygienic measures are observed. Thus, there is no need for isolation of the patients treated with

ParvOryx. However, to discover and appropriately meet the very unlike case of uncontrolled viral replication after administration of ParvOryx, certain measures have been implemented. The in-patient stay is to be continued until first occurrence of H-1PV-specific antibodies in serum or until all shedding samples (feces, urine, and saliva) are tested negative for H-1PV genomes. During each follow-up visit the presence of specific antibodies will be determined. If the antibodies fall below the detection limit, the subject has to be re-admitted to the trial unit and the extent of virus shedding is to be determined. If no viral genomes are shed in any matrix, no further measures are required and the subject may be discharged. Otherwise the subject remains in-patient until re-occurrence of H-1PV-specific antibodies or until all shedding samples are tested negative for viral genomes.

The only a-priori planned safety measure related to environmental safety is that subjects should entirely avoid contact with pregnant women and infants up to 2 months after the first administration of ParvOryx.

Benefit/risk assessment

As discussed above, no satisfying therapeutic options exist for treatment of locally advanced and metastatic pancreatic cancer. The prognosis is dismal with a six-month progression-free survival of approximately 50% and a median survival of about 11 months [5].

The first open, non-randomized clinical trial with ParvOryx, referred to as ParvOryx01, evaluated safety and tolerability as well as antitumor activity and clinical efficacy in patients with progressive primary or recurrent glioblastoma multiforme (GBM). ParvOryx01 was completed in May 2015 [18]. The investigated doses ranged between 1E06 and 5E09 pfu. They were administered as combination of either multiple intravenous infusions or a single intratumoral injection and multifocal intracerebral injections at the end of tumor resection surgery. As in the current trial, the intravenous dose was divided into equal fractions which were given on consecutive days. The interval between the first administration and surgery with subsequent intracerebral injections of the drug was 10 days. In general, ParvOryx was safe and well-tolerated with only one potential serious adverse reaction observed after a combination of direct glioblastoma administration and intracerebral injection at the end of surgery. The clinical symptoms of the above reaction (mainly hydrocephalus and reduced level of consciousness) were strictly confined to the central nervous system, i.e. there was no causal link to the systemically available virus. As the potential underlying pathomechanisms remained unclear, the causal relationship to ParvOryx can neither be confirmed nor excluded. Of note, no comparable clinical events occurred in any of the other patients treated by the same route and with

the same dose of ParvOryx. Since neither of the above routes of administration is used in the current study, there is no risk of similar adverse reactions.

The single intravenous dose at the initial level equals to that investigated at the highest level in ParvOryx01. Since the intravenous administrations are to be performed on four, instead of five consecutive days, the total intravenous dose is reduced to 80% of the dose investigated previously. The starting local, i.e. intrametastatic dose is more than four times lower than the highest doses injected intratumorally and intracerebrally in the foregoing trial. Since the metastatic/hepatic tissue is presumably far less susceptible to any kind of injury than the neuronal tissue of the brain, the chosen approach appears acceptable. Owing to the overall higher dose range investigated in the current study as well as to the planned co-treatment with gemcitabine, the steps of dose-escalation were chosen more conservatively than in the previous trial.

As in the foregoing trial, the treatment of a consecutive subject is only allowed if the treatment was well-tolerated in the previous subject who, as per protocol, underwent a close medical monitoring during the treatment and up to 3 weeks thereafter. This sequential schedule of enrolment minimizes the individual risks for the included patients.

Although H-1PV is non-pathogenic in man, strong preventive hygienic measures were implemented in the ParvOryx01 study [18]. Amongst others, the investigation of virus distribution and excretion belonged to the main objectives of the trial. Considering the fact that no active virus could ever be detected in any body fluid (faeces, urine, and saliva) and taking into account the rapid formation of virus-specific antibodies, the transmission of H-1PV from the trial patients is considered as highly unlikely. Thus, it is well justifiable to omit the strict isolation conditions applied previously and to rely on the general hygienic standards which are routinely applied at the trial center. In case of a surface contamination with ParvOryx, an adequate disinfection is to be carried out. Since H-1PV was shown to have some embryo- and fetotoxic effects in rodents [19, 20], the trial subjects are obliged to strictly avoid contact with pregnant women and newborn infants for the period of 2 months after beginning of the treatment with ParvOryx. This is to be considered an additional safety measure, i.e. there are currently no indications for a predisposition of pregnant women or infants for an infection with H-1PV.

The risk of trial-specific procedural complications related to the intrametastatic administration of ParvOryx, collection of tissue and blood samples is generally very low.

Taken together, the current protocol of ParvOryx02 trial is well justifiable and may be associated with individual benefits for the included patients. Moreover, the trial will yield important information required for further clinical development of ParvOryx, which may have important implications for the general population of patients with pancreatic cancer. Taken together, the individual hazards for study subjects and the environmental risks are well predictable and acceptable.

Statistical analysis

- *Analysis variables*
  Safety and tolerability will be assessed on the basis of the following parameters:
  AEs and SAEs; physical examinations, vital signs, 12-lead ECGs, and chosen laboratory parameters (clinical chemistry, hematology, coagulation); viremia and virus shedding (H-1PV genomes (Vg) and active virus (H-1PV) in body fluids); virus-specific antibodies.
  Efficacy will be assessed on the basis of the following parameters:
  Investigation of the metastatic tissue: findings in general pathological examination, detection of H-1PV by FISH and qPCR, assessment of tumor infiltration with immune cells, determination of quantity and distribution of cytokines and chemokines, determination of H-1PV protein expression (NS-1).
  Parameters derived from blood: determination of absolute and relative abundance of distinct immune cell subsets as determined by FACS, investigation of cellular anti-viral and anti-tumor immunity by ELISPOT.
  Clinical Parameters: progression-free survival (PFS) and overall survival (OS) assessed by RECIST-criteria.
- *Statistical methods*
  Safety analysis: AEs will be summarized by MedDRA system organ class and preferred term. Separate tabulations will be produced for all treatment-emergent AEs, treatment-related AEs (those considered by the Investigator as at least possibly IMP-related), SAEs, and discontinuations due to AEs. Summary tables and by-patient listings will be provided for AEs, SAEs, events leading to discontinuation of treatment, and deaths.
  Summary tables and by-patient listings will be provided for clinical laboratory data and vital signs data, presented as both actual values and changes from baseline relative to each on-study evaluation. Details of any abnormalities will be included in patient listings.
  Efficacy analysis: No confirmatory statistical analyses will be performed. All recorded variables (see above) will be analyzed descriptively by providing by-patient listings as well as calculating

appropriate summary measures as mean, standard deviation, median, minimum and maximum or absolute and relative frequencies, respectively. If appropriate, changes from baseline relative to each on-study evaluation will be considered. For time-to-event endpoints (progression-free survival and overall survival), Kaplan-Meier estimates and summary measures of the survival function will be provided. Additionally, analyses will be performed separately for each particular dose level. The course of variables over time will be depicted for the total analysis population as well as for each subject.

Discussion

Among other emerging biopharmaceuticals, the clinical use of oncolytic viruses appears to be a promising treatment option for various malignancies. Currently, there is a range of mainly genetically modified oncolytic viruses at different stages of clinical development [21–31]. Recently, talimogene laherparepvec (T-vec) received market authorization by the U.S. Food and Drug Administration (FDA) for treatment of melanoma patients with injectable but non-resectable skin and/or lymphatic lesions [32]. In general the tolerability of oncolytic viruses after systemic and/or local administration is very good with none or only mild unspecific adverse reactions such as fatigue, chills or slight fever. There are no indications for major organ toxicities, local tissue damage or induction of adverse immune effects. The oncolytic viruses are used either as monotherapies or in combination with established chemotherapeutics and/or targeted therapies. There are strong indications for anti-tumor activity and clinical efficacy in connection with either approach. However, in most cases the optimum mode of administration, including dosing schedule and type as well as timing of concomitant treatments still needs to be specified. Interestingly, concomitant therapy with oncolytic viruses and checkpoint inhibitors seems not to influence the safety and tolerability of either treatment [33]. This is of high relevance as the combination may enhance individual anti-tumor immune responses with an improvement of clinical outcome.

Recently, ParvOryx was clinically investigated for its safety and tolerability, anti-tumor activity, immunological effects, and clinical efficacy in patients with GBM [18]. In this study the virus was administered intravenously and into the tumor or in the tumor bed directly after resection. The drug was safe and well-tolerated and showed a promising profile of anti-tumor effects and signs of clinical efficacy, i.e. prolonged survival. However, the optimum dose as well as the most appropriate route and schedule of administration have to be further investigated. The current, second trial with ParvOryx, addresses these questions. Since the total dose of the drug will be further escalated, the primary objective is to evaluate the safety and tolerability of the treatment. At the beginning of the trial, i.e. at the first level, the total dose of ParvOryx equals to the highest total dose in the previous trial. Since a relevant part of the total dose has to be administered directly into the liver metastasis, it is indicated to include one up-front patient at this level, in order to obtain first information on the local tolerability of the drug after direct injection in the liver. Considering the fact that in the foregoing study the local tolerability in the neuronal tissue was very good, no safety-related issues are expected in this context. Since the potential hazards for the consecutive patients have to be minimized as far as possible, a sequential, dose escalation design with extended intervals between enrollment of consecutive subjects and rather conservative dose escalation steps was chosen. As in the previous trial, a broad range of different investigational parameters was implemented. Apart from extended safety tests, various measurements enabling insights into the mode and extent of action of ParvOryx, including local virus availability in the tumor, triggering of changes at the tissue level and induction of virus- and PDAC-specific immune responses were included into the current protocol. Moreover, in order to account for presumable time-dependency of pharmacokinetic characteristics, virus disposition in the tumor tissue and related pharmacodynamics, varying intervals were intercalated between the intravenous administrations on the one hand and biopsies of liver metastases, thorough PK-profiles as well as local administrations of ParvOryx on the other hand.

The IMP contains an active, replication-competent parvovirus H-1PV. Although H-1PV is non-pathogenic in humans, biosafety is still considered a relevant issue in the context of administration of ParvOryx. Based on the results from the previous trial, a transmission of H-1PV from trial patients to others is highly unlikely, since general hygienic measures applicable to the handling of chemotherapeutics, consumables and nursing of patients are implemented. Owing to the pre-clinical findings showing an embryo- and fetotoxicity of H-1PV in rodents, patients' contact with pregnant women and infants is restricted as an additional precaution.

In summary, the current trial will provide further crucial information within the clinical development program of ParvOryx. Since there were pronounced antitumor effects of the drug in various preclinical in-vitro and in-vivo models of pancreatic cancer, the trial will hopefully bring clinical benefits for study patients and, in consequence, for the general patient population.

Abbreviations

(N)IMP: (Non-) Investigational Medicinal Product; (S)AE: (Serious) Adverse Event; ADA: Anti-drug Antibodies; AJCC: American Joint Committee on Cancer; ALAT: Alanine aminotransferase; aPTT: activated Partial Thromboplastin Time; ASAT: Aspartate aminotransferase; Beta-HCG: Beta-human Chorionic Gonadotropin; BSA: Body surface area; CA19–9: Carbohydrate antigen 19–9; CRP: C-reactive protein; CT: Computed tomography; DSMB: Data safety monitoring board; ECG: Electrocardiogram; ECOG: Eastern Cooperative Oncology Group; ELISPOT: Enzyme-linked immunospot assay; FACS: Fluorescence-activated cell sorting; FDA: US Food and Drug Administration; FISH: Fluorescence in-situ Hybridization; GBM: Glioblastoma multiforme; H-1PV: Parvovirus H-1; HDACl(s): Histone deacetylase inhibitor(s); INR: International Normalized Ratio; MedDRA: Medical Dictionary for Regulatory Activities; NCDB: US National Cancer Database; NS-1: Non-structural Protein 1; OS: Overall survival; PFS: Progression-free survival; Pfu: Plaque forming units; PK: Pharmacokinetics; PoC: Proof-of-concept; qPCR: quantitative real-time polymerase chain reaction; RECIST: Response Evaluation Criteria in Solid Tumors; VPA: Valproic acid

Acknowledgements
None

Funding
The ParvOryx02 trial is funded by Oryx GmbH & Co KG, Baldham, Germany. The company was involved in the discussion of the trial design and in the preparation of the current study protocol.

Authors' contributions

JH made major contributions to the study design, edited the trial documents, interacted with regulatory bodies and drafted the manuscript, ML made contributions to the study design, reviewed the trial documents and proofread the manuscript. OK made contributions to the study design, reviewed the trial documents and proofread the manuscript. MK was responsible for the statistical concept of the trial and proofread the manuscript. KG made contributions to the study design and reviewed the manuscript. DJ made contributions to the study design and reviewed the manuscript. MD made contributions to the study design and reviewed the manuscript. BH made contributions to the study design and reviewed the manuscript. TS planned the handling of the trial medication and reviewed the manuscript. OS contributed to the implementation of radiological methods and reviewed the manuscript. AS planned and described pathological methodology and reviewed the manuscript. NH planned and described method of immunological tissue investigations and reviewed the manuscript. VD planned and described immunological investigations and reviewed the manuscript. BL planned and described methods of virus determinations in blood and tissue, provided contributions to the trial documents and reviewed the manuscript. AA planned and described methods of virus determinations in tissue, provided contributions to the trial documents and reviewed the manuscript. JR planned and described methods of virus determinations in blood and tissue, provided contributions to the trial documents and reviewed the manuscript. CEE made contributions to the study design, reviewed the trial documents and proofread the manuscript. CS made major contributions to the study design and drafted the manuscript. GU made major contributions to the study design and drafted the manuscript. All authors have read and approved the final version of the manuscript.

Competing interests

The ParvOryx02 trial is funded by Oryx GmbH & Co KG, Baldham, Germany. JH and ML declare no competing interests. OK receives salary from Oryx GmbH & Co KG. MK declares no competing interests. KG holds patents related to H-1PV. DJ declares no competing interests. MD and BH receive salary from Oryx GmbH & Co KG. TS, OS, AS, NH, VD, BL and AA declare no competing interests. JR holds patents related to H-1PV. CE, CS and GU declare no competing interests.

Author details

[1]Coordination Centre for Clinical Trials, University Hospital Heidelberg, Marsilius-Arkaden, Tower West, Im Neuenheimer Feld 130.3, 69120 Heidelberg, Germany. [2]Oryx GmbH & Co KG, Marktplatz 1, 85598 Baldham, Germany. [3]Institute of Medical Biometry and Informatics, University Hospital Heidelberg, Marsilius-Arkaden, Tower West, Im Neuenheimer Feld 130.3, 69120 Heidelberg, Germany. [4]Department of Neurosurgery, Klinikum Darmstadt, Grafenstraße 9, 64283 Darmstadt, Germany. [5]Department of Medical Oncology, National Center for Tumor Diseases (NCT), Im Neuenheimer Feld 460, 69120 Heidelberg, Germany. [6]Central Pharmacy, University Hospital Heidelberg, Im Neuenheimer Feld 670, 69120 Heidelberg, Germany. [7]Department of Radiology, German Cancer Research Center, Im Neuenheimer Feld 280, 69120 Heidelberg, Germany. [8]Department of Pathology, University Hospital Heidelberg, Im Neuenheimer Feld 224, 69120 Heidelberg, Germany. [9]Tissue Imaging & Analysis Center (TIGA), University Heidelberg – BioQuant, Im Neuenheimer Feld 267, 69120 Heidelberg, Germany. [10]Institute of Immunology, Transplantation Immunology, University Hospital Heidelberg, Im Neuenheimer Feld 305, 69120 Heidelberg, Germany. [11]Department of Applied Tumor Virology, German Cancer Research Center, Im Neuenheimer Feld 242, 69120 Heidelberg, Germany.

References

1. Ferlay J, Steliarova-Foucher E, Lortet-Tieulent J, Rosso S, Coebergh JW, Comber H, et al. Cancer incidence and mortality patterns in Europe: estimates for 40 countries in 2012. Eur J Cancer. 2013;49(6):1374–403.
2. Malvezzi M, Bertuccio P, Levi F, La Vecchia C, Negri E. European cancer mortality predictions for the year 2014. Ann Oncol. 2014;25(8):1650–6.
3. Quaresma M, Coleman MP, Rachet B. 40-year trends in an index of survival for all cancers combined and survival adjusted for age and sex for each cancer in England and Wales, 1971-2011: a population-based study. Lancet. 2015;385(9974):1206–18.
4. Bilimoria KY, Bentrem DJ, Ko CY, Ritchey J, Stewart AK, Winchester DP, et al. Validation of the 6th edition AJCC Pancreatic Cancer Staging System: report from the National Cancer Database. Cancer. 2007;110(4):738–44.
5. Conroy T, Desseigne F, Ychou M, Bouche O, Guimbaud R, Becouarn Y, et al. FOLFIRINOX versus gemcitabine for metastatic pancreatic cancer. N Engl J Med. 2011;364(19):1817–25.
6. Von Hoff DD, Ervin T, Arena FP, Chiorean EG, Infante J, Moore M, et al. Increased survival in pancreatic cancer with nab-paclitaxel plus gemcitabine. N Engl J Med. 2013;369(18):1691–703.
7. Saif MW. U.S. Food and Drug Administration approves paclitaxel protein-bound particles (Abraxane(R)) in combination with gemcitabine as first-line treatment of patients with metastatic pancreatic cancer. JOP. 2013;14(6):686–8.
8. Rommelaere J, Cornelis JJ. Antineoplastic activity of parvoviruses. J Virol Methods. 1991;33(3):233–51.
9. Geletneky K, Herrero YC, Rommelaere J, Schlehofer JR. Oncolytic potential of rodent parvoviruses for cancer therapy in humans: a brief review. J Vet Med B Infect Dis Vet Public Health. 2005;52(7–8):327–30.
10. Dupressoir T, Vanacker JM, Cornelis JJ, Duponchel N, Rommelaere J. Inhibition by parvovirus H-1 of the formation of tumors in nude mice and colonies in vitro by transformed human mammary epithelial cells. Cancer Res. 1989;49(12):3203–8.
11. Faisst S, Schlehofer JR, zur Hausen HA. Transformation of human cells by oncogenic viruses supports permissiveness for parvovirus H-1 propagation. J Virol. 1989;63(5):2152–8.
12. Guetta E, Graziani Y, Tal J. Suppression of Ehrlich ascites tumors in mice by minute virus of mice. J Natl Cancer Inst. 1986;76(6):1177–80.
13. Nuesch JP, Rommelaere J. Tumor suppressing properties of rodent parvovirus NS1 proteins and their derivatives. Adv Exp Med Biol. 2014;818:99–124.
14. Angelova AL, Aprahamian M, Grekova SP, Hajri A, Leuchs B, Giese NA, et al. Improvement of gemcitabine-based therapy of pancreatic carcinoma by means of oncolytic parvovirus H-1PV. Clin Cancer Res. 2009;15(2):511–9.
15. Angelova AL, Grekova SP, Heller A, Kuhlmann O, Soyka E, Giese T, et al. Complementary induction of immunogenic cell death by oncolytic parvovirus H-1PV and gemcitabine in pancreatic cancer. J Virol. 2014;88(10):5263 76.

16. Portal A, Pernot S, Tougeron D, Arbaud C, Bidault AT, De La Fouchardière C, et al. Nab-paclitaxel plus gemcitabine for metastatic pancreatic adenocarcinoma after Folfirinox failure: an AGEO prospective multicentre cohort. Br J Cancer. 2015;113(7):989–95.
17. Frese KK, Neesse A, Cook N, Bapiro TE, Lolkema MP, Jodrell DI, et al. nab-Paclitaxel potentiates gemcitabine activity by reducing cytidine deaminase levels in a mouse model of pancreatic cancer. Cancer Discov. 2012;2(3):260–9.
18. Geletneky K, Huesing J, Rommelaere J, Schlehofer JR, Leuchs B, Dahm M, et al. Phase I/IIa study of intratumoral/intracerebral or intravenous/intracerebral administration of Parvovirus H-1 (ParvOryx) in patients with progressive primary or recurrent glioblastoma multiforme: ParvOryx01 protocol. BMC Cancer. 2012;12:99.
19. FERM VH, Kilham L. CONGENITAL ANOMALIES INDUCED IN HAMSTER EMBRYOS WITH H-1 VIRUS. Science. 1964;145:510–1.
20. FERM VH, Kilham L. HISTOPATHOLOGIC BASIC OF THE TERATOGENIC EFFECTS OF H-1 VIRUS ON HAMSTER EMBRYOS. J Embryol Exp Morphol. 1965;13:151–8.
21. Philip PA, Benedetti J, Corless CL, Wong R, O'Reilly EM, Flynn PJ, et al. Phase III study comparing gemcitabine plus cetuximab versus gemcitabine in patients with advanced pancreatic adenocarcinoma: Southwest Oncology Group-directed intergroup trial S0205. J Clin Oncol. 2010;28(22):3605–10.
22. Nakao A, Kasuya H, Sahin TT, Nomura N, Kanzaki A, Misawa M, et al. A phase I dose-escalation clinical trial of intraoperative direct intratumoral injection of HF10 oncolytic virus in non-resectable patients with advanced pancreatic cancer. Cancer Gene Ther. 2011;18(3):167–75.
23. Hamano S, Mori Y, Aoyama M, Kataoka H, Tanaka M, Ebi M, et al. Oncolytic reovirus combined with trastuzumab enhances antitumor efficacy through TRAIL signaling in human HER2-positive gastric cancer cells. Cancer Lett. 2015;356(2 Pt B):846–54.
24. Zeh HJ, Downs-Canner S, McCart JA, Guo ZS, Rao UN, Ramalingam L, et al. First-in-man study of western reserve strain oncolytic vaccinia virus: safety, systemic spread, and antitumor activity. Mol Ther. 2015;23(1):202–14.
25. Chiocca EA, Abbed KM, Tatter S, Louis DN, Hochberg FH, Barker F, et al. A phase I open-label, dose-escalation, multi-institutional trial of injection with an E1B-Attenuated adenovirus, ONYX-015, into the peritumoral region of recurrent malignant gliomas, in the adjuvant setting. Mol Ther. 2004;10(5):958–66.
26. Eisenberg DP, Adusumilli PS, Hendershott KJ, Yu Z, Mullerad M, Chan MK, et al. 5-fluorouracil and gemcitabine potentiate the efficacy of oncolytic herpes viral gene therapy in the treatment of pancreatic cancer. J Gastrointest Surg. 2005;9(8):1068–77.
27. Himeno Y, Etoh T, Matsumoto T, Ohta M, Nishizono A, Kitano S. Efficacy of oncolytic reovirus against liver metastasis from pancreatic cancer in immunocompetent models. Int J Oncol. 2005;27(4):901–6.
28. Galanis E, Carlson SK, Foster NR, Lowe V, Quevedo F, McWilliams RR, et al. Phase I trial of a pathotropic retroviral vector expressing a cytocidal cyclin G1 construct (Rexin-G) in patients with advanced pancreatic cancer. Mol Ther. 2008;16(5):979–84.
29. Kaufman HL, Kim-Schulze S, Manson K, DeRaffele G, Mitcham J, Seo KS, et al. Poxvirus-based vaccine therapy for patients with advanced pancreatic cancer. J Transl Med. 2007;5:60.
30. Hecht JR, Bedford R, Abbruzzese JL, Lahoti S, Reid TR, Soetikno RM, et al. A phase I/II trial of intratumoral endoscopic ultrasound injection of ONYX-015 with intravenous gemcitabine in unresectable pancreatic carcinoma. Clin Cancer Res. 2003;9(2):555–61.
31. Galanis E, Atherton PJ, Maurer MJ, Knutson KL, Dowdy SC, Cliby WA, et al. Oncolytic measles virus expressing the sodium iodide symporter to treat drug-resistant ovarian cancer. Cancer Res. 2015;75(1):22–30.
32. Pol J, Kroemer G, Galluzzi L. First oncolytic virus approved for melanoma immunotherapy. Oncoimmunology. 2016;5(1):e1115641.
33. Pusonov I, Milhem M, Andtabacka R, Minor D, Hamid O, Li A, et al. Survival, safety, and response patterns in a phase 1b multicenter trial of talimogene laherparepvec (T-VEC) and ipilimumab (ipi) in previously untreated, unresected stage IIIB-IV melanoma. J Clin Oncol. 2016;33(15_suppl (May 20 Supplement)):Abstract 9063.

An elevated expression of serum exosomal microRNA-191, − 21, −451a of pancreatic neoplasm is considered to be efficient diagnostic marker

Takuma Goto[1†], Mikihiro Fujiya[1*†], Hiroaki Konishi[1†], Junpei Sasajima[1], Shugo Fujibayashi[1], Akihiro Hayashi[1], Tatsuya Utsumi[1], Hiroki Sato[1], Takuya Iwama[1], Masami Ijiri[1], Aki Sakatani[1], Kazuyuki Tanaka[1], Yoshiki Nomura[1], Nobuhiro Ueno[1], Shin Kashima[1], Kentaro Moriichi[1], Yusuke Mizukami[1], Yutaka Kohgo[2] and Toshikatsu Okumura[1]

Abstract

Background: Pancreatic cancer is associated with an extremely poor prognosis, so new biomarkers that can detect the initial stages are urgently needed. The significance of serum microRNA (miR) levels in pancreatic neoplasm such as pancreatic cancer and intraductal papillary mucinous neoplasm (IPMN) diagnosis remains unclear. We herein evaluated the usefulness of miRs enclosed in serum exosomes (ExmiRs) as diagnostic markers.

Methods: The ExmiRs from patients with pancreatic cancer ($n = 32$) or IPMN ($n = 29$), and patients without neoplasms (controls; $n = 22$) were enriched using ExoQuick-TC™. The expression of ExmiRs was evaluated using a next-generation sequencing analysis, and the selected three miRs through this analysis were confirmed by a quantitative real-time polymerase chain reaction.

Results: The expression of ExmiR-191, ExmiR-21 and ExmiR-451a was significantly up-regulated in patients with pancreatic cancer and IPMN compared to the controls ($p < 0.05$). A receiver operating characteristic curve analysis showed that the area under the curve and the diagnostic accuracy of ExmiRs were 5–20% superior to those of three serum bulky circulating miRs (e.g.; ExmiR-21: AUC 0.826, accuracy 80.8%. Circulating miR-21: AUC 0.653, accuracy 62.3%). In addition, high ExmiR-451a was associated with mural nodules in IPMN ($p = 0.010$), and high ExmiR-21 was identified as a candidate prognostic factor for the overall survival ($p = 0.011$, HR 4.071, median OS of high-ExmiR-21: 344 days, median OS of low-ExmiR-21: 846 days) and chemo-resistant markers ($p = 0.022$).

Conclusions: The level of three ExmiRs can thus serve as early diagnostic and progression markers of pancreatic cancer and IPMN, and considered more useful markers than the circulating miRs (limited to these three miRs).

Keywords: Pancreatic cancer, Exosome, microRNA-21, microRNA-451a, Intraductal papillary mucinous neoplasm, Tumor marker

* Correspondence: fjym@asahikawa-med.ac.jp
†Equal contributors
[1]Division of Gastroenterology and Hematology/Oncology, Department of Medicine, Asahikawa Medical University, 2-1 Midorigaoka-higashi, Asahikawa, Hokkaido 078-8510, Japan
Full list of author information is available at the end of the article

Background

Pancreatic cancer (PC) is a frequent cause of cancer death worldwide [1]. While advances in clinical treatments, including chemotherapy and surgery, have improved the prognosis of PC in the past decades, the early detection of PC remains quite difficult. Thus, the prognosis of PC remains poor, even when using advanced imaging techniques such as computed tomography or positron emission tomography. Carbohydrate antigen 19–9 (CA19–9) is the most sensitive diagnostic marker for PC, but it is not useful for diagnosing early PC [2]. Therefore, new biomarkers that can detect the initial stages of PC are urgently needed.

Intraductal papillary mucinous neoplasm (IPMN) is a pre-cancerous lesion, and 1–2% of IPMN cases progress to PC each year [3]. IPMN progress from a non-invasive to an invasive lesion [4], and the postoperative prognosis of patients with invasive IPMN appears to be considerably worse than that of patients with non-invasive IPMN [5]. This evidence suggests that biological markers able to distinguish invasive IPMN from non-invasive IPMN can improve the survival of PC patients. While the utility of CA19–9 and MUC5AC as serum markers of malignant IPMN has been reported, their sensitivities were not high enough to be indicative factors for resection [6]. Indeed, even when novel imaging procedures are utilized, it is difficult to predict the malignant potential of IPMN [4]. Novel indicators that can predict the malignant potential of IPMN are therefore eagerly awaited.

MicroRNAs (miRs), which are small RNAs that regulate approximately 30% of human genes [7], are secreted into the blood and body fluids [8]. Recent studies have shown that the abnormal expression of extracellular circulating miRs (CmiRs) in serum or plasma was correlated with the prognosis of PC, suggesting that CmiRs may be potential diagnostic or prognostic markers for advanced PC [9].

miR-21 was reported that proportionally increased during the progression from IPMN to PC, but no other miRs have been identified as markers for the detection of IPMN as well as the progression of PC.

miRs have been reported to be stably contained within vesicles called exosomes [10]. Exosomes are small (40–100 nm diameter) vesicles composed of a lipid bilayer and secreted by cells to interact with distant tissues; they may be found in all body fluids, including the serum and plasma [10–12]. miRs and mRNAs were found to be enclosed in exosomes, stabilized from RNase and highly enriched compared to the serum [11, 12], and the expressions of these exosomal microRNAs (ExmiRs) were dysregulated in several types of cancer patients [10]. ExmiRs are therefore expected to be useful as non-invasive diagnostic biomarkers in cancer patients.

We herein assessed for the first time the expression of ExmiRs in patients with IPMN and PC using a next-generation sequencing analysis, and revealed that three ExmiRs were upregulated in IPMN and PC. In addition, the expression of these ExmiRs was correlated with poor prognosis in PC patients and the high-risk cases in the IPMN group, respectively.

Methods

Patients

Thirty-two patients with newly diagnosed PC and 29 with IPMN (no prior treatment) at Asahikawa Medical University Hospital from April 2013 to December 2015 were respectively enrolled in the PC group and IPMN group in this study. Twenty-two patients without malignant or neoplastic lesions were registered in the control group; these patients were recruited from patients who visited the Division of Gastroenterology and Hematology/Oncology in Asahikawa Medical University during the study period. The characteristics of the patients in the control group are shown in Table 1. Six cases complaining of abdominal pain and 1 case complaining of nausea were included. Patients with other cancers or neoplasms were excluded from this study. All patients with PC and IPMN underwent enhanced computed tomography from the chest to the abdominal region for tumor staging, according to either the TNM criteria or the IPMN guidelines. Informed consent was obtained from all of the participants regarding

Table 1 Characteristics of the control, IPMN, and PC groups

Characteristic		Control	IPMN	PC
Total, n		22	29	32
Sex, n (%)	Female	8 (36.4)	16 (55.2)	15 (46.9)
	Male	14 (63.6)	13 (44.8)	17 (53.1)
Age (mean ± SD)		57.5 ± 15.3	73.8 ± 7.8	64.0 ± 10.1
Stage (UICC) I / IIa / IIb / III / IV		–	–	2 / 7 / 4 / 5 / 14
Fukuoka criteria FN / WF / HRS		–	14 / 11 / 4	–
Clinical information		GBP 4		
		Chronic gastritis 3		
		Gallbladder stone 2		
		ADM 2		
		Liver cyst 1		
		IBS 1		
		Accessory spleen 1		
		Only symptom 7		

SD standard deviation, *IPMN* intraductal papillary mucinous neoplasm, *PC* pancreatic cancer, *FN* Fukuoka negative, *WF* worry-some Feature, *HRS* high-risk stigmata, *GBP* gallbladder cholesterol polyp, *ADM* adenomyomatosis, *IBS* irritable bowel syndrome

the use of their blood samples in this study. The study was approved by the Medical Ethics Committee of Asahikawa Medical University.

Serum samples
A blood examination and sampling were performed before treatment, which included surgery, chemotherapy, and radiotherapy. The peripheral blood from patients was collected and then centrifuged at 5000 rpm (rpm) for 10 min at 4 °C. The serums were then transferred to fresh tubes and stored at – 80 °C. Before analysis, the serum samples were filtrated through a 0.45-μm pore membrane (Millipore, Billerica, MA, USA). The amount of serum used in all of this study was unified in 250 μl according to the Manufacture.

Isolation of the exosomes from the serum and MicroRNA isolation from the exosomes
Exosomes were collected from the serum using ExoQuick Exosome Precipitation Solution (System Biosciences, Mountain View, CA, USA) in accordance with the manufacturer's instructions. Exosomal RNAs were isolated by using Trizol (Invitrogen, Grand Island, NY, USA) and purified using a mirVana miRNA isolation kit (Life Technologies, Carlsbad, CA, USA). The purity and concentration of all RNA samples were quantified spectrophotometrically using the NanoDrop ND-1000 system (NanoDrop, Wilmington, DE, USA). Exosomes were quantified using a CD63 ExoELISA kit (System Biosciences) in accordance with the manufacturer's instructions.

Selection of MicroRNA in the exosome using a next-generation sequencer
Five patients were randomly selected from each groups to examine the expression of their exosomal miR. The volumes of the RNA samples (collected from 250-μl serum samples) was normalized. RNA libraries were generated using an Ion Total RNA-Seq Kit v2 (Life Technologies) in accordance with the manufacturer's instructions. The RNA libraries were then processed for the emulsion PCR using an Ion OneTouchTM system and an Ion OneTouch 200 Template kit v2 (Life Technologies). Template-positive Ion SphereTM particles were enriched and purified for the sequencing reaction with an Ion OneTouchTM ES system (Life Technologies). The template-positive Ion SphereTM Particles were then applied to Ion PI™ Chips (Life Technologies), and the next-generation sequencing reaction was carried out using an Ion Proton™ Semiconductor sequencer (Life Technologies). All of the sequencing data were mapped on a miR sequence using the CLC Genomics Workbench software program (CLC Bio, Aarhus, Denmark), and an expression analysis was performed for each sample.

MicroRNA detection by quantitative real-time polymerase chain reaction
miRs were reverse-transcribed, and their expressions were determined by quantitative real-time polymerase chain reaction (qRT-PCR) using TaqMan microRNA assay kits in accordance with the manufacturer's instructions (Applied Biosystems, Foster City, CA, USA). The Ct values were used in the analysis of the qRT-PCR data.

Statistical analysis
The expression of miR and CD63 in serum samples was compared using the Mann-Whitney U test (for two groups) or the Kruskal-Wallis test followed by Dunn's test (for three groups). There was no adjustment for multiple comparisons in the subgroup or multiple miRs analysis. The diagnostic performance was confirmed by Receiver Operating Characteristic (ROC) curve analysis. The cutoff point was determined by the following formula: Distance = $(1-sensitivity)^2 + (1-specificity)^2$.

In survival analyses, the probability of overall survival (OS) was determined by the Kaplan-Meier method with a log-rank test and Cox's proportional-hazards regression model. The statistical analysis was performed using the Graph Pad PRISM (Version 5.0a; GraphPad Software, Inc. La Jolla, CA, USA), SPSS and R software programs. The level of significance was set at $p < 0.05$.

Results
Characteristics of the control, IPMN and PC groups
The subjects comprised 32 patients with PC, 29 patients with IPMN and 22 patients without malignant or neoplastic lesions (Control group). Among the 32 PC patients, 12 underwent surgical resection and 28 received chemotherapy. All of the patients in the IPMN group were diagnosed with branched-duct type (BD)-IPMN. Among the 29 IPMN patients, 15 with Fukuoka Negative (FN) and 11 with Worrisome Features (WF) were conservatively observed, and four cases with High-risk Stigmata (HRS) underwent surgical resection. The conditions of the patients in the Control group ($n = 22$) included gallbladder cholesterol polyp ($n = 4$), chronic gastritis ($n = 3$), gallbladder stone or adenomyomatosis (n = 2), and liver cyst or irritable bowel syndrome or accessory spleen ($n = 1$), the remaining seven only had symptoms and were not diagnosed with any disease. The median age in the IPMN group (73.8 ± 7.8 years) was older than that in the PC (64.0 ± 10.1 years) and control groups (57.5 ± 15.3 years), but no significant difference were noted in gender among the groups (Table 1).

Serum exosomes were not markedly different between the control, IPMN and PC groups

First, we assessed the concentration of serum exosomes in each group. The control ($N = 20$), IPMN ($N = 29$) and PC groups ($N = 31$) were subjected to this assay. Exosomes were isolated from 250 μL serum using ExoQuick solution and the yields were measured by a CD63, a component of the exosome layer, ExoELISA kit (System Biosciences). No significant differences were noted in the optical density (OD) of CD63 among the groups, indicating no marked differences in the concentration of serum exosomes (Additional file 1: Figure S1).

ExmiR-191, – 21, and -451a, significantly up-regulated in PC and IPMN, were sensitive diagnostic markers

We analyzed the ExmiR profiles of each group using an exosomal microRNA sequence analysis with next-generation sequencing ($N = 5$ each). Among a total of 347 detected ExmiRs, the expression of ExmiR-191, ExmiR-21 and ExmiR-451a was significantly increased in both the IPMN or PC groups by the Kruskal-Wallis test (Table 2). These three candidates were further evaluated using a qRT-PCR targeting all cases. The expressions of ExmiR-191, – 21 and -451a were significantly higher in PC and IPMN patients than in controls (Fig. 1a). Of note, the expression of CmiR-191, CmiR-21, and CmiR-451a, which are bulky serum miRs including not only ExmiRs but also other serum miRs, did not differ markedly among the groups (Fig. 1b). Since the IPMN patients were significantly older, the age-adjusted differences were evaluated; no significant interaction was found between any of the ExmiRs and age (ExmiR-191, $p = 0.932$; ExmiR-21, $p = 0.478$; ExmiR-451a, $p = 0.357$).

To evaluate the diagnostic performance of three ExmiRs, ROC curve analysis was performed. The ROC analysis between control and IPMN (Fig. 2a) or PC (Fig. 2b) showed that the area under the curve (AUC), diagnostic accuracy and specificity of the three ExmiRs were superior to those of the three CmiRs. The accuracy of the ExmiRs was almost 5–20% higher than that of the CmiRs. Among the three ExmiRs, ExmiR-21 showed the largest AUC and highest diagnostic accuracy (IPMN diagnosis: accuracy = 78.0%, PC diagnosis: accuracy = 80.8%). These

Table 2 ExmiR-191, −21 and -451a were identified as candidates for biological markers of IPMN and PC by next-generation sequencing analysis

Candidate ExmiR	P value	Fold change (Control vs IPMN)	Fold change (Control vs PC)
ExmiR-191	0.0036	3.171	34.571
ExmiR-21	0.0417	12.222	25.556
ExmiR-451a	0.0477	1.819	11.662

results indicated that ExmiRs were more sensitive markers for diagnosing IPMN and PC than CmiRs.

ExmiR-191, ExmiR-21, and ExmiR-451a were good diagnostic markers for IPMN and early-stage PC

We identified three ExmiRs as biological markers for diagnosing early-stage pancreatic tumorigenesis. We next compared the diagnostic performance of the three ExmiRs with those of carcinoembryonic antigen (CEA) and carbohydrate antigen 19–9 (CA19–9), which are traditional markers for PC. The levels of CA19–9 were significantly higher in the PC group than in the control or IPMN groups (Fig. 3a).

In the ROC analysis between control and IPMN, the AUC and diagnostic accuaracy of ExmiRs were superior to those of CA19–9 and CEA (Fig. 3b). In addition, ROC analysis between control and earlier stages of PCs including patients with stage I and IIa showed that the accuracy of the ExmiRs was preferable to that of CEA. There was no significant difference in comparison to CA19–9; however, the positive detection rate was approximately 10% higher (Fig. 3c). On the other hand, CA19–9 was the best parameter for the diagnosis of advanced-stage PC (stage ≥IIb) (AUC 0.893, accuracy 90%). The ExmiR's, which were somewhat inferior to CA19–9, showed a good AUC value and accuracy (ExmiR-21, AUC 0.862, accuracy 83.7%) (Fig. 3d). Taken together, our results suggested that ExmiR-191, ExmiR-21 and ExmiR-451a were good diagnostic markers for IPMN and early-stage PC, but that CA19–9 was still superior for the diagnosis of advanced cancer.

The expression of ExmiR-451a was associated with mural nodules of IPMN.

The international consensus guideline 2012 for IPMN describes the indication criteria for resection, known as the Fukuoka Criteria. According to the Fukuoka Criteria, IPMNs are categorized as FN, WF and HRS, and these three categories are generally said to reflect progression from benign IPMN to malignant IPMN. The Kruskal-Wallis test revealed no significant differences in the expression levels of ExmiR-191, ExmiR-21 and ExmiR-451a among FN, WF and HRS (Fig. 4a). However, the ExmiR-451a level appeared to gradually increase; we therefore decided to evaluate the associations between ExmiR-451a and each of the factors in the Fukuoka criteria (cyst diameter, presence of mural nodules, presence of main pancreatic duct dilatation, progression of cyst diameter). The expression of ExmiR-451a was significantly higher in the patients with mural nodules than in those without them (Fig. 4b). Although there were no other significant differences, ExmiR-451a also seemed to be high in the IPMN patients with large cyst diameter and main

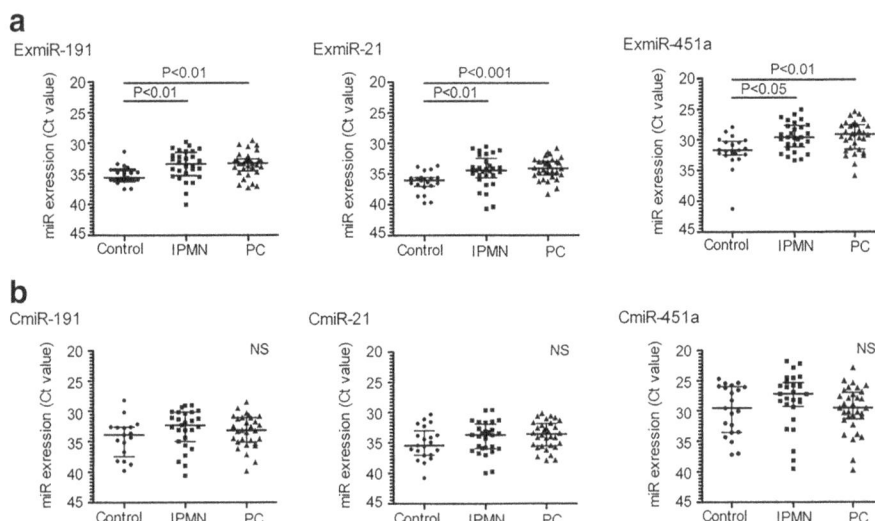

Fig. 1 ExmiR-191, – 21 and -451a were significantly up-regulated in PC and IPMN. The three candidate miRs extracted with next-generation sequencing analysis were further evaluated using a qRT-PCR targeting all cases. **a, b** The expressions of ExmiR-191 (**a**, left panel), ExmiR-21 (**a**, middle panel), ExmiR-451a (**a**, right panel), CmiR-191 (**b**, left panel), CmiR-21 (**b**, middle panel) and CmiR-451a (**b**, right panel) were plotted (median with interquartile range was also shown). The expression of ExmiR-191, ExmiR-21, and ExmiR-451a were significantly higher in PC ($n = 32$) and IPMN patients ($n = 29$) than in controls ($n = 22$), while the expressions of these CmiRs did not differ significantly among the groups

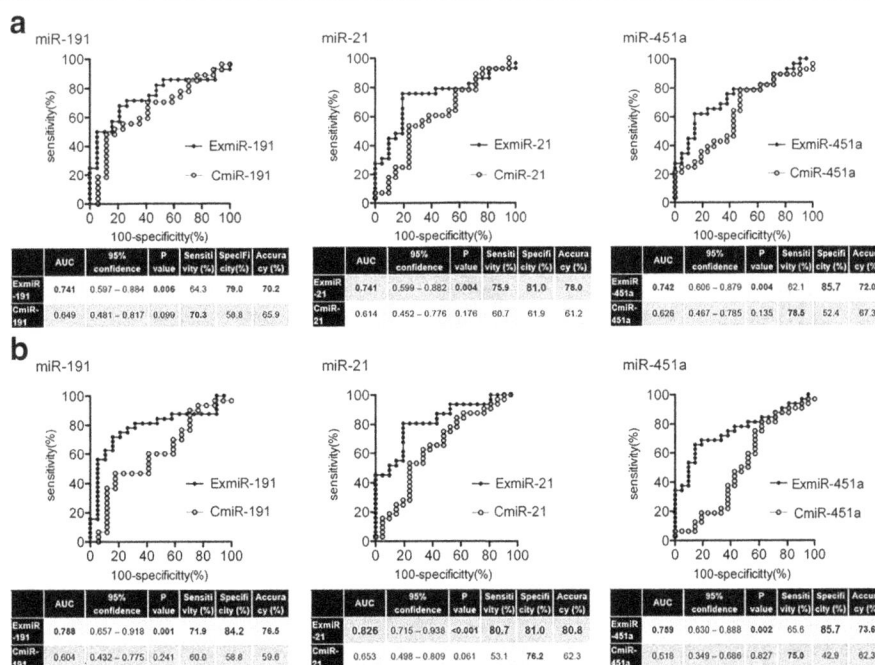

Fig. 2 Three ExmiRs were more sensitive markers for diagnosing IPMN and PC than CmiRs. **a,b** The ROC analysis between control and IPMN (**a**) or PC (**b**) was showed, as follows: miR-191 (left panel), miR-21 (middle panel), and miR-451a (right panel). The AUC, specificity and diagnostic accuracy of three ExmiRs were superior to those of three CmiRs. Among the three ExmiRs, ExmiR-21 showed the highest diagnostic accuracy (IPMN diagnostic accuracy = 78.0%, PC diagnostic accuracy = 80.8%)

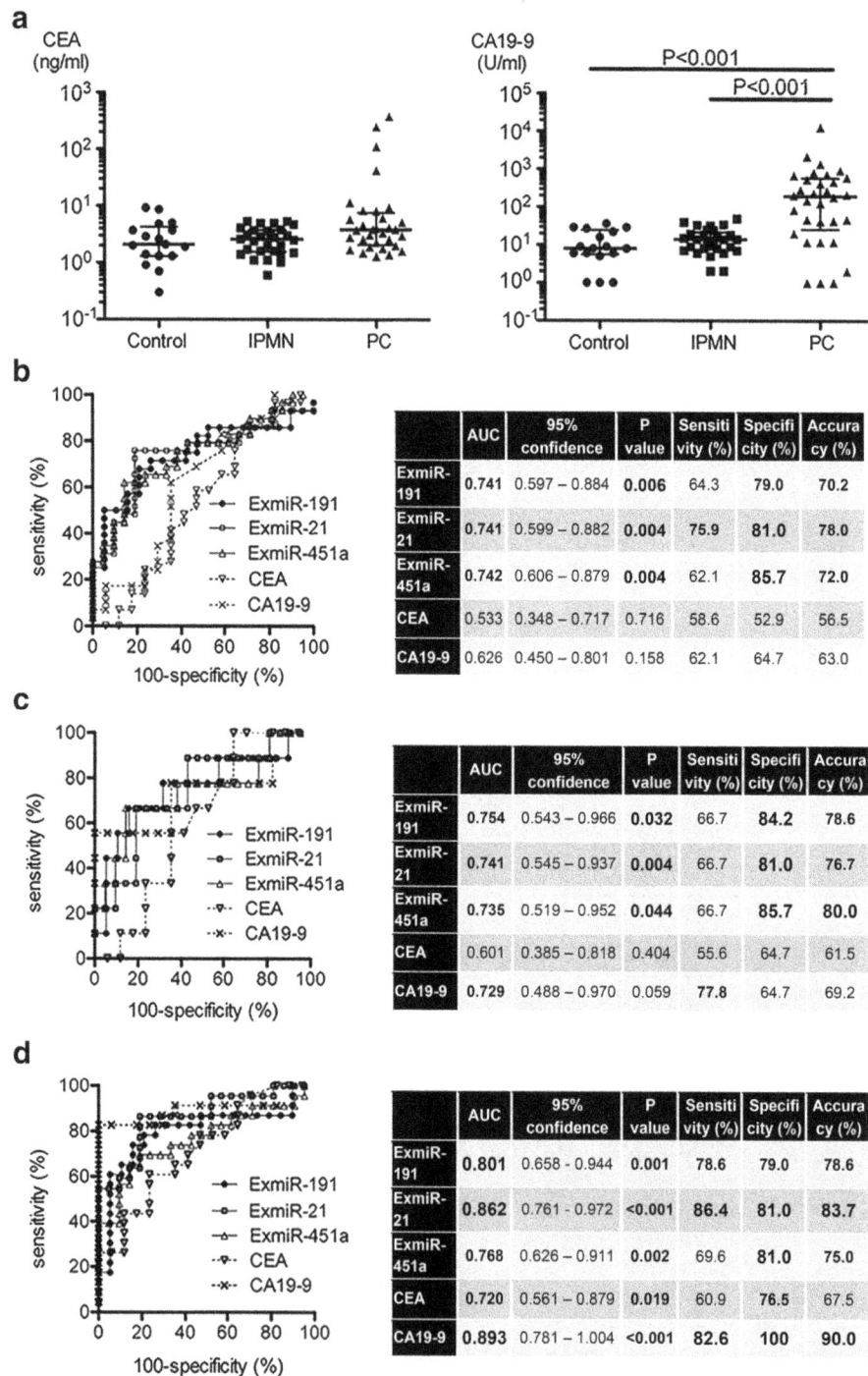

Fig. 3 ExmiR-191, ExmiR-21, and ExmiR-451a were good diagnostic markers for IPMN and early-stage PC. **a** The levels of CEA (left) and CA19–9 (right) were plotted (median with interquartile range was also shown). CA19–9 was significantly higher in the PC group than in the control or IPMN groups. **b** The ROC analysis between control and IPMN was shown. The AUC and diagnostic accuracy of three ExmiRs were clearly superior to traditional markers. **c** The ROC analysis between control and early stage of PC including only patients with stage I or IIa showed. The diagnostic accuracy of three ExmiRs were superior to CEA, and tended to be better than CA19–9. **d** The ROC analysis between the control group and the advanced-stage PC group (stage ≥IIb). The AUC values and accuracy of the three ExmiRs were superior to CEA, but they were not as useful as CA19–9

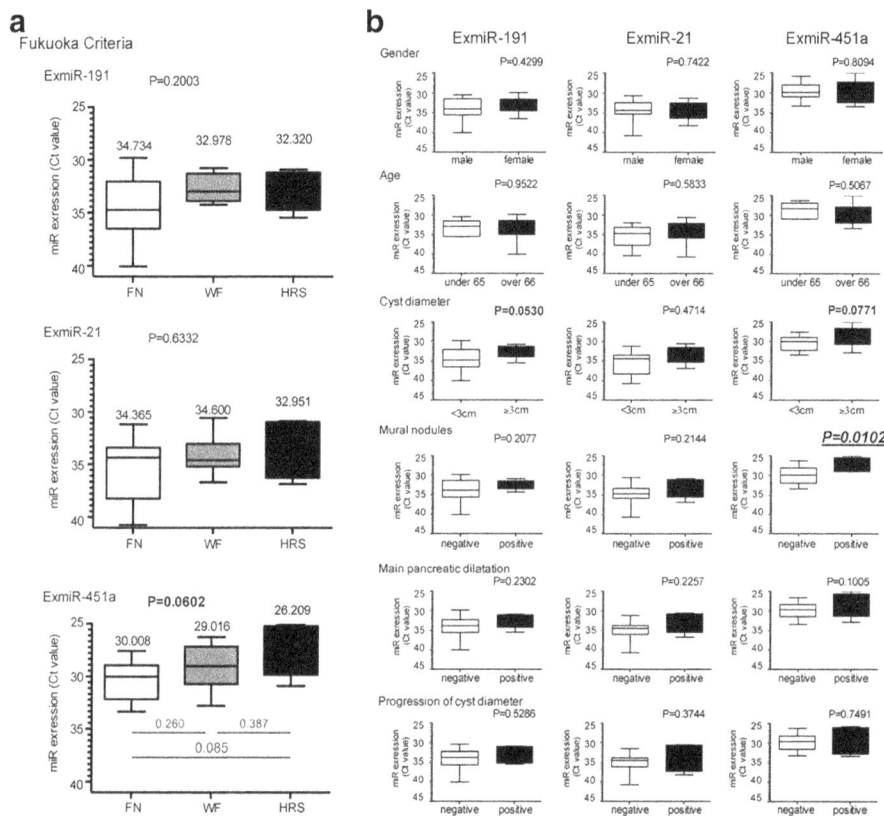

Fig. 4 ExmiR-451a was correlated with the Clinical Features of IPMN, and might be able to diagnose high risk cases. **a** The correlation between the expression levels of the three ExmiRs and the Fukuoka criteria. There were no significant differences in the expression of ExmiR-191, ExmiR-21 or ExmiR-451a between FN, WF and HRS. However, the ExmiR-451a level appeared to be gradually increasing ($p = 0.0602$). **b** The association between the expressions of three ExmiRs and clinical features, gender, age, cyst diameter, mural nodules, main pancreatic dilatation and Progression of cyst diameter, in IPMN group was assessed. The ExmiR expressions were plotted and those median with interquartile range was also shown. The expression of ExmiR-451a was significantly higher in the patients with mural nodules. Although there were no other significant differences, ExmiR-451a also seemed to be high with a large cyst diameter and main pancreatic dilatation

pancreatic dilatation. ExmiR-451a might be strongly associated with the malignant progression of IPMN.

ExmiR-21 was a candidate prognostic factor for the survival of PC patients

We finally focused on the PC group and evaluated the association between the three ExmiRs and the clinical outcomes in PC patients. For the survival analysis, PC patients were categorized into high- and low-ExmiR expression groups using the median miR value as the cut-off point. Survival curves of the three ExmiRs estimated by the Kaplan-Meier method are shown in Fig. 5a. The overall survival in the high-ExmiR-21 expression group (median: 344 days) was significantly shorter than that in the low-ExmiR-21 expression group (median: 846 days), but ExmiR-191 and ExmiR-451a did not affect the survival of PC patients. With regard to the other factors, UICC4 was a significant prognostic factor ($p = 0.0232$, median OS of UICC1,2,3: 1330 days, median OS of UICC4:

388.5 days). We also performed a multivariate survival analysis using Cox's proportional-hazards regression model to assess the relationship between the overall survival and the following candidate prognostic factors that were identified as significant by the Kaplan–Meier method (Fig. 5b). Both UICC stage IV (hazard ratio: 3.902, 95% CI: 1.416–10.750) and the high expression of ExmiR-21 (hazard ratio: 4.071, 95%CI: 1.382–11.996) were identified as independent prognostic factors for the overall survival.

In addition, we also evaluated the association between the clinical outcome of chemotherapy and the three ExmiRs. The expression of ExmiR-21 and ExmiR-451a in the group with progression disease (PD) was significantly higher than in the groups with complete response (CR), partial response (PR), or stable disease (SD) ($p = 0.022$, $p = 0.043$, respectively) (Fig. 5c). This result might suggest that ExmiR-21 and ExmiR-451a reduced the disease control rate in PC patients.

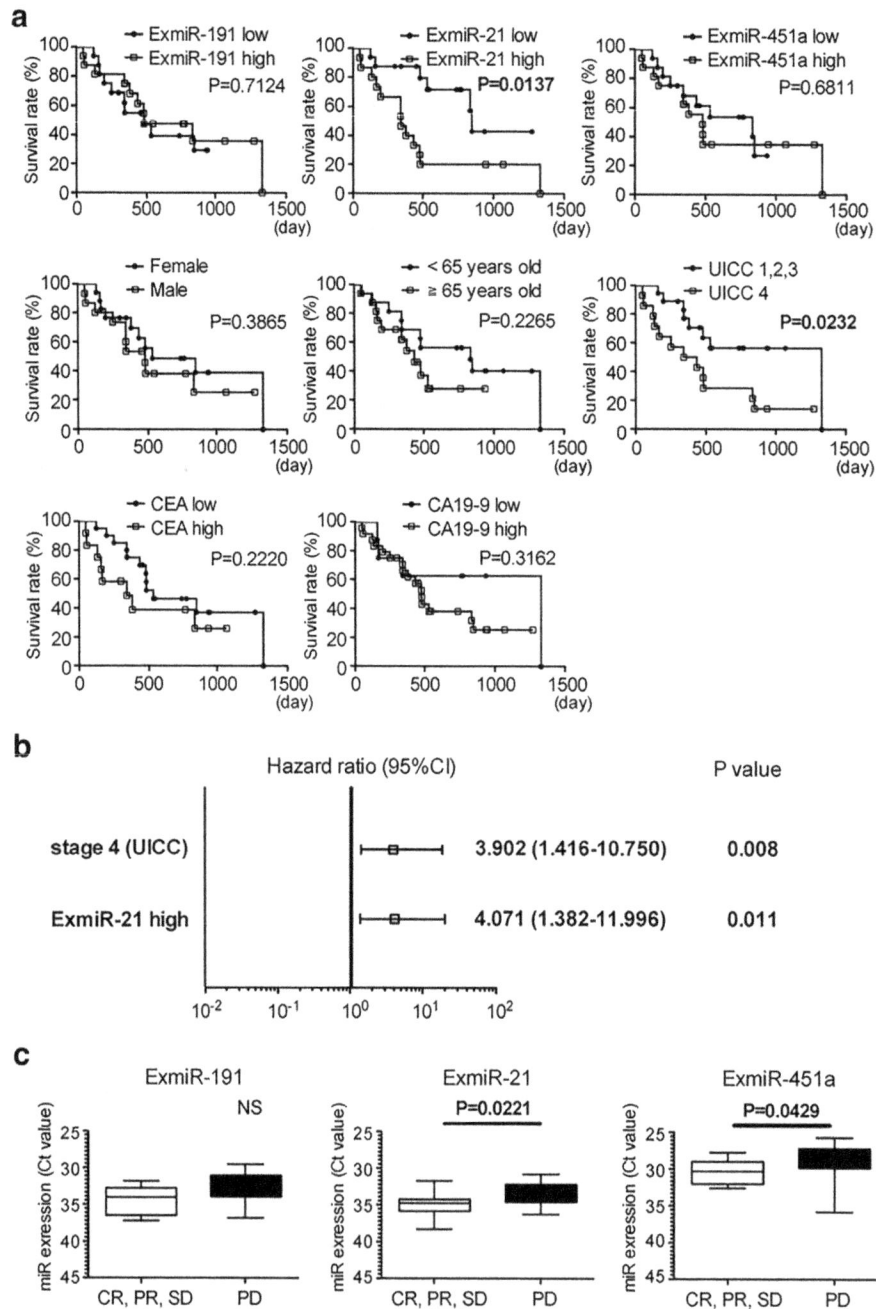

Fig. 5 ExmiR-21 was a candidate prognostic factor for the survival of PC patients. The association between the three ExmiRs and the clinical outcomes in PC patients was evaluated. **a, b** PC patients were categorized into high- and low-ExmiR expression groups using the median miR value as the cut-off point. **a** The survival analysis by Kaplan-Meier method with a log-rank test was shown. The overall survival in the high-ExmiR-21 expression group was significantly shorter than that in the low-ExmiR-21 expression group (p = 0.0137, median OS of low-ExmiR-21 expression group: 846 days, median OS of high-ExmiR-21 expression group: 344 days), but ExmiR-191 and ExmiR-451a were not associated with the survival of PC patients. With regard to the other factors, UICC4 was a significant prognostic factor (p = 0.0232, median OS of UICC1,2,3: 1330 days, median OS of UICC4: 388.5 days). **b** Multivariate survival analysis using Cox's proportional-hazards regression model was performed to assess the relationship between the overall survival and the following candidate prognostic factors that were found to be significant by the Kaplan–Meier method: UICC stage (stage IV) and ExmiR-21. UICC stage IV (hazard ratio: 3.902, 95% CI: 1.416–10.750) and the high expression of ExmiR-21 (hazard ratio: 4.071, 95%CI: 1.382–11.996) were identified as independent prognostic factors. **c** The association between the expressions of three ExmiRs and the clinical outcome of chemotherapy was also assessed. The ExmiR expressions were plotted and those median with interquartile range was also shown. The expression of ExmiR-21 and ExmiR-451a in the group with disease progression (PD) was significantly higher than in the group with complete response (CR), partial response (PR), or stable disease (SD) (p = 0.0221, p = 0.0429, respectively)

Discussion

The present study analyzed for the first time the serum ExmiRs in PC and IPMN patients using a next-generation sequencing, resulting that ExmiR-191, ExmiR-21, and ExmiR-451a were identified as candidate miRs which are dysregulated in IPMN and PC patients. The qRT-PCR confirmed that the expressions of ExmiR-191, ExmiR-21, and ExmiR-451a were increased in the patients with PC and IPMN.

Previous reports have suggested that CmiRs are useful for detecting or determining the prognosis of PC, invasive IPMNs, and other cancers [12, 13]. In the present study, we showed that the expressions of ExmiR-191, ExmiR-21 and ExmiR-451a were significantly up-regulated in PC and IPMN. However, of note: the expressions of CmiR-191, CmiR-21, and CmiR-451a were not markedly changed between the control, IPMN, and PC groups, illustrating the utility of ExmiRs as detection makers of PC and IPMN over CmiRs. CmiRs have been reported to be stabilized in vesicles such as exosomes [14], and the exosomes in serum are highly enriched in miRs [11]. Tanaka et al. also showed that circulating miR-21 originated from exosomes, as the miR-21 expression was significantly higher in exosomes than in the serum remaining after exosome extraction [12]. These present and previous findings therefore suggest that ExmiRs are more useful as markers for tumor detection than CmiRs.

It should be noted that the current established tumor markers were elevated in the advanced cancers, but not in IPMN, while the ExmiRs were upregulated in both IPMN and PC, including both early and advanced phases. The diagnostic performance estimated by the ROC curve analysis favorable AUC and accuracy as compared to CEA and CA19–9 in IPMN and early stage of PC, suggesting the levels of ExmiR-191, ExmiR-21, and ExmiR-451a can thus serve as early diagnostic markers of pancreatic neoplasms.

miR-191 has been reported to be up-regulated in a wide range of human cancers, including PC [15]. miR-191 might be responsible for the abnormal expression of many target genes such as CDK9, NOTCH2, and RPS6KA3 [16], as these genes have been reported to be direct targets of miR-191 and regulators of proliferation. In addition, miR-191 was found to regulate cell invasion and differentiation, facilitate extracellular matrix formation, and encourage metastasis [15]. miR-191 was also found to up-regulate p53 deletion and inhibit the expression of the tumor-suppressive mRNA, C/EBPβ, thereby enhancing the tumor progression in colorectal cancer [17]. Taken together, the findings from these previous studies show the oncogenic features of miR-191, which supports our finding that ExmiR-191 is a candidate diagnostic marker of pancreatic neoplasms.

miR-21 is also considered an oncogenic miR because it is up-regulated in various cancers and targets the tumor-suppressive mRNAs [18]. Previous reports of basic studies have stated that overexpression of miR-21 promoted cellular proliferation, survival, and invasion and migration of cancer cells, including PC cells [19, 20]. The overexpression of miR-21 down-regulated the expression of tumor suppressors such as PDCD4 and TIMP3 and promoted cell proliferation, leading to the development of PC [21, 22]. Conversely, the suppression of miR-21 reduced cancer cell survival and tumor growth in a murine xenograft model [23]. Indeed, clinical studies have shown that miR-21 was up-regulated in invasive IPMN compared with noninvasive IPMN [24] and was up-regulated in noninvasive IPMN compared to normal pancreatic tissue. In the present study, ExmiR-21 was identified as an early diagnostic marker of pancreatic neoplasms, a finding which is consistent with those of previous studies. Recent studies have indeed reported that miR-21 reduced the sensitivity of cancer cells to anticancer drugs such as gemcitabine and 5-FU-based chemotherapy [25], and the suppression of miR-21 increased sensitivity to gemcitabine and induced apoptosis in PC patients [26]. Furthermore, the overexpression of miR-21 correlates with a poor prognosis after PC resection, independent of other clinicopathologic factors [27]. Interestingly, ExmiR-21 was also identified as a chemo-sensitive marker and a prognostic factor for the overall survival in this study. Taken together, these present and previous findings suggest that miR-21 plays a role in pancreatic carcinogenesis.

miR-451a is located on chromosome 17q11.2 in humans and has been reported to suppress cell proliferation and colony formation by targeting the Ywhaz (14–3-3zeta) gene, RAB14 protein, and activating transcription factor 2 (ATF2). It is therefore considered to be a tumor-suppressive miR in several human malignancies [28, 29]. In addition, a clinical study showed that miR-451a expression was down-regulated in cancer tissue, and low miR-451a expression tends to be associated with metastasis and shorter survival duration [30]. These findings suggest that miR-451a acts as a tumor suppressor. In our analysis, ExmiR-451a expression was significantly increased in both the IPMN and PC groups. A high expression of ExmiR-451a might be induced by a positive feedback system due to the progression of the pancreatic tumor. Further analyses of the miR-451a expression in IPMN and PC cells will be needed to fully clarify the role of miR-451a in the development of PC.

The present study was associated with some limitations. We investigated biomarkers using serum samples from 32 patients with PC, 29 patients with IPMN and 22 healthy volunteers as a discovery cohort. To validate the efficacy of three ExmiRs, further studies should be conducted using large cohorts. In addition, the present study focused on IPMN and PC, and did not include cases with other pancreatic cystic neoplasms. A further analysis that includes patients with cystic neoplasms as well as those with non-neoplasms should be performed to identify biomarkers that can be used to distinguish IPMN from other cystic lesions.

Conclusions

In summary, the present study revealed that serum levels of ExmiR-191, ExmiR-21, and ExmiR-451a are up-regulated in PC and IPMN patients. These findings encourage the development of a novel non-invasive strategy for diagnosing pancreatic neoplasm by determining the expressions of ExmiR-191, – 21 and -451a enclosed in exosomes.

Abbreviations
ATF2: activating transcription factor 2; AUC: Area under the curve; CmiR: Circulating microRNA; CR: Complete response; ExmiR: Exosomal microRNA; FN: Fukuoka negative; HRS: High-risk stigmata; IPMN: Intraductal papillary mucinous neoplasm; miR: microRNA; OD: Optical density; OS: Overall survival; PC: Pancreatic cancer; PD: Progression disease; PR: Partial response; ROC: Receiver operating characteristic; rpm: Revolutions per minute; SD: Stable disease; WF: Worrisome feature

Acknowledgements
We wish to express our deepest gratitude to Yasuaki Saijo, a professor of social medicine at Asahikawa Medical University, who advised us on various aspects of the statistical analyses.

Funding
This study was supported by Grants-in-Aid for Scientific Research from Japan Society for the Promotion of Science (15 K19305). The funding body had no role in the design of the study and collection, analysis, or interpretation of data or in writing the manuscript.

Authors' contributions
Conception and Design: TG, HK, JS, MF, YK. Provision of Study Material or Patients: TG, JS, SF, AH, TU, HS, TI, MI, AS, KT, YN, NU, SK. Collection and Assembly of Data: TG, HK, JS, SF, AH, TU, HS, KM, YM. Data Analysis and Interpretation: TG, HK, JS, MF, KM, YM, YK, TO. Manuscript Writing: TG, HK, JS, MF. Provided valuable opinions in manuscript; HK, JS, MF, YN, NU, SK, KM, YM, YK, TO. Critical revision of the manuscript; JS, MF, KM, YM, YK, TO. Final Approval of Manuscript: All the authors.

Competing interests
All authors have read the journal's policy on conflicts of interest and the journal's authorship agreement. The authors declare that they have no competing interests.

Author details
[1]Division of Gastroenterology and Hematology/Oncology, Department of Medicine, Asahikawa Medical University, 2-1 Midorigaoka-higashi, Asahikawa, Hokkaido 078-8510, Japan. [2]Department of Gastroenterology, International University of Health and Welfare Hospital, Nasushiobara, Japan.

References
1. Siegel RL, Miller KD, Jemal A. Cancer statistics, 2015. CA Cancer J Clin. 2015;65:5–29.
2. Ballehaninna UK, Chamberlain RS. The clinical utility of serum CA 19-9 in the diagnosis, prognosis and management of pancreatic adenocarcinoma: an evidence based appraisal. Journal Of Gastrointestinal Oncology. 2012;3:105–19.
3. Uehara H, Nakaizumi A, Ishikawa O, Iishi H, Tatsumi K, Takakura R, et al. Development of ductal carcinoma of the pancreas during follow-up of branch duct intraductal papillary mucinous neoplasm of the pancreas. Gut. 2008;57(11):1561–5.
4. Maguchi H, Tanno S, Mizuno N, Hanada K, Kobayashi G, Hatori T, et al. Natural history of branch duct intraductal papillary mucinous neoplasms of the pancreas: a multicenter study in Japan. Pancreas. 2011;40:364–70.
5. Nagai K, Doi R, Kida A, Kami K, Kawaguchi Y, Ito T, et al. Intraductal papillary mucinous neoplasms of the pancreas: clinicopathologic characteristics and long-term follow-up after resection. World J Surg. 2008;32:271–8.
6. Tanaka M, Castillo C F-d, Adsay V, Chari S, Falconi M, et al. International consensus guidelines 2012 for the management of IPMN and MCN of the pancreas. Pancreatology. 2012;12:183–97.
7. Lim LP, Lau NC, Garrett-Engele P, Grimson A, Schelter JM, Castle J, et al. Microarray analysis shows that some microRNAs downregulate large numbers of target mRNAs. Nature. 2005;433:769–73.
8. Calin GA, Croce CM. MicroRNA signatures in human cancers. Nat Rev Cancer. 2006;6(11):857–66.
9. Le Large TY, Meijer LL, Mato Prado M, Kazemier G, Frampton AE, Giovannetti E. Circulating microRNAs as diagnostic biomarkers for pancreatic cancer. Expert Rev Mol Diagn. 2015;15(12):1525–9.
10. Zöller M. Pancreatic cancer diagnosis by free and exosomal miRNA. World J Gastrointest Pathophysiol. 2013;4(4):74–90.
11. Gallo A, Tandon M, Alevizos I, Illei GG. The majority of microRNAs detectable in serum and saliva is concentrated in exosomes. PLoS One. 2012;7:e30679.
12. Tanaka Y, Kamohara H, Kinoshita K, Kurashige J, Ishi T, Iwatsuki M, et al. Clinical impact of serum exosomal microRNA-21 as a clinical biomarker in human esophageal squamous cell carcinoma. Cancer. 2013;119(6):1159–67.
13. Giovannetti E, Funel N, Peters GJ, Del Chiaro M, Erozenci LA, Vasile E, et al. MicroRNA-21 in pancreatic cancer: correlation with clinical outcome and pharmacologic aspects underlying its role in the modulation of gemcitabine activity. Cancer Res. 2010;70:4528–38.
14. Köberle V, Pleli T, Schmithals C, Augusto Alonso E, Haupenthal J, Bonig H, et al. Differential stability of cell-free circulating microRNAs: implications for their utilization as biomarkers. PLoS One. 2013;8(9):e75184.
15. Song Z, Ren H, Gao S, Zhao X, Zhang H, Hao J. The clinical significance and regulation mechanism of hypoxia-inducible factor-1 and miR-191 expression in pancreatic cancer. Tumor Biol. 2014;35:11319–28.
16. Polioudakis D, Abell NS, Iyer VR. MiR-191 regulates primary human fibroblast proliferation and directly targets multiple oncogenes. PLoS One. 2015;10(5): e0126535.
17. Zhang XF, Li KK, Gao L, Ii SZ, Chen K, Zhang JB, et al. miR-191 promotes tumorigenesis of human colorectal cancer through targeting C/EBPβ. Oncotarget. 2015;6(6):4144–58.
18. Pan X, Wang ZX, Wang R. MicroRNA-21: a novel therapeutic target in human cancer. Cancer Biol Ther. 2010;10:1224–32.
19. Moriyama T, Ohuchida K, Mizumoto K, Yu J, Sato N, Nabae T, et al. MicroRNA-21 modulates biological functions of pancreatic cancer cells including theirproliferation, invasion, and chemoresistance. Mol Cancer Ther. 2009;8:1067–74.
20. Kadera BE, Li L, Toste PA, Wu N, Adams C, Dawson DW, et al. MicroRNA-21 in pancreatic ductal adenocarcinoma tumor-associated fibroblasts promotes metastasis. PLoS One. 2013;8:e71978.
21. Hiyoshi Y, Kamohara H, Karashima R, Sato N, Imamura Y, Nagai Y, et al. MicroRNA-21 regulates the proliferation and invasion in esophageal squamous cell carcinoma. Clin Cancer Res. 2009;15:1915–22.
22. Nagao Y, Hisaoka M, Matsuyama A, Kanemitsu S, Hamada T, Fukuyama T, et al. Association of microRNA-21 expression with its targets, PDCD4 and TIMP3, in pancreatic ductal adenocarcinoma. Mod Pathol. 2012;25:112–21.
23. Frezzetti D, De Menna M, Zoppoli P, Guerra C, Ferraro A, Bello AM, et al. Upregulation of miR-21 by Ras in vivo and its role in tumor growth. Oncogene. 2011;30:275–86.
24. Matthei H, Wylie D, Lloyd M, Dal Molin M, Kemppainen J, Mayo SC, et al. MicroRNA biomarkers in cyst fluid augment the diagnosis and management of pancreatic cysts. Clin Can Res. 2012;18:4713–24.

25. Hong L, Han Y, Zhang Y, Zhang H, Zhao Q, Wu K, et al. MicroRNA-21: a therapeutic target for reversing drug resistance in cancer. Expert Opin Ther Targets. 2013;17(9):1073–80.

26. Park JK, Lee EJ, Esau C, Schmittgen TD. Antisense inhibition of microRNA-21 or –221 arrests cell cycle, induces apoptosis, and sensitizes the effects of gemcitabine in pancreatic adenocarcinoma. Pancreas. 2009;38:e190–e199.

27. Frampton AE, Krell J, Jamieson NB, Gall TM, Giovannetti E, Funel N, et al. microRNAs with prognostic significance in pancreatic ductal adenocarcinoma: a meta-analysis. Eur J Cancer. 2015;51(11):1389–404.

28. Wang R, Wang ZX, Yang JS, Pan X, De W, Chen LB. MicroRNA-451 functions as a tumor suppressor in human non-small cell lung cancer by targeting ras-related protein 14 (RAB14). Oncogene. 2011;30:2644–58.

29. Li Y, Wang J, Dai X, Zhou Z, Liu J, Zhang Y, et al. miR-451 regulates FoxO3 nuclear accumulation through Ywhaz in human colorectal cancer. Am J Transl Res. 2015;7(12):2775–85.

30. Su Z, Zhao J, Rong Z, Geng W, Wang Z. MiR-451, a potential prognostic biomarker and tumor suppressor for gastric cancer. Int J Clin Exp Pathol. 2015;8(8):9154–60.

Treatment of pancreatic ductal adenocarcinoma with tumor antigen specific-targeted delivery of paclitaxel loaded PLGA nanoparticles

Shu-ta Wu[1], Anthony J. Fowler[2], Corey B. Garmon[2], Adam B. Fessler[2], Joshua D. Ogle[2], Kajal R. Grover[1], Bailey C. Allen[1], Chandra D. Williams[3], Ru Zhou[1], Mahboubeh Yazdanifar[1], Craig A. Ogle[2] and Pinku Mukherjee[1]*[ID]

Abstract

Background: Pancreatic ductal adenocarcinoma (PDA) remains the most aggressive cancers with a 5-year survival below 10%. Systemic delivery of chemotherapy drugs has severe side effects in patients with PDA and does not significantly improve overall survival rate. It is highly desirable to advance the therapeutic efficacy of chemotherapeutic drugs by targeting their delivery and increasing accumulation at the tumor site. MUC1 is a membrane-tethered glycoprotein that is aberrantly overexpressed in > 80% of PDA thus making it an attractive antigenic target.

Methods: Poly lactic-co-glycolic acid nanoparticles (PLGA NPs) conjugated to a tumor specific MUC1 antibody, TAB004, was used as a nanocarrier for targeted delivery into human PDA cell lines in vitro and in PDA tumors in vivo. The PLGA NPs were loaded with fluorescent imaging agents, fluorescein diacetate (FDA) and Nile Red (NR) or isocyanine green (ICG) for in vitro and in vivo imaging respectively or with a chemotherapeutic drug, paclitaxel (PTX) for in vitro cytotoxicity assays. Confocal microscopy was used to visualize internalization of the nanocarrier in vitro in PDA cells with high and low MUC1 expression. The in vivo imaging system (IVIS) was used to visualize in vivo tumor targeting of the nanocarrier. MTT (3-(4,5-Dimethylthiazol-2-yl)-2,5-Diphenyltetrazolium Bromide) assay was used to determine in vitro cell survival of cells treated with PTX-loaded nanocarrier. One-sided t-test comparing treatment groups at each concentration and two-way ANOVAs comparing internalization of antibody and PLGA nanoparticles.

Results: In vitro, TAB004-conjugated ICG-nanocarriers were significantly better at internalizing in PDA cells than its non-conjugated counterpart. Similarly, TAB004-conjugated PTX-nanocarriers were significantly more cytotoxic in vitro against PDA cells than its non-conjugated counterpart. In vivo, TAB004-conjugated ICG-nanocarriers showed increased accumulation in the PDA tumor compared to the non-conjugated nanocarrier while sparing normal organs.

Conclusions: The study provides promising data for future development of a novel MUC1-targeted nanocarrier for direct delivery of imaging agents or drugs into the tumor microenvironment.

Keywords: PLGA, Nanoparticles, Mucin 1, Anti-MUC1 antibody, Targeted delivery, Paclitaxel, Pancreatic ductal adenocarcinoma

* Correspondence: pmukherj@uncc.edu
[1]Department of Biological Sciences, University of North Carolina at Charlotte, Charlotte, NC 28223, USA
Full list of author information is available at the end of the article

Background

Pancreatic Cancer is a highly aggressive disease with a 5-year relative survival rate of $\sim 9\%$ [1]. Greater than 90% of all pancreatic cancers arise in the epithelial ducts of the pancreas and are designated pancreatic ductal adenocarcinomas (PDA). Only 18-20% of patients diagnosed with PDA are eligible for surgical resection followed by chemo and radiation therapies. For majority of PDA patients, chemo and radiation therapies are the only choices. However, due to chemo-resistance, the overall survival rate with or without surgical resection remains dismal [2]. It is established that one of the reasons for failed therapy is the inefficient delivery of chemotherapy drugs to the tumor site, likely due to the dense stroma and deficient vascular network in the pancreatic tissue microenvironment [3, 4]. Therefore, there is a pressing need to develop a novel drug delivery system for PDA that can increase the drug accumulation and uptake in a tumor specific manner [5].

Nanoparticles (NPs) modified to degrade in the tumor microenvironment or target tumor antigens are promising platforms for the targeted delivery of therapeutic drugs to specific cells and tissues [6–9]. NPs formulated from biodegradable and biocompatible polymers, such as Poly lactic-co-glycolic acid (PLGA), are being utilized increasingly in research due to their excellent systemic characteristics [10]. PLGA NPs allow for the encapsulation of a variety of hydrophobic chemotherapeutics or imaging agents, and can thereby facilitate the systemic delivery of these otherwise insoluble compounds with localization at the tumor site. This localization is the result of the enhanced permeability and retention effect (EPR), which is caused by the vasculature permeability in tumors being greater than in normal tissues, and thus provide a mechanism of selection for the NPs, as they do not penetrate into neighboring normal tissue [11, 12]. The unorganized structure of the tumor and lack of lymphatic drainage prolong the retention of NPs after they escape from the leaky vasculature [13]. PLGA NPs with polyethylene glycol (PEG) displayed at the surface have been shown to increase circulatory half-lives of the NPs, while surface modification with targeting agents have been shown to aid in localization of the NPs selectively at targeted tissues [14–17]. Novel chemotherapeutic agents and combinations like FOLFIRINOX (5-fluorouracil, oxaliplatin, irinotecan, and leucovorin) or Abraxane (nab-paclitaxel, an albumin-coated formulation of paclitaxel) have been developed and have seen some success [18, 19]. The combination of gemcitabine and nab-paclitaxel has been shown to increase the intratumor concentration of gemcitabine by roughly three-fold in xenograft models [20, 21]. Paclitaxel, a taxane agent, (PTX) is one of the most widely used anticancer drugs approved for the treatment of many types of cancer. PTX interferes with cell division by interacting with the polymer form of tubulin and promoting microtubulin assembly. This stabilizes the polymers against depolymerization, which induces M-phase cell cycle arrest and cell death [22, 23]. Targeted NPs consisting of PLGA encapsulated PTX will provide a drug delivery system that would increase delivery of PTX to the tumor site, due to the EPR effect [24]. Systemic administration of the drug loaded NPs, however, have many problems associated with it. For instance, if the NP is too large, issues can arise that prevent them from reaching the tumor site, as the NPs have to cross through several biological barriers, such as blood vessels, tissues, organs, and cells. Without any specificity for the tumor site, it may be necessary to use fairly high doses of NPs and drugs to achieve sufficient local concentrations. In PDA, due to poor vascularization and despoplasia, non-targeted NPs may not suitable. Conjugating the NPs with tumor targeting moieties could possibly overcome some of these challenges.

Mucin-1 (MUC1), is a transmembrane protein with an extracellular domain that is heavily glycosylated [25]. It is normally expressed on epithelial cells of the mammary gland, esophagus, stomach, duodenum, uterus, prostate, lung, and pancreas [26]. In healthy tissues, the negatively charged glycosylated extracellular domain of MUC1 creates a physical barrier and an anti-adhesive surface, preventing pathogenic colonization [27]. In over 80% of PDA, MUC1 is hypoglycosylated and overexpressed [28] which in turn is also associated with higher metastasis and poor prognosis [29, 30]. These characteristics ranked MUC1 as one of the best tumor antigens for targeted therapy [31]. We have developed a novel monoclonal antibody, TAB004 (OncoTAb, Inc., Charlotte, NC), which specifically targets the hypoglycosylated form MUC1 (tMUC1) [32–34].

This study was aimed at investigating the targeting ability of TAB004 conjugated PLGA NPs in vitro and in vivo. NR, FDA, and ICG were used as the imaging agents and PTX as the chemotherapeutic drug. We hypothesized that the conjugation of TAB004 to the surface of PLGA NPs will increase their accumulation and duration at the tumor site and thereby increase the overall therapeutic index of the treatment. For this purpose, PTX, ICG, or FDA&NR were encapsulated in PEGylated PLGA NPs and then conjugated to TAB004. Unconjugated particles were used as controls. Internalization, retention, and therapeutic efficacy were evaluated in vitro in several MUC1 high and low expressing human PDA cell lines.

Methods

Materials

All chemical reagents used for the study were of analytical grade. Poly(DL-lactide-co-glycolide) M_W 20,000 (PLGA) (50:50) PolySciences, Inc. (Warrington, PA). Polyethylene glycol M_w 1000 (PEG$_{1000}$), Poly(vinyl alcohol) M_W 6000 (PVA) (80 mol% hydrolyzed), 1,1'-carbonyldiimidazole (CDI), 1,3-diaminopropane (DAP), Dextrose were purchased from Sigma Aldrich (St. Louis, MO). Paclitaxel was purchased from Matrix Scientific (Columbia, SC), ICG was purchased from Chem-Impex (Wood Dale, IL). TAB004 monoclonal antibody was obtained from OncoTAb, Inc. (Charlotte, NC, USA).

Cell culture

Human PDA cell lines including BxPC3, HPAC, HPAFII, and MIA PaCa-2 were purchased from ATCC (Manassas, VA). Murine PDA cell line, KCM was generated in our lab [35]. KCM, HPAC, HPAF II, and MIA PaCa-2 were maintained in Dulbecco's modified Eagle's medium (DMEM, 11965-092, Gibco). BxPC3 cell lines were maintained in RPMI medium 1640 (RPMI, 11875-093, Gibco). Growth media for these cell lines were supplemented with 10% fetal bovine serum (FBS, Gibco), 3. 4 mM L-glutamine, 90 units (U) per ml penicillin, and 90 µg/ml streptomycin (Cellgro).

Determination of NP loading

For the paclitaxel NP (PTX) formulation a 20 mg sample of was dissolved into 600 µl of DMSO-$d6$ and the concentration of the respective cargo determined using ^{1}H NMR at 25 °C by comparing unique resonances of the cargo to the methylene residue of PLGA at [5.2 ppm]. For the fluorescein diacetate (FDA), indocyanine green (ICG), and Nile red (NR) NP formulations, a sample of nanomaterial (2-4 mg) was dissolved into DMSO and the amount of cargo quantified by UV-Vis.

$$Encapsulation\ Efficiency = \frac{Amount\ of\ cargo\ encapsulated}{Amount\ of\ cargo\ used} \times 100$$

Determination of NP size and polydispersity

Particle size, polydispersity index (PDI), along with zeta potential were determined by dynamic light scattering (Zetasizer Nano, Malvern Instruments) Table 1.

Table 1 Structural Properties of PTX, FDA, NR, and ICG Nanomaterials

Nanomaterial	HD (nm)	PDI	ZP (Ω)
PTX NPs	141.8 ± .6	.155 ± .009	−7.6 ± .2
FDA NPs	171.3 ± 1.2	.129 ± .004	−6.4 ± .2
NR NPs	209.3 ± .6	.175 ± .007	−6.7 ± .1
ICG NPs	180.7 ± .9	.076 ± .006	−6.8 ± .1

HD Hydrodynamic Diameter, *PDI* Polydispersity Index, *ZP* Zeta Potential

Cargo release profiles

Release profiles of NPs were modeled using FDA NPs. The release characteristics of these particles were characterized in phosphate buffered saline (PBS) at pH 7.4.

Synthesis of PCL$_{14K}$-PEG$_{1000}$

PCL$_{14K}$-PEG$_{1000}$ was prepared according to the following procedure. Polycaprolactone (2 g, M_w ~ 14,000) was added to a 50 ml oven dried round-bottom flask fitted with a claisen adapter and equipped with a magnetic stir bar, a rubber septum, and a reflux condenser with attached drying tube. To this was added 20 ml of thionyl chloride via syringe, and the rubber septum replaced with a ground-glass stopper, and the resulting solution heated to reflux for 3 h. The thionyl chloride was then removed under reduced pressure using a rotary evaporator. The resulting residue was placed under a nitrogen atmosphere and 50 ml of freshly distilled tetrahydrofuran (THF) was added by cannula followed by PEG$_{1000}$-diol (2.9 g, 20 equivalent) and triethylamine (2 ml, 14.35 mmol). The resulting solution was left to stir for 18 h at room temperature. This solution was then poured into 500 ml of DI water under vigorous stirring to precipitate the desired product and remove unreacted PEG$_{1000}$ diol. The precipitate was isolated by filtration, re-dissolved into THF (50 ml), and precipitated as before. This process was repeated three times. Finally, the isolated product was dried under vacuum at 25 °C for 72 h. The desired product was isolated as a solid white material (1.13 g, 53%). ^{1}H NMR (500 MHz CDCl$_3$): δ 1.36 (m, -CH$_2$CH$_2$CH$_2$-), 1.63 (m, -CH$_2$CH$_2$CH$_2$-), 2.28 (t, -C(O)CH$_2$-), 3.62 (s, -OCH$_2$CH$_2$-), 4.04 (t, -OCH$_2$).

Synthesis of PCL$_{14K}$-PEG$_{1000}$-NH2

PCL$_{14K}$-PEG$_{1000}$-NH2 was prepared by the according to the following procedure. PCL$_{14K}$-PEG$_{1000}$ (1 g) was added to a 50 ml oven dried 2-neck round-bottom flask equipped with a magnet stir bar and a rubber septum with nitrogen inlet. To this was added 20 ml of dry methylene chloride (DCM) followed by 1,1'-carbonyldiimidazole (100 mg, .62 mmol) and the resulting solution left to stir for 6 h at room temperature. To this was added 1,3-diaminopropane (1 ml, 12.19 mmol) and the resulting solution left to stir for 12 h at room temperature. The DCM was then removed under reduced pressure using a rotary evaporator. The resulting viscous yellow liquid was dissolved into THF (20 ml) and precipitated by pouring the solution into 250 ml of vigorously stirred DI water. The precipitate was isolated by filtration, re-dissolved into THF (20 ml), and precipitated as before. This process was repeated three times. Finally, the isolated product was dried under vacuum at 25 °C for 72 h. The desired product was isolated as a yellow solid (.5 g, 50%). Although the resonances for the end-group -C(O)NHCH$_2$CH$_2$CH$_2$NH$_2$- are not assigned due to obfuscation of these resonances by the polymer backbone, the polymer tested positive for the presence of primary amines using the Kaiser test [36]. H NMR (500 MHz CDCl$_3$): δ 1.37 (m, -CH$_2$CH$_2$CH$_2$-), 1.64 (m, -CH$_2$CH$_2$CH$_2$-), 2.29 (t, -C(O)CH$_2$-), 3.63 (s, -OCH$_2$CH$_2$-), 4.05 (t, -OCH$_2$).

Nanoparticle preparation: General method

Nanoparticles (NPs) were prepared by the nanoprecipitation according to the method of Langer et al. [37]. Briefly; 100 mg of PLGA (50:50, M$_w$ ~ 20 K), 5 mg of PCL-PEG$_{1000}$, 1 mg PCL-PEG$_{1000}$-NH2, and 1 - 5 mg of cargo was dissolved into 10 ml of acetone. This solution was then added dropwise via syringe into a stirred solution of 1% PVA (20 ml) at a rate of 90 ml/hr. controlled using a syringe pump. The resulting colloidal suspension was then transferred to a 100 ml round-bottom flask, and the acetone removed under reduced pressure using a rotary evaporator. NPs were then purified by centrifugation (25 min, 30,000×g) using three successive washes of sterile filtered 18 Ω water at 4 °C. The resulting NP pellet was then resuspended into sterile filtered 18 Ω water (10 ml), whereupon dextrose (10 mg) was added as a lyoprotectant. This colloidal suspension was then flash frozen in liquid nitrogen then lyophilized at 25 °C and 50 mTorr for 24 - 48 h resulting in a flocculent solid. Paclitaxel (PTX), Fluorescein Diacetate (FDA), and Nile Red (NR) were all prepared according to the general method described above. See Table 2 for the amount of cargo used in the preparation of the respective nanomaterials.

ICG preparation

ICG NP's were prepared similarly using a modified nanoprecipitation method according to procedure reported by Cai [38]. Briefly; 100 mg of PLGA (50:50, M$_w$ ~ 20 K), 5 mg of PCL-PEG$_{1000}$, 1 mg PCL-PEG$_{1000}$-NH2 was dissolved into 9 ml of acetonitrile. Meanwhile 1 mg of ICG was dissolved into 1 ml of sterile filtered 18 Ω water. The two solutions were then mixed, and vortexed rapidly for 2 min. The resulting solution was then added dropwise via syringe into a stirred solution of 1% PVA (20 ml) at a rate of 90 ml/hr. controlled using a syringe pump. The resulting colloidal suspension was then transferred to a 100 ml round-bottom flask, and the acetonitrile removed

under reduced pressure using a rotary evaporator. NPs were then purified by centrifugation (25 min, 30,000×g) using three successive washes of sterile filtered 18 Ω water at 4 °C. The resulting NP pellet was then resuspended into sterile filtered 18 Ω water (10 ml), whereupon dextrose (10 mg) was added as a lyoprotectant. This colloidal suspension was then flash frozen in liquid nitrogen, and lyophilized at 25 °C and 50 mTorr for 24 - 48 h resulting in a flocculent green solid.

FDA release profiles

1 ml Solutions of FDA NPs (1 mg/ml) in PBS (pH 7.4) were incubated with constant stirring at 37 °C over 72 h. 100 μl samples were taken at the indicated time-points and centrifuged (16,000 x g) to pellet out the remaining NPs. 50 μl of NP free buffer was removed carefully so as not to disturb the pellet, and 20 μl of 5% NaOH added to hydrolyze the liberated FDA. Absorbance measurements were recorded at 490 nm. These values were compared to a control sample having been dissolved in a 50:50 acetonitrile (CAN):H$_2$O solution to liberate the entire sample of FDA from the NPs, and hydrolyzed as above.

SEM imaging

Lyophilized nanoparticles were re-suspended in H$_2$O at 0.01 mg/mL concentrations and sonicated for 10 s. Samples were placed on SPI 5 × 5 silicon chips and dried overnight at 40 °C. Scanning electron microscopy (SEM) images were obtained with a Raith 150 microscope operated at 10 kV.

Generation of BxPC3.MUC1, BxPC3.Neo, and KCM-Luc

Full-length MUC1 gene was cloned into the pLNCX.1 vector consisting of the neomycin resistance gene for retroviral infection. GP2-293 cells were transfected with MUC1 pLNCX.1 and pVSV-G vectors and the resulting viral supernatant used to infect a MUC1-null human PDA cell line, BxPC3. These cells were designated BxPC3.MUC1 cells. BxPC3.MUC1 serves as MUC1-high positive control. BxPC3.Neo represent BxPC3 cells that express the empty vector and therefore serves as the MUC1-negative controls [30]. KCM cell line was generated from spontaneous PDA tumors arising in the PDA.MUC1 triple transgenic mice. This cell line is syngeneic to the C57/Bl6 mouse background and expresses human MUC1 [34, 35]. Retroviral transduction of KCM cells with MSCV Luciferase PGK-Hygro (MSCV Luciferase PGK-hygro was a gift from Scott Lowe, Addgene plasmid # 18782) was performed by transfecting GP2-293 cells with the MSCV Luciferase PGK-Hygro and pVSV-G vectors and using the subsequent viral supernatant to infect KCM cells.

Table 2 Cargo Loading of PTX, FDA, NR, and ICG into Nanomaterials

Nanomaterial	Cargo Loading (mg)	Amount Encapsulated (mg/100 mg NPs)	EE (%)
PTX NPs[a]	5	2.3 ± .1	46.7 ± 1.8
FDA NPs[b]	5	1.7 ± .1	34.2 ± .9
NR NPs[b]	2	.26 ± .01	13.1 ± .6
ICG NPs[b]	1.75	.39 ± .01	22.1 ± .3

EE Encapsulation Efficiency. [a]Determined by 1H NMR. [b]Determined by UV-Vis

Conjugation of TAB004 to PLGA NPs

TAB004 conjugation to PLGA nanoparticles was performed using NuLink conjugation kit (NuChemie). PLGA nanoparticles were weighed out into an appropriate Eppendorf tube. To a vial containing 1 mg of the NuLink© bis-electrophile thioester was added 1 drop of DMSO to assist with dissolution, then 500 μl of 18 Ω H_2O was added. The solution was vortexed until all of the labeling reagent was dissolved. The PLGA nanoparticles were re-suspended in 200 μl of 18 Ω H_2O. The labeling solution was added dropwise to the nanoparticles while under a gentle vortex and allowed to incubate at room temperature (how long time) after mixing. The labeled nanoparticles were centrifuged at 21,000 rcf and 4 °C to pellet them. The supernatant was removed and the labeled nanoparticles re-suspended in 200 μl of 18 Ω H_2O. 30 μg of TAB004 at mg/ml conc (in azide free buffer) was then added to the labeled NP solution in one portion. The next day, the nanoparticles were centrifuged at 21,000 rcf and 4 °C to pellet them and the supernatant discarded. Nanoparticles were re-suspended into desired working volume of PBS. Successful TAB004 conjugation to the PLGA nanoparticle was confirmed using FACS (BD Fortessa) and an anti-mouse IgG_1-FITC secondary antibody.

Cell viability assays

Cell viability assays were performed using MTT (3-(4,5-Dimethylthiazol-2-yl)-2,5-Diphenyltetrazolium Bromide) (Fisher Scientific, USA). Optimal number of cells per cell line were plated into 96-well tissue culture plates to ensure cells would not be over confluent after 48 h post treatment. 24 h after cells were plated, they were treated with corresponding concentrations of dimethyl sulfoxide (DMSO), PTX, blank PLGA nanoparticles, PTX loaded PLGA nanoparticles, and TAB004 conjugated PTX loaded PLGA nanoparticles for 1.5 h. After 1.5 h the treatments were washed off with 1× PBS and 200 μl of fresh media was added to the wells and cell lines were incubated for 48 h at 37 °C, > 90% humidity, and 5% CO_2 conditions. Following the 48 h incubation, the media was replaced with 100 μl of phenol red free media and 10 μl of MTT was added to each well. Plates were incubated at 37 °C, > 90% humidity, and 5% CO_2 conditions for 4 h, after which the media and MTT were removed, 100 μl of DMSO added, and incubated at 37 °C for 10 min. The plates were then read using a ThermoFisher Scientific MultiScan GO. Cell viability data for each treatment group (PTX, NP loaded with PTX, and TAB004 conjugated to NPs loaded with PTX) was normalized to their own vehicle control cell viabilities (DMSO and Blank NPs).

Internalization of NPs

Cell lines were plated into 4-chamber well slides (154, 917, LAB-TEK) at optimal concentration to ensure cells would not be over confluent after 24 h. 24 h after cells were plated, they were treated with fluorescein (20 μg/ml), or fluorescein diacetate and Nile Red containing PLGA nanoparticles at 1 mg/ml concentration for 1.5 h at 37 °C, > 90% humidity, and 5% CO_2 conditions. After treatment, cells were washed with PBS for 5 min (3×) and fixed with 4% formaldehyde. Prolong Gold Antifade reagent with DAPI (P36935, Molecular Probes) was applied to mount coverslips. Images were acquired on an Olympus Fluoview FV 1000 confocal microscope.

Specificity and internalization of TAB004

TAB004 conjugation to pHrodo Red was performed using the pHrodo Red, succinimidyl ester (pHrodo Red, SE) kit (P36600, Molecular Probes). TAB004 conjugation to indocyanine green (ICG) was performed using the ICG Labeling Kit –NH_2 (LK31-10, Dojindo Molecular Technologies, Inc.). All conjugations were performed using manufacturer protocols. Cell lines were plated into 4-chamber well slides (154,917, LAB-TEK) at optimal concentration to ensure cells would not be over confluent after 24 h. 24 h after cells were plated, they were treated with 5 μl of TAB004-pHrodo Red conjugation solution for various time points at 37 °C, > 90% humidity, and 5% CO_2 conditions. During the last 5 min of treatment, Wheat Germ Agglutinin-Alexa Fluor 488 conjugate (W11261, Molecular Probes), was added to each chamber at 5 μg/ml. The cells were washed with PBS for 5 min (3×) and fixed with 4% formaldehyde. Prolong Gold Antifade reagent with DAPI (P36935, Molecular Probes) was applied to mount coverslips. Images were acquired on a GE Healthcare Life Sciences DeltaVision Elite Imaging microscope.

Mouse strains

C57Bl/6 mice were purchased from Jackson Laboratory and housed at UNC Charlotte's vivarium.

Orthotopic tumor model

C57/Bl6 female mice were injected in the pancreas with 5×10^5 KCM-Luc cells and allowed to recuperate for 7 days before any experiments were performed. This study and all procedures were performed after approval from the Institutional Animal Care and Use Committee of UNC Charlotte.

Visualization of KCM-Luc orthotopic tumors, TAB004-ICG, and TAB004 conjugated PLGA NPs with ICG

Orthotopic KCM-Luc tumor bearing C57/Bl6 mice were injected with 125 μl of Redijet D-Luciferin (760,504, Perkin Elmer) intraperitoneally and imaged 25 min later with a Perkin Elmer IVIS Spectrum. Orthotopic KCM-Luc tumor bearing C57/Bl6 mice were injected with 25 μg of TAB004-ICG, 50 mg/kg of NP w/ICG, or 50 mg/kg of TAB004-NP w/ICG intraperitoneally and imaged at various time points with a Perkin Elmer IVIS Spectrum. Mice were euthanized at the end of imaging studies. All procedures were conducted in accordance to the Institutional Animal Care and Use Committee of UNC Charlotte. All mice and organ images and region of interests (ROIs) were acquired and processed in Living Imagine 4.3.1 (Caliper Life Sciences, Waltham, MA).

Results

Nanoparticle preparation and characterization

We evaluated the size and release profile of PLGA NPs to determine an optimal size for use (Fig. 1a). As shown, PCL_{14K}-PEG_{1K} and PCL_{14K}-PEG_{1K}-NH_2 partitions into the aqueous environment during self-assembly of the nanoparticles, thereby generating a nanoparticle having a pegylated surface with a small percentage of nucleophilic amines available for chemical modification. During self-assembly the cargo is encapsulated in the hydrophobic core. The functionalization of the NP surface was performed using the NuLink bis-electrophile (Fig. 1b).

Fluorescein Diacetate (FDA) PLGA NPs were used as a model system to investigate the size and release profile of the NP platform described (Fig. 2a, b). In vitro cargo release of the NPs was evaluated in PBS at pH 7.4. FDA was steadily released over the course of 120 h. The percent of FDA released at 24, 48, 72, and 96 h was 24%, 37%, 50%, 59%, and 70% respectively (Fig. 2b).

PLGA NPs internalize into BxPC3.MUC1 and BxPC3.Neo human PDA cell lines

We determined whether the PLGA NPs internalizes into a human PDA cell line. Wild-type BxPC3 cells have minimal expression of endogenous MUC1. We generated BxPC3. MUC1 cells that stably express full-length MUC1. As control, we generated BxPC3.Neo that expresses the empty vector. BxPC3.MUC1 cells express high levels of MUC1 while BxPC3.Neo cells express minimal levels of MUC1 [30]. In the later experiments, this will enable us to assess the specificity of the TAB004 antibody in an otherwise genetically identical PDA cell line. BxPC3. MUC1 and BxPC3.Neo cell lines were treated for 1.5 h with FDA and Nile Red loaded NPs. This matched the total treatment time of PDA cell lines in the cell viability assay. After 1.5 h, FDA and NR loaded PLGA NPs internalized through endocytosis into both BxPC3.MUC1 and BxPC3.Neo cell lines equally (Fig. 3) suggesting that internalization is independent of MUC1 expression levels. Punctate green fluorescence, from the hydrolysis of FDA in the NPs, can be seen within the cytoplasm of the cells, indicating internalization of the NPs (Fig. 3). Fluorescence is only observed if FDA is hydrolyzed within the cells [39]. Although we detect a slight trend of increased endocytosis in the BxPC3.MUC1 versus BxPC3.Neo cells, the difference is not statistically significant.

TAB004 antibody internalizes into PDA cell lines that express tMUC1

Next we determined the specificity of TAB004 to MUC1 and quantified the internalization of TAB004 antibody by fluorescent microscopy (Fig. 4). The presence and uptake of TAB004 was visualized by conjugating the antibody to pHrodo Red, which is non-fluorescent outside the cell, but fluoresces red only post endocytosis (Fig. 4a). The green fluorescence is wheat germ agglutinin that stains the cell membrane. The fluorescent signal from TAB004 is significantly increased in BxPC3.MUC1 when compared

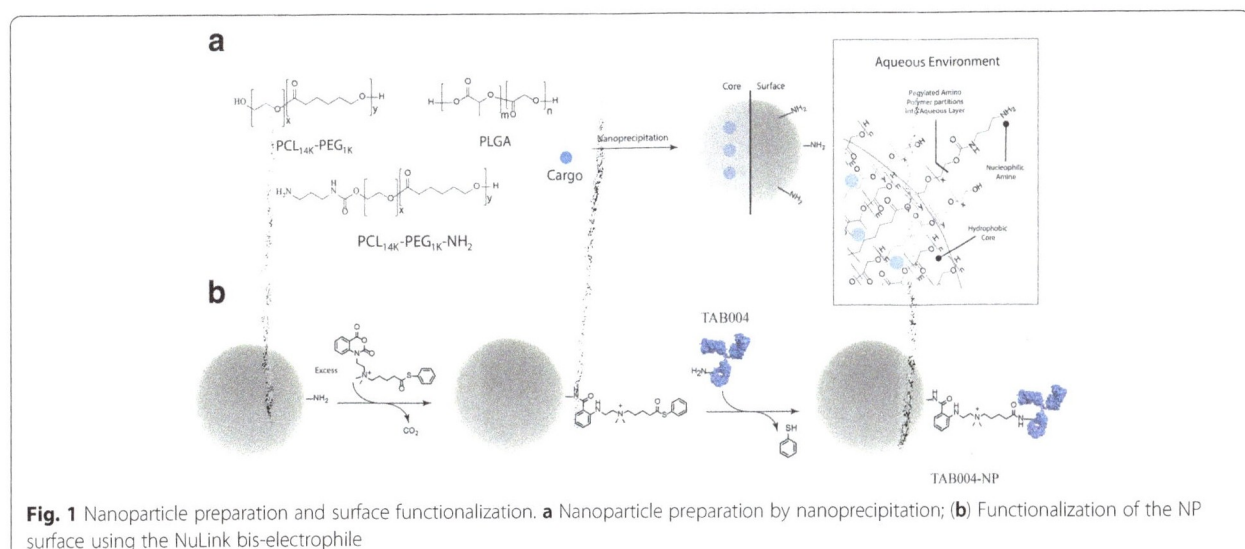

Fig. 1 Nanoparticle preparation and surface functionalization. **a** Nanoparticle preparation by nanoprecipitation; (**b**) Functionalization of the NP surface using the NuLink bis-electrophile

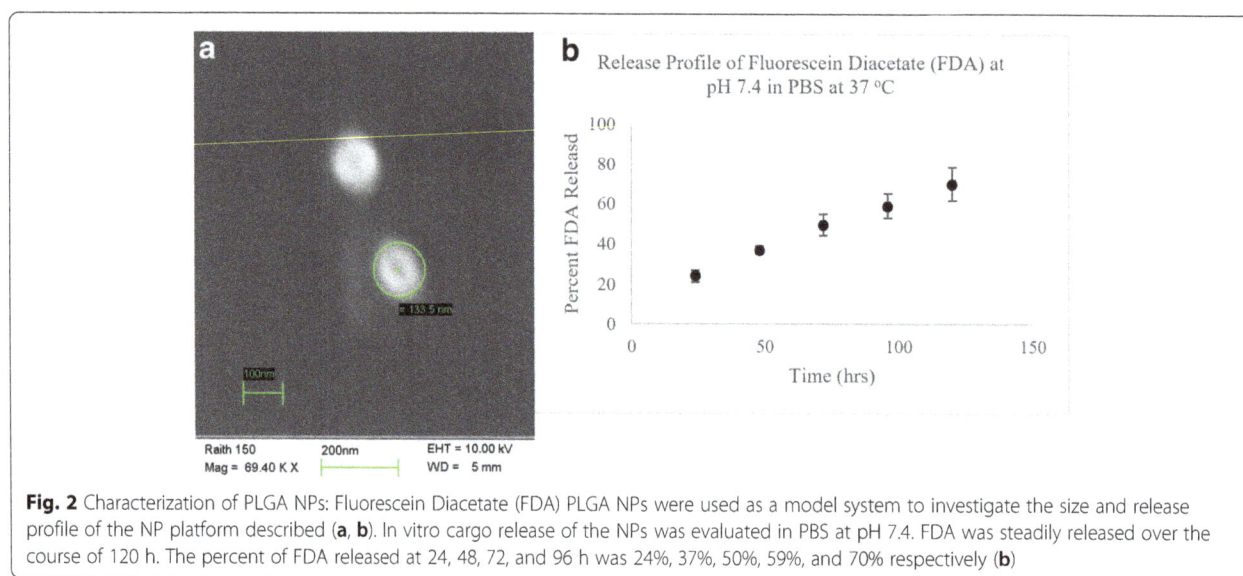

Fig. 2 Characterization of PLGA NPs: Fluorescein Diacetate (FDA) PLGA NPs were used as a model system to investigate the size and release profile of the NP platform described (**a**, **b**). In vitro cargo release of the NPs was evaluated in PBS at pH 7.4. FDA was steadily released over the course of 120 h. The percent of FDA released at 24, 48, 72, and 96 h was 24%, 37%, 50%, 59%, and 70% respectively (**b**)

to BxPC3.Neo cells at all time points (Fig. 4b). There is some internalization observed in BxPC3 Neo, which can be caused by the very low level of endogenous MUC1 that is present, or by non-specific endocytosis as PDA cells have been shown to actively swallow their surroundings through macropinocytosis [40, 41].

TAB004 conjugated PTX loaded PLGA NPs are specific for and inhibit growth of tMUC1 expressing cells

The successful conjugation of TAB004 to the surface of the NPs (T-NPs) was determined by flow cytometry (Additional file 1: Figure S1). The linking reagent, a thioester, was tested and was successful in linking TAB004 to the NPs (Additional file 1: Figure S1B). Flow cytometry data shows a shift in fluorescence when NPs are conjugated to TAB004 and labeled with FITC conjugated anti-mouse IgG1. Unconjugated NPs did not display any shift in fluorescence (Additional file 1: Figure S1A). NPs without the linking reagent but incubated with TAB004, or FITC anti-mouse IgG1, or both also served as controls and as expected did not show any shift in fluorescence signal. This suggests that the thioester linker was successful in conjugating TAB004 to the NPs.

We compared the internalization of unconjugated NPs to TAB004 conjugated NPs (T-NPs) in MUC1 high BxPC3.MUC1 versus MUC1 low BxPC3.Neo cells.

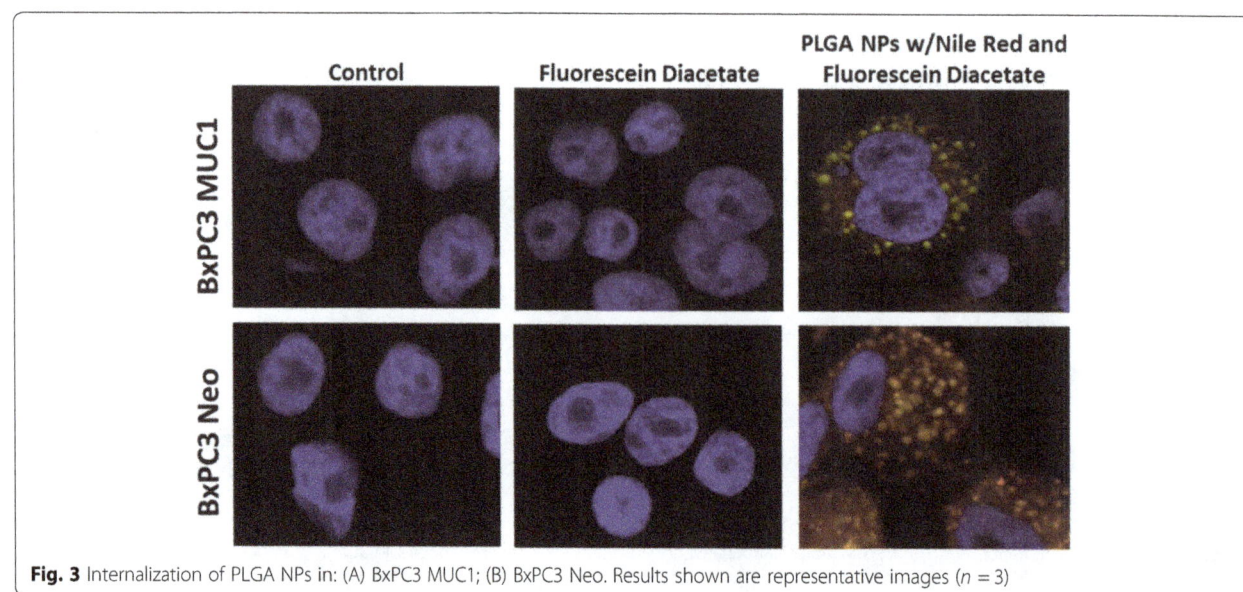

Fig. 3 Internalization of PLGA NPs in: (A) BxPC3 MUC1; (B) BxPC3 Neo. Results shown are representative images (*n* = 3)

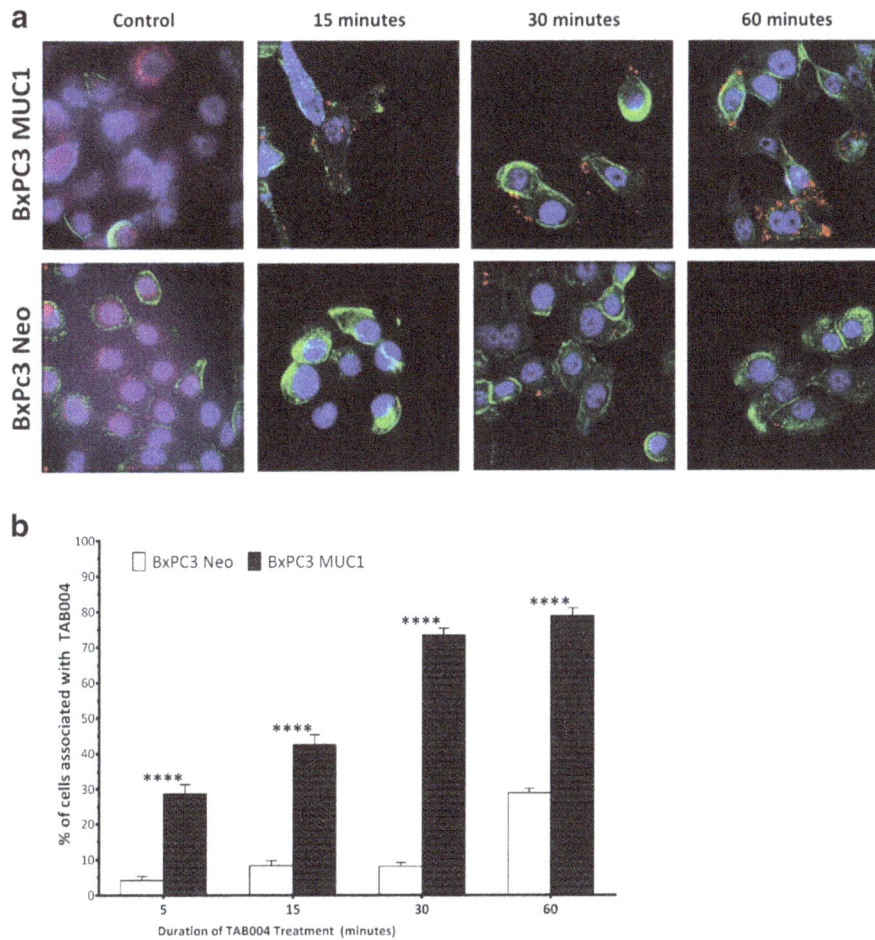

Fig. 4 Specificity and internalization of TAB004 in BxPC3 MUC1 and Neo: (**a**) representative images cells treated with TAB004 conjugated to pHRodo red (*n* = 3); (**b**) quantification of images determine by the number of cells associated with TAB004 divided by total number of cells. Data shown is mean ± SEM (*n* = 3) and determine by two-way ANOVA and Bonferroni's post-hoc test, *p < 0.05, **p < 0.01, ***p < 0.001, ****p < 0.0001

BxPC3.MUC1 and BxPC3.Neo cells were treated with FDA loaded NPs or T-NPs and fluorescence signal quantified over time (Fig. 5). There was no significant increase in fluorescence between T-NPs and NPs in the MUC1-low BxPC3.Neo cells (Fig. 5c). However, a significant increase in fluorescence was detected in BxPC3. MUC1 cells treated with T-NPs compared to when treated with NPs. This significant increase in fluorescence was observed at 60 and 90 min post treatment. The data indicates that linking TAB004 to the NPs was highly effective in longer term retention of the NPs within the MUC1-high cells compared to NPs alone and that this retention was antigen specific.

Therefore, we next determined the cytotoxicity of PTX loaded T-NPs compared to PTX loaded NPs in the same cells (BxPC3.Neo and BxPC3.MUC1) as well as in a panel of other human PDA cell lines with varying levels of MUC1 expression and sensitivity to PTX (Fig. 6). The comparison we were interested in was between the treatment groups (NP and T-NPs) and not necessarily

between the various cell lines. We selected a single dose of PTX for each cell line where at least 90% of cells remained viable post PTX treatment (~IC$_{10}$). We determined if there was any added cytotoxic effect of NPs or T-NPs loaded with PTX at the same concentration as the PTX alone. There was no difference in viability between PTX, NP-PTX or T-NP-PTX treated BxPC3. Neo cells (Fig. 6). This was expected based on Fig. 5c where no difference in internalization and retention was observed in BxPC3.Neo cells between NPs and T-NPs. On the other hand, in MUC1-expressing BxPC3 MUC1, MiaPaca2, and HPAC cells, we observed a significant decrease in cell viability between NP-PTX versus T-NP-PTX at a single dose (Fig. 6). This decrease was not noted in HPAF-II cell even though these cells express high levels of MUC1 (Fig. 6). The reasons for the lack of responsiveness to T-NPs in HPAF-II cells are not currently known. Although the effect of T-NPs versus NPs is modest, it is highly significant because of PDA's high resistance to chemotherapy.

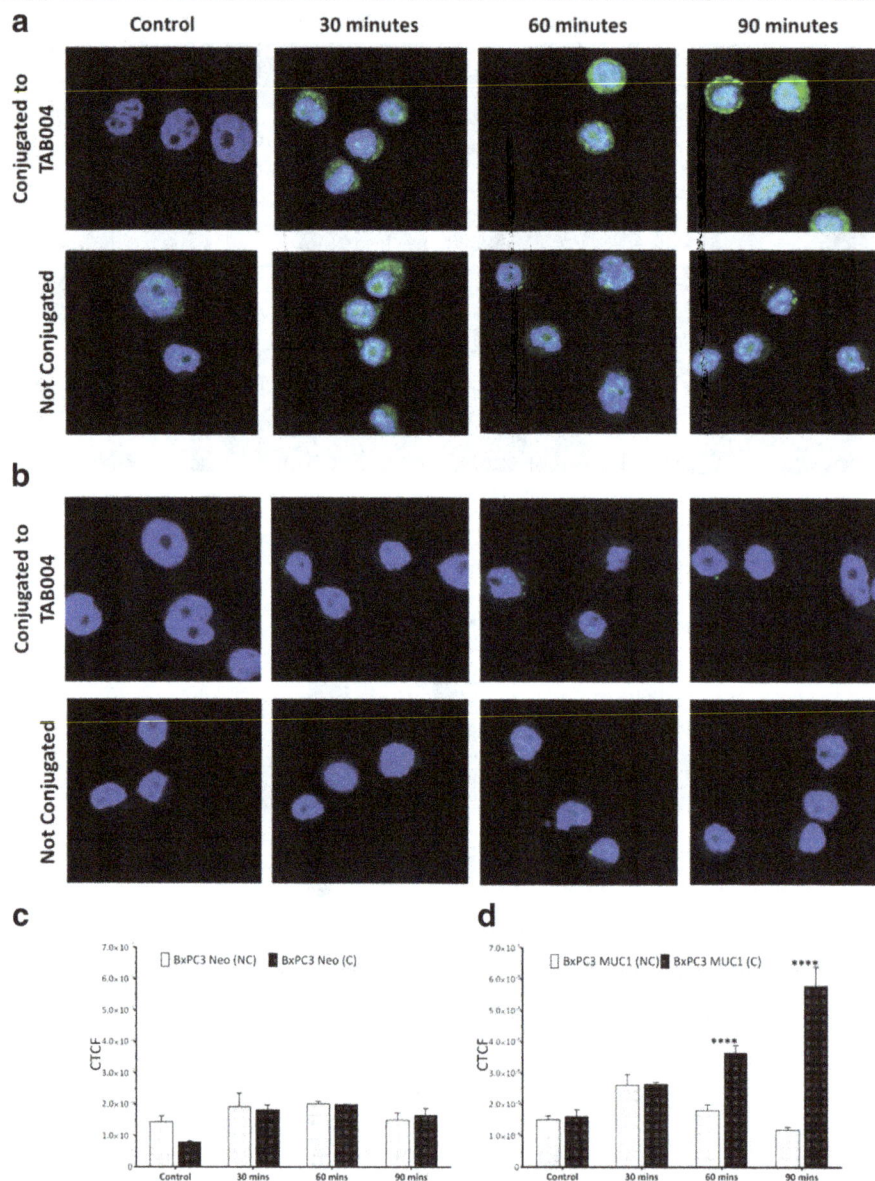

Fig. 5 Internalization of TAB004 conjugated NPs loaded with fluorescein diacetate (FDA): (**a**) representative images of BxPC3 MUC 1 ($n = 3$) treated with T-NPs; (**b**) representative images of BxPC3 Neo ($n = 3$) treated with T-NPs; (**c**) and (**d**) quantification of fluorescence using Image J to determine corrected total cell fluorescence (CTCF). Data shown is mean ± SEM ($n = 3$) and determined by a one-sided t-test, *$p < 0.05$, **$p < 0.01$, ***$p < 0.001$, ****$p < 0.0001$

TAB004 accumulates at the tumor site and its conjugation to PLGA NPs appears to increase their accumulation in an Orthotopic PDA tumor model

We demonstrated the specificity of TAB004 in vitro, but the same needed to be determined in vivo. C57BL/6 immune competent mice bearing murine syngeneic orthotopic KCM tumors [35] were injected intraperitoneally with TAB004 conjugated with ICG and imaged 24 h post injection. The KCM cells stably expressed the luciferase gene and thus bioluminescent tumors could be visualized by IVIS post luciferin injection. TAB004 localizes and persists specifically at the tumor site 24 h later (Fig. 7a-d). Images of

4 representative mice are shown. It is clear that the TAB004-ICG localizes only to the bioluminescent pancreatic tumors. The fluorescent radiant efficiency values for region of interests (ROIs) around the tumor site were acquired for TAB004-ICG injected mice and displayed significant increase over tumor bearing control mice that were not injected with TAB004-ICG (Fig. 7e).

Next, we tested ICG loaded NPs and ICG loaded T-NPs in mice bearing the same KCM bioluminescent orthotopic tumors to determine if TAB004 can increase the accumulation of NPs at the tumor site (Additional file 2: Figure S2). ICG loaded NPs appear to clear from the mouse between

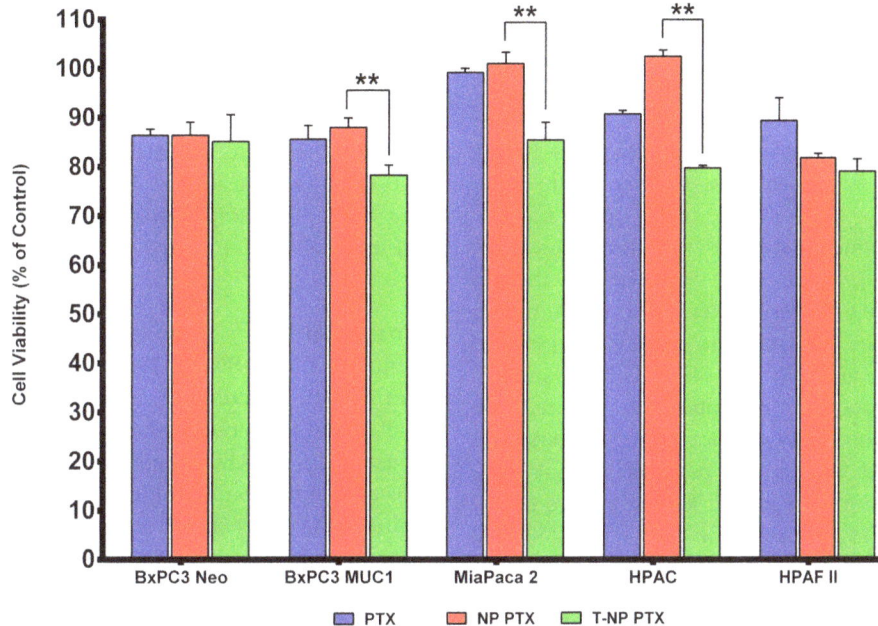

Fig. 6 Cell viability of PDA cell lines treated with PTX, PTX loaded NPs and PTX loaded TAB004 conjugated NPs. Concentration of PTX is 3.05×10^{-3} µg/ml. Data shown is mean ± SEM ($n = 3$) and determine by a one-sided t-test comparing treatment groups at each concentration, $*p < 0.05$, $**p < 0.01$, $***p < 0.001$, $****p < 0.000$

24 and 48 h post injection (Additional file 2: Figure S2), similar to the biodistribution profile of ICG loaded NPs injected in non-tumor bearing mice (data not shown). However, ICG loaded T-NPs appeared to accumulate and persist at the tumor site 24 and 48 h post injection (Additional file 2: Figure S2B). Ex vivo images of the tumor and liver of the mice were taken 48 h post injection and ICG loaded T-NPs seem to accumulate and persist in

the tumor while ICG load NPs cannot be detected in the tumor post 48 h. We noted that the fluorescence in the liver was identical for ICG loaded T-NPs and ICG loaded NPs (Additional file 2: Figure S2C) suggesting that the tumor localization is extremely high for T-NPs versus NPs. Thus, TAB004 conjugated NPs may be developed as a potential platform for targeted delivery of not only PTX, but other drugs and imaging agents directly to the

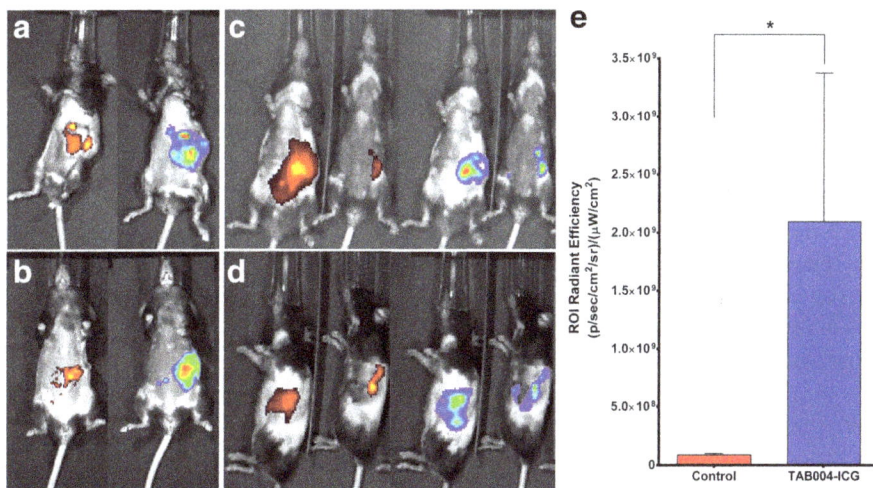

Fig. 7 In vivo imaging of TAB004-ICG in orthotopically injected bioluminescent tumor bearing mice (ICG - red/yellow, tumor (luciferase-expressing) – rainbow, $n = 4$): (**a**) mouse 1; (**b**) mouse 2; (**c**) mouse 3 and 4 ventral view; (**d**) mouse 3 and 4 side view; (**e**) quantification of fluorescent radiant efficiency values in TAB004-ICG injected and control mice, $*p < 0.05$

pancreatic tumor while reducing toxicity to other major organs. Future studies will evaluate the in vivo anti-tumor efficacy in several models of PDA.

Discussion

The ability to target drug-loaded nanoparticles to the tumor site would greatly enhance efficacy of the drug and reduce toxicity. PLGA is one of the most effective biodegradable polymers used to construct polymeric nanoparticles (NPs). It has been approved by the US FDA for use in drug delivery systems due to controlled and sustained- release properties, low toxicity, and biocompatibility with tissue and cells [42–44]. PEG-functionalized PLGA NPs are especially desirable, as pegylated-NP platforms have demonstrated significantly reduced systemic clearance compared with similar particles without PEG. This design parameter is important for the passive targeting of nanocarrier to tumor by the EPR effects [45]. To enhance tumor-specific targeting, in this study, we aimed to investigate PEG-functionalized PLGA NPs conjugated to monoclonal antibody TAB004. TAB004 specifically recognizes the hypoglycosylated tumor form of MUC1 [32, 46, 47] while sparing recognition of MUC1 on normal epithelial cells. Over 80% of PDA expresses this tumor form of MUC1 and is an established target for immunotherapy [48, 49]. In Fig. 4, we show that TAB004 specifically internalizes in the BxPC3.MUC1 ells but not in BxPC3.Neo cells. Further, we showed that compared to the unconjugated NPs, TAB004 conjugated NPs had significantly enhanced and prolonged cellular accumulation in the BxPC3.MUC1 versus BxPC3.Neo cells confirming antigen specific targeted internalization (Fig. 5). This enhanced cellular internalization and accumulation of T-NPs over NPs is most likely due to the specific binding of TAB004 to tumor form of MUC1 expressed on BxPC3. MUC1 cells thus enabling the NPs to readily internalize through a process of macropinocytosis [50]. Although modest, PTX-loaded T-NPs showed significantly enhanced cytotoxicity (Fig. 6) in an antigen specific manner. The modest enhancement of cytotoxicity may be attributed to the limited time (1.5 h) of exposure of cells to the drug. Longer incubation with the nanoparticles caused degradation of the NPs, which then interfered with the OD values in the survival assay. It is well established that the antitumor effect of PTX results from its intracellular accumulation over time [51]. In vivo in an immune compromised mouse model, we observed specific localization and accumulation of TAB004 only to the orthotropic BxPC3.MUC1 tumors generated in the pancreas (Fig. 7) but not in MUC1-negative tumors or in normal epithelial organs [34]. In a pilot in vivo experiment using immune competent mice, we showed that compared to ICG-NPs, TAB004 conjugated ICG-NPs accumulated in the KCM tumor while unconjugated ICG-NPs failed to accumulate

in the tumor (Additional file 2: Figure S2). Thus, we believe that the modest cytotoxic advantage observed in vitro will be significantly enhanced in vivo. Future studies will evaluate the in vivo efficacy of various drug loaded TAB004-NPs in several PDA models. Taken together the data validates the tumor specificity of TAB004 and that loaded NPs conjugated to TAB004 may be a promising nanocarrier for targeted therapy and imaging of PDA.

Conclusion

Conjugation of NPs to TAB004 greatly enhanced the internalization, retention, and targeting ability of NPs in vitro and in vivo in orthotopic models of human and mouse PDA. TAB004 conjugated PTX loaded NPs showed modest but significant increase in cytotoxicity against PDA cells in vitro. The anti-tumor efficacy of chemotherapeutic drugs in vivo will need to be investigated using this delivery platform.

Additional files

Additional file 1: Figure S1. Confirmation of TAB004 conjugation to PLGA NPs with FACS. Blank NPs were treated with: (A) control (red), TAB004 (blue), anti-mouse IgG$_1$ FITC (green), and both TAB004 and anti-mouse IgG$_1$ FITC (orange/yellow); (B) control (red), NHS Ester linking reagent (blue), and NHS Ester linking reagent,TAB004, and anti-mouse IgG$_1$ FITC (green).

Additional file 2: Figure S2. In vivo imaging of ICG loaded NPs and ICG loaded T-NPs orthotopically injected bioluminescent tumor bearing mice (ICG - red/yellow, tumor – rainbow, $n = 3$): (A) ICG loaded NPs injected into tumor bearing mouse; (B) ICG loaded T-NPs injected into tumor bearing mouse; (C) ex vivo imaging of liver and tumor from (A) and (B).

Abbreviations
ACN: Acetonitrile; CDI: 1,1'-carbonyldiimidazole; DAP: 1,3-diaminopropane; DCM: Dry methylene chloride; DMSO: Dimethyl sulfoxide; EE: Encapsulation efficiency; EPR: Enhanced permeability and retention effect; FACS: Fluorescence-activated cell sorting; FBS: Fetal bovine serum; FDA: Fluorescein diacetate; FOLFIRINOX: 5-fluorouracil, oxaliplatin, irinotecan, and leucovorin; HD: Hydrodyamic diameter; ICG: Indocyanine green; IVIS: In vivo imaging system; MTT: 3-(4,5-dimethyathiazol-2-yl)-2,5diphenyltetrazolium bromide; MUC1: Mucin-1; NPs: Nanoparticles; NR: Nile Red; OD: Optical density; PBS: Phosphate-buffered salin; PCL: Polycaprolactone; PDA: Pancreatic ductal adenocarcinoma; PDI: Polydispersity index; PEG: Polyethylene glycol; PLGA: Poly(lactic-co-glycolic acid); PTX: Paclitaxel; PVA: Poly(vinyl alchohol); SEM: Scanning electron microscopy; THF: Tetrahydrofuran (oxolane); tMUC1: Tumor-associated MUC1; T-NPs: TAB004 conjugated to PLGA NPs; ZP: Zeta potential

Acknowledgements
This work was supported by the CPCP Levine UNCC Pancreatic Cancer Pilot Project, National Institutes of Health, National Cancer Institute (NIH-NIC Grant RO1 CA118944-01A1), UNC Charlotte Faculty Research Grant, and UNC Charlotte, The Williams States Lee College of Engineering, Center for Biomedical Engineering and Science IVIS Imaging System Award. The authors thank Laura J. Moore and the UNC Charlotte's Vivarium staff, A. Perez and H. Gordils, for their support in caring for the animals. We also thank OncoTAb, Inc., for supplying TAB004 that was used in this research, and NuChemie LLC for the labeling reagents used in this study.

Funding

CPCP Levine UNCC Pancreatic Cancer Pilot Project, National Institutes of Health, National Cancer Institute (NIH-NIC Grant RO1 CA118944-01A1), UNC Charlotte Faculty Research Grant, and UNC Charlotte, The Williams States Lee College of Engineering, Center for Biomedical Engineering and Science IVIS Imaging System Award.

Authors' contributions

The manuscript was written through contributions of all authors. All authors have given approval to the final version of the manuscript. SW designed and performed all biological assays and authored this manuscript. AJF provided the schema for NP assembly and along with, CBG, JDO and ABF constructed and characterized the PLGA NPs. KRG, BCA, and MY assisted with certain biological assays. RZ contributed to in vitro experimental design. CDW provided in vivo experimental design and performed surgeries on the mice.

Competing interests

The authors declare the following competing interests:
PM is co-founder and Chief Scientific Officer of OncoTab, Inc.

Author details

[1]Department of Biological Sciences, University of North Carolina at Charlotte, Charlotte, NC 28223, USA. [2]Department of Chemistry, University of North Carolina at Charlotte, Charlotte, NC 28223, USA. [3]Department of Animal Laboratory Resources, University of North Carolina at Charlotte, Charlotte, NC 28223, USA.

References

1. Siegel RL, Miller KD, Jemal A. Cancer statistics, 2015. CA Cancer J Clin. 2015;65(1):5–29.
2. Winter JM, et al. Survival after resection of pancreatic adenocarcinoma: results from a single institution over three decades. Ann Surg Oncol. 2012;19(1):169–75.
3. Fokas E, et al. Pancreatic ductal adenocarcinoma: from genetics to biology to radiobiology to oncoimmunology and all the way back to the clinic. Biochim Biophys Acta. 2015;1855(1):61–82.
4. Erkan M, et al. The role of stroma in pancreatic cancer: diagnostic and therapeutic implications. Nat Rev Gastroenterol Hepatol. 2012;9(8):454–67.
5. Durymanov MO, Rosenkranz AA, Sobolev AS. Current approaches for improving Intratumoral accumulation and distribution of nanomedicines. Theranostics. 2015;5(9):1007–20.
6. Du JZ, et al. Tumor extracellular acidity-activated nanoparticles as drug delivery systems for enhanced cancer therapy. Biotechnol Adv. 2014;32(4):789–803.
7. Muthu MS, et al. Nanotheranostics - application and further development of nanomedicine strategies for advanced theranostics. Theranostics. 2014;4(6):660–77.
8. Yang T, et al. Anti-tumor efficiency of lipid-coated cisplatin nanoparticles co-loaded with MicroRNA-375. Theranostics. 2016;6(1):142–54.
9. Xing L, et al. Ultrasound-mediated microbubble destruction (UMMD) facilitates the delivery of CA19-9 targeted and paclitaxel loaded mPEG-PLGA-PLL nanoparticles in pancreatic Cancer. Theranostics. 2016;6(10):1573–87.
10. Bose RJ, Lee SH, Park H. Lipid-based surface engineering of PLGA nanoparticles for drug and gene delivery applications. Biomater Res. 2016;20:34.
11. Bertrand N, et al. Cancer nanotechnology: the impact of passive and active targeting in the era of modern cancer biology. Adv Drug Deliv Rev. 2014;66:2–25.
12. Dong X, Mumper RJ. Nanomedicinal strategies to treat multidrug-resistant tumors: current progress. Nanomedicine. 2010;5(4):597–615.
13. Hollis CP, et al. Biodistribution and bioimaging studies of hybrid paclitaxel nanocrystals: lessons learned of the EPR effect and image-guided drug delivery. J Control Release. 2013;172(1):12–21.
14. Okamura Y, et al. Prolonged hemostatic ability of polyethylene glycol-modified polymerized albumin particles carrying fibrinogen gamma-chain dodecapeptide. Transfusion. 2007;47(7):1254–62.
15. Moghimi SM, Hunter AC, Murray JC. Long-circulating and target-specific nanoparticles: theory to practice. Pharmacol Rev. 2001;53(2):283–318.
16. Danhier F, et al. PLGA-based nanoparticles: an overview of biomedical applications. J Control Release. 2012;161(2):505–22.
17. Dreau D, et al. Mucin-1-antibody-conjugated mesoporous silica nanoparticles for selective breast Cancer detection in a Mucin-1 transgenic murine mouse model. J Biomed Nanotechnol. 2016;12(12):2172–84.
18. Cooper AB, et al. Does the use of neoadjuvant therapy for pancreatic adenocarcinoma increase postoperative morbidity and mortality rates? J Gastrointest Surg. 2015;19(1):80–6. discussion 86-7
19. Von Hoff DD, Goldstein D, Renschler MF. Albumin-bound paclitaxel plus gemcitabine in pancreatic cancer. N Engl J Med. 2014;370(5):479–80.
20. Von Hoff DD, et al. Gemcitabine plus nab-paclitaxel is an active regimen in patients with advanced pancreatic cancer: a phase I/II trial. J Clin Oncol. 2011;29(34):4548–54.
21. Frese KK, et al. Nab-paclitaxel potentiates gemcitabine activity by reducing cytidine deaminase levels in a mouse model of pancreatic cancer. Cancer Discov. 2012;2(3):260–9.
22. He L, Orr GA, Horwitz SB. Novel molecules that interact with microtubules and have functional activity similar to Taxol. Drug Discov Today. 2001;6(22):1153–64.
23. Herbst RS, Khuri FR. Mode of action of docetaxel - a basis for combination with novel anticancer agents. Cancer Treat Rev. 2003;29(5):407–15.
24. Kolishetti N, et al. Engineering of self-assembled nanoparticle platform for precisely controlled combination drug therapy. Proc Natl Acad Sci U S A. 2010;107(42):17939–44.
25. Hattrup CL, Gendler SJ. Structure and function of the cell surface (tethered) mucins. Annu Rev Physiol. 2008;70:431–57.
26. Gendler SJ. MUC1, the renaissance molecule. J Mammary Gland Biol Neoplasia. 2001;6(3):339–53.
27. Yolken RH, et al. Human milk mucin inhibits rotavirus replication and prevents experimental gastroenteritis. J Clin Invest. 1992;90(5):1984–91.
28. Burdick MD, et al. Oligosaccharides expressed on MUC1 produced by pancreatic and colon tumor cell lines. J Biol Chem. 1997;272(39):24198–202.
29. Patton S, Gendler SJ, Spicer AP. The epithelial mucin, MUC1, of milk, mammary gland and other tissues. Biochim Biophys Acta. 1995;1241(3):407–23.
30. Roy LD, et al. MUC1 enhances invasiveness of pancreatic cancer cells by inducing epithelial to mesenchymal transition. Oncogene. 2011;30(12):1449–59.
31. Cheever MA, et al. The prioritization of Cancer antigens: a National Cancer Institute pilot project for the acceleration of translational research. Clin Cancer Res. 2009;15(17):5323–37.
32. Curry JM, et al. The use of a novel MUC1 antibody to identify cancer stem cells and circulating MUC1 in mice and patients with pancreatic cancer. J Surg Oncol. 2013;107(7):713–22.
33. Moore LJ, et al. Antibody-guided in vivo imaging for early detection of mammary gland tumors. Transl Oncol. 2016;9(4):295–305.
34. Wu ST, et al. Early detection of pancreatic cancer in mouse models using a novel antibody, TAB004. PLoS One. 2018;13(2):e0193260.
35. Besmer DM, et al. Pancreatic ductal adenocarcinoma mice lacking mucin 1 have a profound defect in tumor growth and metastasis. Cancer Res. 2011;71(13):4432–42.
36. Sarin VK, et al. Quantitative monitoring of solid-phase peptide synthesis by the ninhydrin reaction. Anal Biochem. 1981;117(1):147–57.
37. Farokhzad OC, et al. Targeted nanoparticle-aptamer bioconjugates for cancer chemotherapy in vivo. Proc Natl Acad Sci U S A. 2006;103(16):6315–20.
38. Zheng C, et al. Indocyanine green-loaded biodegradable tumor targeting nanoprobes for in vitro and in vivo imaging. Biomaterials. 2012;33(22):5603–9.
39. Amin ML, Kim D, Kim S. Development of hematin conjugated PLGA nanoparticle for selective cancer targeting. Eur J Pharm Sci. 2016;91:138–43.
40. Kamphorst JJ, et al. Human pancreatic cancer tumors are nutrient poor and tumor cells actively scavenge extracellular protein. Cancer Res. 2015;75(3):544–53.
41. Sousa CM, Kimmelman AC. The complex landscape of pancreatic cancer metabolism. Carcinogenesis. 2014;35(7):1441–50.

42. Mahapatro A, Singh DK. Biodegradable nanoparticles are excellent vehicle for site directed in-vivo delivery of drugs and vaccines. J Nanobiotechnology. 2011;9:55.

43. Nobs L, et al. Poly(lactic acid) nanoparticles labeled with biologically active Neutravidin for active targeting. Eur J Pharm Biopharm. 2004;58(3):483–90.

44. Sadat Tabatabaei Mirakabad F, et al. PLGA-based nanoparticles as cancer drug delivery systems. Asian Pac J Cancer Prev. 2014;15(2):517–35.

45. Guo J, et al. Aptamer-functionalized PEG-PLGA nanoparticles for enhanced anti-glioma drug delivery. Biomaterials. 2011;32(31):8010–20.

46. Roy LD, et al. A tumor specific antibody to aid breast cancer screening in women with dense breast tissue. Genes Cancer. 2017;8(3-4):536–49.

47. Mukherjee P. Tumor specific antibodies and uses therefor. 2016, Google Patents.

48. Zhou R, et al. A novel association of neuropilin-1 and MUC1 in pancreatic ductal adenocarcinoma: role in induction of VEGF signaling and angiogenesis. Oncogene. 2016;35(43):5608–18.

49. Steentoft C, et al. Glycan-directed car-t cells. Glycobiology. 2018; https://doi.org/10.1093/glycob/cwy00.

50. Hisatsune A, et al. Internalization of MUC1 by anti-MUC1 antibody from cell membrane through the macropinocytotic pathway. Biochem Biophys Res Commun. 2009;388(4):677–82.

51. Fonseca C, Simões S, Gaspar R. Paclitaxel-loaded PLGA nanoparticles: preparation, physicochemical characterization and in vitro anti-tumoral activity. J Control Release. 2002;83(2):273–86.

A phase II study to evaluate LY2603618 in combination with gemcitabine in pancreatic cancer patients

Berta Laquente[1], Jose Lopez-Martin[2], Donald Richards[3], Gerald Illerhaus[4], David Z. Chang[5], George Kim[6], Philip Stella[7], Dirk Richel[8], Cezary Szcylik[9], Stefano Cascinu[10], G. L. Frassineti[11], Tudor Ciuleanu[12], Karla Hurt[13], Scott Hynes[13], Ji Lin[13], Aimee Bence Lin[13], Daniel Von Hoff[14] and Emiliano Calvo[15*]

Abstract

Background: The aim of this study was to determine whether checkpoint kinase 1 inihibitor (CHK1), LY2603618, and gemcitabine prolong overall survival (OS) compared to gemcitabine alone in patients with unresectable pancreatic cancer.

Methods: Patients with Stage II-IV locally advanced or metastatic pancreatic cancer were randomized (2:1) to either 230 mg of LY2603618/1000 mg/m^2 gemcitabine combined or 1000 mg/m^2 gemcitabine alone. OS was assessed using both a Bayesian augment control model and traditional frequentist analysis for inference. Progression-free survival (PFS), overall response rate (ORR), duration of response, pharmacokinetics (PK), and safety (Common Terminology Criteria for Adverse Events [AEs] v 3.0) were also evaluated.

Results: Ninety-nine patients ($n = 65$, LY2603618/gemcitabine; $n = 34$, gemcitabine) were randomized (intent-to-treat population). The median OS (months) was 7.8 (range, 0.3–18.9) with LY2603618/gemcitabine and 8.3 (range, 0.8-19.1+) with gemcitabine. Similarly, in a Bayesian analysis, the study was not positive since the posterior probability that LY2603618/gemcitabine was superior to gemcitabine in improving OS was 0.3, which did not exceed the prespecified threshold of 0.8. No significant improvements in PFS, ORR, or duration of response were observed. Drug-related treatment-emergent AEs in both arms included nausea, thrombocytopenia, fatigue, and neutropenia. The severity of AEs with LY2603618/gemcitabine was comparable to gemcitabine. The LY2603618 exposure targets (AUC$_{(0-\infty)}$ $\geq$21,000 ng hr/mL and C$_{max}$ $\geq$2000 ng/mL) predicted for maximum pharmacodynamic response were achieved after 230 mg of LY2603618.

Conclusions: LY2603618/gemcitabine was not superior to gemcitabine for the treatment of patients with pancreatic cancer.

Keywords: CHK1, cancer, gemcitabine, phase II, LY2603618

* Correspondence: emiliano.calvo@start.stoh.com
[15]START Madrid-CIOCC, Centro Integral Oncológico Clara Campal, Medical Oncology Division, Hospital Universitario Madrid Norte Sanchinarro, Calle Oña, 10, 28050 Madrid, Spain
Full list of author information is available at the end of the article

Background

Pancreatic cancer is the fourth leading cause of cancer-related deaths in the United States [1]. Current therapeutic strategies for pancreatic cancer have a modest impact on disease course and prognosis [2]. The 5-year survial rate remains low (<5%) [3]. Until recently, gemcitabine was the standard of care for patients with advanced/metastatic pancreatic cancer. FOLFIRINOX (oxaliplatin, irinotecan, leucovorin, and 5-FU) and gemcitabine plus *nab*-paclitaxel (Abraxane®) are novel therapeutic regimens demonstrating survival advantages in patients with advanced pancreatic cancer [4–8]. Although these recent advances are promising, there is still a need for novel therapeutic targets to further improve and sustain clinical response in pancreatic cancer patients.

Checkpoint kinase 1 (CHK1) is a protein kinase involved in the DNA damage response. Activation of CHK1 initiates cell cycle arrest allowing for DNA repair and replication. Inhibition of CHK1 allows cells to enter mitosis without DNA repair, eventually leading to apoptosis [9]. Furthermore, inhibition of CHK1 sensitizes tumor cells to DNA-damaging agents making CHK1 a unique target for cancer therapy. Azorsa and colleagues recently identified CHK1 as a therapeutic target for sensitizing pancreatic cancer cells to gemcitabine therapy using a synthetic lethal RNAi screening approach [10].

LY2603618, a selective CHK1 inhibitor, enhances the activity of cytotoxic chemotherapy agents, including gemcitabine, in in vitro and in vivo nonclinical efficacy studies [11, 12]. Phase I of this Phase I/II study determined the recommended Phase II dose to be 230 mg [13]. Phase II, as presented here, determined if the overall survival (OS) in patients with Stage II-IV unresectable pancreatic cancer who were administered LY2603618 and gemcitabine exceeded the OS of patients treated with gemcitabine alone.

Methods

Study objectives

The primary objective of this Phase II study was to compare OS with LY2603618/gemcitabine to gemcitabine alone in patients with Stage II-IV unresectable pancreatic cancer. Secondary objectives included characterizing the safety and toxicity profile of LY2603618/gemcitabine and gemcitabine; estimating progression-free survival (PFS), duration of response, and change in tumor size; assessing response rates; evaluating the pharmacokinetics (PK) of LY2603618; investigating biomarker responses; and performing an exploratory assessment of Fridericia's heart rate-corrected QT interval (QTcF).

Patients

Adult patients who had given informed consent had adequate hematological, liver, and renal functions; histological or cytological evidence of a diagnosis of Stage II or III adenocarcinoma of the pancreas not amenable to resection with curative intent or Stage IV disease; and an Eastern Cooperative Oncology Group performance status (ECOG PS) 0–2. Patients with previous radical surgery for pancreatic cancer were eligible after progression was documented. Exclusion criteria included known hypersensitivity to gemcitabine; females who were pregnant or lactating; prior radiotherapy involving >25% of marrow-producing area; and treatment with any non-approved drug within 30 days of enrollment. Patients may have received previous adjuvant treatment with gemcitabine.

Study design and treatment plan

Prior to enrollment, the study protocol, patient informed consent, and any other written study documentation were approved by an ethics committee. This trial was conducted in accordance with the Declaration of Helsinki and the Good Clinical Practice Guidelines of the International Conference on Harmonization. Phase II of this open-label, multicenter, randomized, 2-arm, Phase I/II trial was conducted in patients with locally advanced or metastatic pancreatic cancer. Patients were randomized (2:1) to either LY2603618/gemcitabine or gemcitabine. Gemcitabine (1000 mg/m^2) was given as a 30-min infusion on days 1, 8, and 15 of a 28-day cycle. LY2603618 (230 mg) was administered as a 1-h infusion ~24 h after administration of gemcitabine. Patients continued on treatment until disease progression, unacceptable toxicity, or patient unwillingness to participate.

Statistical analysis

The primary objective was a comparison of OS on the intent-to-treat (ITT) population using a Bayesian posterior probability for the superiority of the combination over gemcitabine. Ninety-nine patients were planned, resulting in a frequentist design with ~60% power (1-sided, 0.2 type I error, no interim analysis) to detect a 2-month improvement in survival (7 months gemcitabine vs. 9 months LY2603618/gemcitabine). The Bayesian model [14, 15] incorporated historical gemcitabine data [16, 17] with prospective gemcitabine data to compare survival between the treatment arms and increase the power compared to the frequentist design. LY2603618 and gemcitabine would be considered superior to gemcitabine if the posterior probability of superiority exceeded 0.8. Simulation resulted in estimated power of 0.76 and type I error rate of 0.15. In addition to the Bayesian model, frequentist analysis of OS was also performed as a sensitivity analysis. The definition of secondary efficacy variables was consistent with standard conventions per RECIST (v 1.1) [18].

Exploratory analyses included: change from baseline in tumor size and carbohydrate antigen 19–9 (CA19-9) levels, and changes in QTcF from electrocardiograms (ECG) obtained at baseline and after LY2603618 administration on days 2 and 16 during cycle one.

Safety

All patients who received at least one dose of study drug were evaluated for safety and toxicity. AE severity was graded using the Common Terminology Criteria for AEs (CTCAE) v 3.0.

Pharmacokinetic/pharmacodynamic analysis

LY2603618 concentrations were quantified using a validated high-pressure liquid chromatography/mass spectrometry/mass spectrometry method. Whole blood samples were collected following the LY2603618 infusion on days 2 and 16 of cycle 1 before the start (<10 min) of infusion; immediately prior to the end of infusion (<5 min); and at 1, 3, and 24 h after the end of infusion. LY2603618 PK parameters were computed from the plasma concentration versus time data by standard noncompartmental analyses (Phoenix WinNonlin version 6.3, Pharsight, A Certara Company®; Princeton, NJ, USA). The PK parameters of maximum plasma concentration (C_{max}) and area under the plasma concentration time-curve from time 0 to the time of the last measurable plasma concentration ($AUC_{[0\text{-}tlast]}$) or infinity ($AUC_{[0\text{-}\infty]}$) on days 2 and 16 of cycle one were calculated, as well as the terminal elimination half-life ($t_{1/2}$), volume of distribution at steady-state (V_{ss}), systemic clearance (CL), percentage of $AUC_{[0\text{-}\infty]}$ extrapolated ($\%AUC_{[tlast\text{-}\infty]}$), and the intra- and intercycle accumulation ratios (R_A).

Biomarker response

A nucleoside analog deoxyribonucleic acid (DNA) incorporation assay method measured the amount of gemcitabine incorporated into genomic DNA [19]. A sample for CA–19–9 analysis was collected at the start of each cycle.

Results

Patient disposition

Of the 107 enrolled patients, a total of 99 patients ($n = 65$, LY2603618/gemcitabine; $n = 34$, gemcitabine alone) were randomized and included in the ITT population. The first patient was enrolled on 26 February 2009. Patient demographics and disease characteristics at baseline are summarized in Table 1. The majority of the patient population (mean age, 64 years) presented with Stage IV disease (76.8%) and more than 90% had an ECOG PS 0–1 at study entry (Table 1). The primary reasons for study discontinuation in the LY2603618/gemcitabine arm and gemcitabine alone arm, respectively, included: progressive disease (70.8%; 61.8%), AE (12.3%; 17.6%), subject decision (4.6%; 14.7%), investigator decision (6.2%; 2.9%), death (4.6%; 2.9%), and protocol violation (1.5%; 0).

Table 1 Patient demographics and disease characteristics at baseline

Parameter	LY2603618/ gemcitabine	Gemcitabine
	($n = 65$)	($n = 34$)
Age, years		
Mean (SD)	64.3 (8.3)	64.4 (10.1)
Median	64.0	65.5
Range	47–83	39–90
Gender, n (%)		
Female	23 (35.4)	14 (41.2)
Male	42 (64.6)	20 (58.8)
Race, n (%)		
White	62 (95.4)	32 (94.1)
Black or African American	2 (3.1)	2 (5.9)
American Indian or Alaska Native	1 (1.5)	0
BSA at baseline (m^2)		
Mean (SD)	1.8 (0.2)	1.8 (0.2)
Median	1.8	1.7
Range	1.3–2.5	1.4–2.5
Disease stage, n (%)		
II	6 (9.2)	3 (8.8)
III	8 (12.3)	5 (14.7)
IV	50 (76.9)	26 (76.5)
Unknown	1 (1.5)	0
ECOG PS, n (%)		
0	28 (43.1)	14 (41.2)
1	31 (47.7)	17 (50)
2	6 (9.2)	3 (8.8)

BSA body mass index; *ECOG PS* Eastern Cooperative Oncology Group performance status; *LY2603618/gemcitabine* LY2603618 (230 mg flat dose) combined with gemcitabine 1000 mg/m^2; m^2 meters squared; *mg* milligrams; *n* number of patients; *SD* standard deviation

Clinical efficacy

The Bayesian model was applied to compare OS between treatments. The posterior probability of superiority of LY2603618/gemcitabine over gemcitabine alone was 0.33, which did not exceed the pre-specified threshold of 0.8. These findings were confirmed by the frequentist analysis. The median OS was 7.8 months (range, 0.3–18.9 months) for LY2603618/gemcitabine and 8.3 months (range, 0.8–19.1+ months) for gemcitabine alone (Fig. 1a).

Overall, LY2603618/gemcitabine was not statistically superior to gemcitabine alone when PFS, duration of response, ORR, and clinical benefit rate were assessed (Table 2). The median PFS was 3.5 months (range, 0–15.9 months) for LY2603618/gemcitabine and 5.6 months (range, 0–17.4 months) for gemcitabine (Table 2; Fig. 1b). No complete response (CR) was observed with either treatment. Although not statistically significant, a

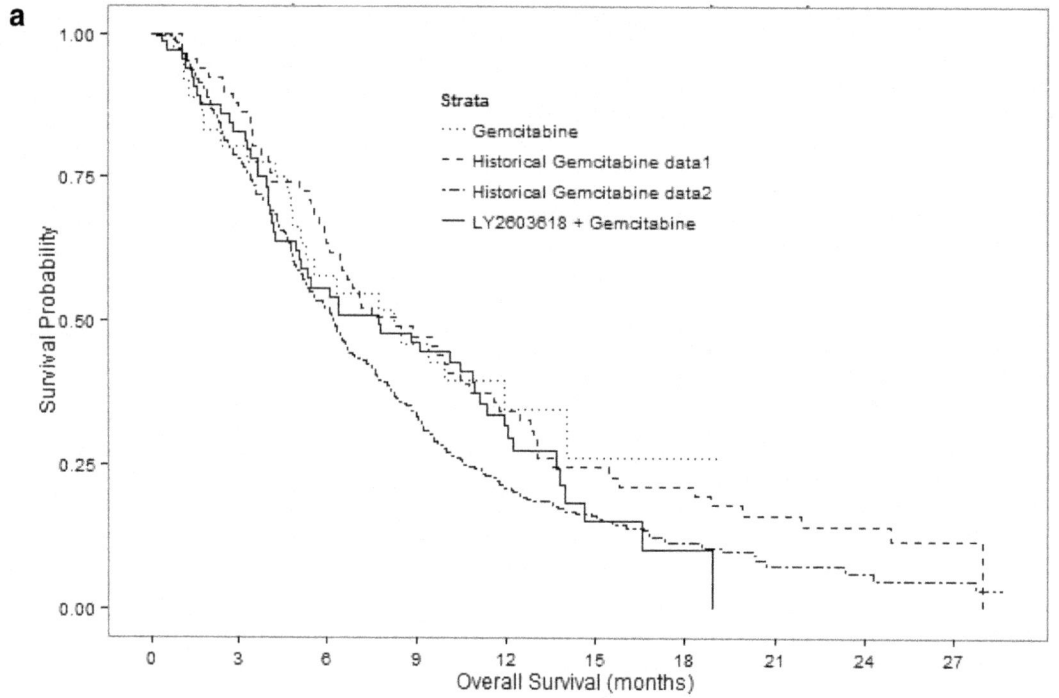

LY2603618 + Gemcitabine	68	52	35	29	15	5	1	0	0	0
Historical Gemcitabine data2	278	212	140	92	55	35	18	8	5	3
Historical Gemcitabine data1	66	58	41	29	21	15	13	9	6	2
Gemcitabine	39	29	20	15	7	2	1	0	0	0

Numbers at risk

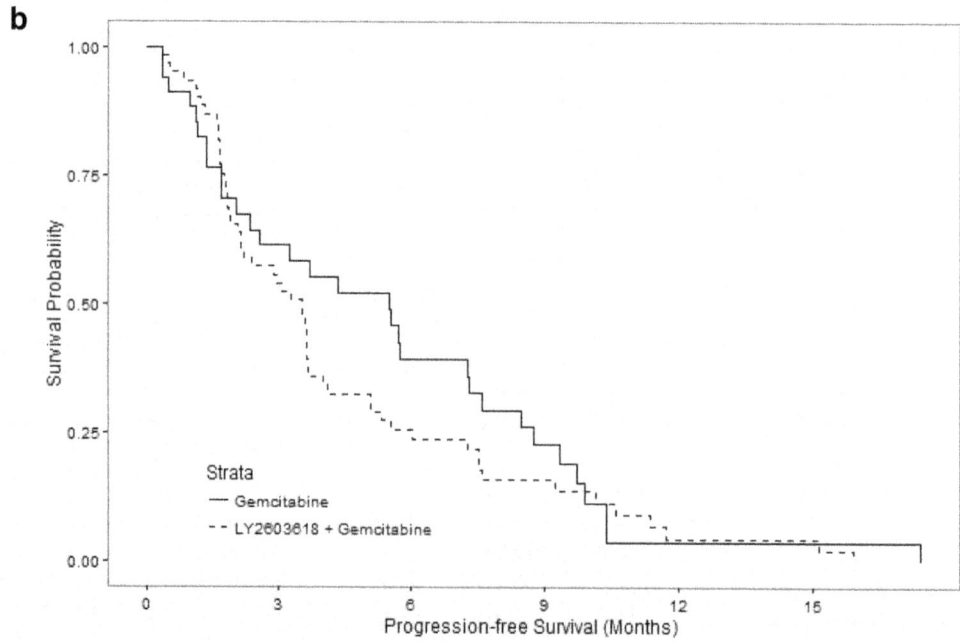

| LY2603618 + Gemcitabine | 68 | 33 | 14 | 7 | 2 | 2 |
| Gemcitabine | 39 | 20 | 12 | 7 | 1 | 1 |

Numbers at risk

Fig. 1 (See legend on next page.)

(See figure on previous page.)
Fig. 1 a Overall survival. Kaplan Meier survival curves of patients treated with LY2603618/gemcitabine combination therapy compared with historical gemcitabine studies. [[1]Jänne PA, Paz-Ares L, Oh Y, Eschbach C, Hirsh V, Enas N, Brail L, von Pawel J. Randomized, double-blind, phase II trial comparing gemcitabine-cisplatin plus the LTB4 antagonist LY293111 versus gemcitabine-cisplatin plus placebo in first-line non-small-cell lung cancer. J Thorac Oncol. 2014;9:126–31. [2]Oettle H, Richards D, Ramanathan RK, van Laethem JL, Peeters M, Fuchs M, Zimmerman A, John W, Von Hoff D, Arning M, Kindler HL. A phase III trial of pemetrexed plus gemcitabine versus gemcitabine in patients with unresectable or metastatic pancreatic cancer. Ann Oncol. 2005;16:1639–45.] **b** Progression-free survival. Kaplan Meier survival curves of patients treated with LY2603618/gemcitabine compared with gemcitabine monotherapy

numerically higher percentage of patients had a partial response (PR) in the LY2603618/gemcitabine arm (21.5%; 95% confidence intervals [CI], 12.3–33.5) than in the gemcitabine arm (8.8%; 95% CI, 1.9–23.7). No distinguishing baseline characteristics were noted among patients with a response. Due to the overlapping confidence intervals, the clinical significance of the difference in response rates is unknown. The clinical benefit rate was 55.4% (95% CI, 42.5–67.7) and 64.7% (95% CI, 46.5–80.3) in the LY2603618/gemcitabine and gemcitabine arms, respectively. No significant difference in the change in tumor size (the sum of target lesions, per RECIST) from baseline to 8 weeks was observed between treatments ($P = .6726$).

Safety

The median number of cycles completed was 2.0 (range, 0–16 cycles) for LY2603618/gemcitabine and 2.5 (range, 0–18 cycles) for gemcitabine. As shown in Table 3, study drug-related treatment-emergent AEs (TEAEs) were comparable between LY2603618/gemcitabine (89.2%) and gemcitabine (91.2%). The most frequently observed TEAEs in both arms were nausea, thrombocytopenia, fatigue, and neutropenia. Fewer patients experienced anemia with LY2603618/gemcitabine (13.8%) than with

gemcitabine (26.5%). In contrast, a higher incidence of vomiting, decreased appetite, and stomatitis was observed for LY2603618/gemcitabine than for gemcitabine. For each arm, neutropenia and thrombocytopenia were the most common grade 3/4 TEAEs possibly related to treatment, in addition to anemia, which was also common to gemcitabine (Table 4). Serious adverse events (SAE) related to study treatment were reported among 13.8% and 23.5% of patients in the LY2603618/gemcitabine and gemcitabine arms, respectively.

Fourteen patients ($n = 8$, LY2603618/gemcitabine; $n = 6$, gemcitabine) discontinued the study due to AEs. Of the eight patients who discontinued in the LY2603618/gemcitabine arm, four events (grade 4 cerebrovascular accident, grade 1 left bundle branch block, grade 3 acute pulmonary oedema, and grade 3 atrial fibrillation) were possibly related to treatment. Of the six patients who discontinued in the gemcitabine arm, four possibly related events occurred (grade 3 thrombotic microangiopathy, grade 4

Table 2 Secondary efficacy endpoints

	LY2603618/ gemcitabine	Gemcitabine
	($n = 65$)	($n = 34$)
Progression-free survival, mos.		
Median (range)	3.5 (0–15.9)	5.6 (0–17.4)
Duration of response, mos.		
Median (range)	3.5 (1.5–14.1)	6.0 (3.7–6.8)
Best Overall Response, n (%; 95% CI)		
CR	0	0
PR	14 (21.5%; 12.3–33.5)	3 (8.8%; 1.9–23.7)
SD	22 (33.8%; 22.6–46.6)	19 (55.9%; 37.9–72.8)
Clinical Benefit Rate, n (%; 95% CI)	36 (55.4%; 42.5–67.7)	22 (64.7%; 46.5–80.3)

CI confidence interval; *CR* complete response; *LY2603618/gemcitabine* LY2603618 (230 mg flat dose) combined with gemcitabine 1000 mg/m²; *mos* months; *n* number of patients; *PR* partial response; *SD* stable disease

Table 3 Study drug-related treatment-emergent adverse events in ≥10% of the safety population

Preferred Term, n (%)	LY2603618/gemcitabine	Gemcitabine
	($n = 65$)	($n = 34$)
Patients with ≥1 TEAE	58 (89.2)	31 (91.2)
Thrombocytopenia	21 (32.3)	14 (41.2)
Nausea	22 (33.8)	8 (23.5)
Fatigue	16 (24.6)	10 (29.4)
Neutropenia	14 (21.5)	9 (26.5)
Anemia	9 (13.8)	9 (26.5)
Vomiting	14 (21.5)	3 (8.8)
Decreased appetite	12 (18.5)	3 (8.8)
Diarrhea	11 (16.9)	3 (8.8)
Pyrexia	9 (13.8)	5 (14.7)
Asthenia	7 (10.8)	5 (14.7)
Constipation	9 (13.8)	3 (8.8)
Leukopenia	7 (10.8)	5 (14.7)
Stomatitis	10 (15.4)	1 (2.9)
Alopecia	6 (9.2)	4 (11.8)
Oedema peripheral	7 (10.8)	2 (5.9)

LY2603618/gemcitabine LY2603618 (230 mg flat dose) combined with gemcitabine 1000 mg/m²; *n* number of patients; *TEAE* treatment-emergent adverse events

Table 4 Grade 3/4 study drug-related treatment-emergent adverse events in ≥5% of the safety population

Preferred Term, n (%)	LY2603618/gemcitabine (n = 65)		Gemcitabine (n = 34)	
	Grade 3	Grade 4	Grade 3	Grade 4
Patients with ≥1 TEAE	25 (38.5)	6 (9.2)	19 (55.9)	3 (8.8)
Decreased hemoglobin	2 (3.1)	0	4 (11.8)	0
Decreased leukocytes	5 (7.7)	0	1 (2.9)	1 (2.9)
Decreased neutrophils/				
Decreased platelets	7 (10.8)	0	3 (8.8)	1 (2.9)
Thrombotic microangiopathy	0	0	2 (5.9)	0
Fatigue	1 (1.5)	1 (1.5)	3 (8.8)	0
Dehydration	0	0	2 (5.9)	0
Hyponatremia	2 (3.1)	0	2 (5.9)	0

LY2603618/gemcitabine LY2603618 (230 mg flat dose) combined with gemcitabine 1000 mg/m^2; *n* number of patients; *TEAE* treatment-emergent adverse events

acute renal failure, grade 2 thrombocytopenia, and grade 3 hemolytic uraemic syndrome). Four deaths were reported during the study; three due to disease progression and one due to a non-related peripheral arterial ischemia event.

Pharmacokinetic/pharmacodynamic analyses

LY2603618 demonstrated consistent PK parameters after single (day 2) and repeat administration (day 16) during cycle 1 (Table 5). The LY2603618 plasma systemic exposure targets (i.e., $AUC_{(0-\infty)}$ ≥21,000 ng hr/mL and C_{max} ≥2000 ng/mL) that correlate with maximal pharmacodynamic (PD) effect observed in nonclinical HT-29 xenograft models (data on file) were achieved on a mean cohort basis after 230 mg of LY2603618 (Table 5). More specifically, 87% and 73% of the individual PK profiles on days 2 and 16 of cycle 1 were above the targets for C_{max} and $AUC_{(0-\infty)}$, respectively.

For the PD analyses, dFdC was incorporated into DNA following gemcitabine administration, with the levels declining to almost baseline by the end of each treatment cycle. The highest levels of dFdC incorporation were observed on days 8 and 15 across all doses. The increases in the amount of dFdC incorporation did not correspond to increasing doses of LY2603618.

Of the patients who had baseline CA19-9 levels > upper limit of normal, a similar percentage of patients (65.4% LY2603618/gemcitabine; 64% gemcitabine) experienced a >50% reduction from baseline in CA19-9 levels.

QTcF assessment

In a time-point exploratory QTcF assessment, no clinically significant trends in ECG parameter changes were reported. Five patients had a change in QTcF from baseline between 30 and 60 milliseconds (msec); no patients had a change in QTcF >60 msec.

Discussion

The current study was part of a Phase I/II study designed to compare the OS of LY2603618/gemcitabine to gemcitabine alone. This study used a Bayesian augmented control design to incorporate historical gemcitabine data, which

Table 5 Summary of LY2603618 noncompartmental pharmacokinetic parameter estimates

Parameter	Geometric Mean (CV%) 230 mg LY2603618	
	Cycle 1	
	Day 2 (n = 58)	Day 16 (n = 48)
C_{max} (ng/mL)	3170 (50)	3410 (50)
t_{max} [a] (h)	1.00 (0.88–1.38)	1.00 (0.88–1.83)
$C_{av,24}$ (ng/mL)	966 (68) [d]	987 (60) [e]
$AUC_{(0-24)}$ (ng*h/mL)	23200 (68) [d]	23700 (60) [e]
$AUC_{(0-\infty)}$ (ng*h/mL)	29400 (84) [d]	29100 (74) [e]
$AUC_{(tlast-\infty)}$ (%)	14.3 (131) [d]	12.0 (152) [e]
CL (L/h)	7.79 (84) [d]	7.87 (74) [e]
V_{ss} (L)	104 (48) [d]	95.1 (42) [e]
$t_{1/2}$ (h)	9.67 (48) [d]	8.86 (48) [e]
R_A [b]	–	108 (32) [f]
R_A [c]	–	–

$AUC_{(0-\infty)}$ area under the plasma concentration time-curve from time 0 to infinity; $AUC_{(0-24)}$ area under the plasma concentration time-curve from time 0 to 24 h; $AUC_{(tlast-\infty)}$ fraction of $AUC_{(0-\infty)}$ extrapolated from the time of the last measurable plasma concentration (t_{last}) to infinity; $C_{av,24}$ average plasma concentration over 24 h calculated using $AUC_{(0-24)}$; *CL* systemic clearance; C_{max} maximum plasma concentration; *CV%* percent coefficient of variation; m^2 meters squared; *mg* milligrams; *n* number of pharmacokinetic observations; *NC* not calculated; R_A accumulation ratio; t_{max} time of maximum observed plasma concentration; V_{ss} volume of distribution at steady state following intravenous (IV) administration; $t_{1/2}$ elimination half-life
[a]Median (range)
[b]Intracycle accumulation ratio [Cycle 1 Day 16 $AUC_{(0-\infty)}$/Cycle 1 Day 2 $AUC_{(0-\infty)}$]
[c]Intercycle accumulation ratio [Cycle 2 Day 2 $AUC_{(0-\infty)}$/Cycle 1 Day 2 $AUC_{(0-\infty)}$]
[d]n = 54
[e]n = 42
[f]n = 38

minimized the number of patients needed for the treatment to be evaluated. Stage II or III patients not amenable to resection with curative intent or Stage IV disease were included in the current study to match the populations used in the historical studies used as reference data. The OS of LY2603618/gemcitabine was not superior to gemcitabine alone in patients with locally advanced or metastatic pancreatic cancer by either the Bayesian or frequentist approach. In addition, no significant differences between arms in any of the secondary endpoints were observed.

The safety profiles were comparable between arms, indicating that the addition of LY2603618 did not significantly change the safety profile of gemcitabine. This is consistent with the CHK1 inhibitor MK8776 [20], but in contrast to the data reported with the CHK1 selective inhibitors GDC-0425 and AZD7762 [21, 22]. In a Phase 1 study with AZD7762, unpredictable cardiac toxicity was observed [21]. Although it was demonstrated safe and feasible to administer GDC-0425 with gemcitabine, the CHK1 inhibitor appeared to increase some of the toxicities associated with gemcitabine [22].

A trend towards a lower LY2603618 systemic exposure and more rapid CL associated with a larger interpatient variability in Phase II (Table 5) compared to Phase I was observed [13]. This is likely a result of the more limited PK sampling schedule (sampling to only 24 h post dose) used in the Phase II study (i.e., larger $AUC_{(tlast-\infty)}$ (%) values; Table 5), thereby limiting the capability of the conventional PK analysis method to accurately quantify the terminal elimination phase of LY2603618 and resulting in an underestimate of $AUC_{(0-\infty)}$ and overestimate of CL. In contrast, the LY2603618 PK profiles over the first 24 h from Phase II demonstrated a high degree of concordance with the PK profiles from Phase I. The average $t_{1/2}$ following administration of 230 mg LY2603618 was consistent with a $t_{1/2}$ suitable for achieving and maintaining the desired target human exposures while minimizing the intra- and intercycle accumulation (Table 5). Gemcitabine did not appear to affect the PK of LY2603618, as the PK parameters reported in this study were similar to the PK parameters calculated after LY2603618 monotherapy [23].

The study had inherent limitations that may have contributed to the negative clinical outcome observed. In addition, due to the lack of a clinically-validated PD marker to quantify direct CHK1 inhibition by LY2603618, the magnitude and duration of CHK1 target inhibition at 230 mg is neither known nor has it been correlated to clinical responses. Therefore, it is possible the PK surrogate targets (i.e., $AUC_{(0-\infty)} \geq 21,000$ ng•hr/mL and $C_{max} \geq 2000$ ng/mL) derived from nonclinical xenograft models for maximal PD response were not appropriate thresholds to predict clinical responses in humans. In addition,

inclusion of only patients with Stage IV disease may have yielded a more favorable clinical outcome.

One Phase III randomized trial comparing gemcitabine with FOLFIRINOX reported statistically significant improvements in OS (hazard ratio [HR] 0.57, $P < .0001$), PFS (HR 0.47, $P < .0001$), and ORR ($P = .0001$) in chemonaïve patients with ECOG PS 0 and 1 [5]. Despite the clinical efficacy observed with FOLFIRINOX, this treatment was associated with more frequent and more severe toxicity [5]. As a result, only patients with an adequate PS are typically eligible for FOLFIRINOX treatment. Recent meta-analyses have reported that patients with poorer performance had less OS benefit from combined therapies for metastatic pancreatic cancer [24, 25]. Since FOLFIRINOX emerged as a treatment option during the conduct of this study, there was concern that a greater proportion of patients with low PS status who were not eligible for FOLFIRINOX would be included. However, only 9.2% and 8.8% of patients on the experimental arm and control arm, respectively, were PS 2 and so this consideration was unlikely to have affected the outcome.

The Metastatic Pancreatic Adenocarcinoma Clinical Trial (MPACT) demonstrated improved clinical efficacy with gemcitabine/*nab*-paclitaxel than gemcitabine (median OS, 8.5 months vs. 6.7 months, respectively); however, fatigue, neuropathy, and neutropenia were more common among patients receiving combination therapy than monotherapy [4, 8]. Interestingly, the overall incidence of grade III/IV study drug-related TEAEs in the current study was not increased in the LY2603618/gemcitabine arm compared with the gemcitabine arm, except for the incidence of grade 3 leukocytes and platelets, which was higher in the LY2603618/gemcitabine arm.

Conclusion

OS was not improved with the addition of LY2603618/gemcitabine compared with gemcitabine alone. The safety and PK profiles were comparable between treatment arms. As a result of this finding, LY2603618/gemcitabine will not be further developed for the treatment of patients with pancreatic cancer.

Abbreviations

%$AUC_{[tlast-\infty]}$: Percentage of $AUC_{[0-\infty]}$ extrapolated; 5-FU: Fluorouracil; AE: Adverse event; $AUC_{[0-tlast]}$: Area under the plasma concentration time-curve from time 0 to the time of the last measurable plasma concentration; $AUC_{[0-\infty]}$: Area under the plasma concentration time-curve from time 0 to infinity; $AUC_{(0-24)}$: Area under the plasma concentration time-curve from time 0 to 24 h; $AUC_{(tlast-\infty)}$: Fraction of $AUC_{(0-\infty)}$ extrapolated from the time of the last measurable plasma concentration (t_{last}) to infinity; CA19-9: Carbohydrate antigen 19–9; C_{av24}: Average plasma concentration over 24 h calculated using $AUC_{(0-24)}$; CHK1: Checkpoint kinase 1; CI: Confidence intervals; CL: Systemic clearance; C_{max}: Maximum plasma concentration; CR: Complete response; CTCAE: Common terminology criteria for adverse events; CV%: Percent coefficient of variation; dFdC 2′: 2′-difluorodeoxycytidine; DNA: Deoxyribonucleic acid; ECG: Electrocardiogram; ECOG PS: Eastern cooperative oncology group performance status; FOLFIRINOX: Oxaliplatin, irinotecan, leucovorin, and 5-FU; ITT: Intent-to-treat; m²: Meters squared; mg: Milligram; MPACT: Metastatic pancreatic adenocarcinoma clinical trial; msec: Millisecond; NC: Not calculated; ORR: Overall response rate; OS: Overall survival; PD: Pharmacodynamic; PFS: Progression-free survival; PK: Pharmacokinetics; PR: Partial response; PS: Performance status; QTcF: Fridericia's heart rate-corrected QT interval; R_A: Intra- and intercycle accumulation ratios; RNAi: Ribonucleic acid interference; SAE: Serious adverse event; $t_{1/2}$: Terminal elimination half-life; TEAE: Treatment-emergent AEs; t_{max}: Time of maximum observed plasma concentration; V_{ss}: Volume of distribution at steady-state

Acknowledgements
The authors wish to acknowledge Chastity Bradley, PhD for her medical writing assistance, Elizabeth Kumm for statistical support, Ignacio Garcias-Ribas and Eric Westin for their contributions to the CHK1 clinical program, and Rodney L. Decker for his assistance with the PK analysis. We wish to also thank the patients who participated in this trial and the study coordinators, nurses, nurse practitioners, clinical research assistants, and doctors who assisted with the research.

Funding
The study was sponsored by Eli Lilly and Company. Eli Lilly and Company was responsible for all aspects of this study, including study concept/design, data analysis, and the interpretation and writing of the manuscript with the use medical writing resources.

Authors' contributions
As per ICMJE guidelines, all authors were involved in the study design, research, analysis, and/or interpretation of the data; likewise, all authors shared the responsibility of writing/editing the submitted manuscript and are fully accountable for the integrity of the data. In addition, all authors have read and approved the manuscript. The individual contributions of each author have been outlined below: Conception of the work: DVH. Design of the work: KH, SH, GK. Acquisition of data for the work: BL, JL-M, DRichards, GI, DZC, GK, PS, DRichel, CS, SC, GLF, TC, DVH, EC, KH. Analysis of data for the work: SH, JL, ABL, GK, DZC, DVH, TC. Interpretation of data for the work: BL, JL-M, KH, SH, JL, ABL, GK, EC, DZC, DVH, TC. Drafting of the manuscript: SH, JL, SC, TC. Critical revision of the manuscript for important intellectual content: BL, JL-M, DRichards, GI, DZC, GK, PS, DRichel, CS, GLF, KH, SH, ABL, DVH, EC.

Competing interests
P. Stella is employed by a for-profit health care company, Physician Resource Management, and is the president as well as part-owner and founder of the company. D. Von Hoff is currently a consultant for Eli Lilly and Company. K. Hurt, S. Hynes, J. Lin, and A. Bence Lin are employees of Eli Lilly and Company and own Eli Lilly and Company stock. All remaining authors have declared no conflicts of interest.

Author details
[1]Institut Català d'Oncologia-IDIBELL (Institut d'Investigació Biomèdica de Bellvitge), Barcelona, Spain. [2]University Hospital and Research Institute, Madrid, Spain. [3]US Oncology Research, Tyler, USA. [4]Hematology, Onkology, and Palliative Care, Klinikum Stuttgart, Stuttgart, Germany. [5]Virginia Oncology Associates, Eastern Virginia Medical School, US Oncology Research, Hampton, VA, USA. [6]21st Century Oncology, University of Florida Health Oncology, Jacksonville, USA. [7]St. Joseph Mercy Hospital, Ypsilanti, MI, USA. [8]Academic Medical Center, Amsterdam, Netherlands. [9]Department of Oncology, Military Institute of Medicine, Warsaw, Poland. [10]Department of Oncology and Hematology, Universitá di Modena e Reggio Emilia, Policlinico di Modena, Modena, Italy. [11]Department of Oncology, Istituto Scientifico Romagnolo per lo Studio e la Cura dei Tumori (IRST) IRCCS, Meldola, Italy. [12]Institute of Oncology Ion Chiricuta, University of Medicine and Pharmacy Iuliu Hatieganu, Cluj Napoca, Romania. [13]Eli Lilly and Company, Indianapolis, IN, USA. [14]Translational Genomics Research Institute (TGen) and HonorHealth Research Institute, Phoenix, AZ, USA. [15]START Madrid-CIOCC, Centro Integral Oncológico Clara Campal, Medical Oncology Division, Hospital Universitario Madrid Norte Sanchinarro, Calle Oña, 10, 28050 Madrid, Spain.

References
1. American Cancer Society. American Cancer Society Cancer Facts & Figures. 2014. http://www.cancer.org/acs/groups/content/@research/documents/webcontent/acspc-042151.pdf. accessed 18 Aug 2015.
2. Puleo F, Maréchal R, Demetter P, Bali M, Calomme A, Closset J, Bachet JB, Deviere J, Van Laethem JL. New challenges in perioperative management of pancreatic cancer. World J Gastroenterol. 2015;21:2281–93.
3. Kuhlmann KF, de Castro SM, Wesseling JG, ten Kate FJ, Offerhaus GJ, Busch OR, van Gulik TM, Obertop H, Gouma DJ. Surgical treatment of pancreatic adenocarcinoma; actual survival and prognostic factors in 343 patients. Eur J Cancer. 2004;40:549–58.
4. Von Hoff DD, Ramanathan RK, Borad MJ, Laheru DA, Smith LS, Wood TE, Korn RL, Desai N, Trieu V, Iglesias JL, Zhang H, Soon-Shiong P, Shi T, Rajeshkumar NV, Maitra A, Hidalgo M. Gemcitabine plus nab-paclitaxel is an active regimen in patients with advanced pancreatic cancer: a phase I/II trial. J Clin Oncol. 2011;29:4548–54.
5. Conroy T, Desseigne F, Ychou M, Bouché O, Guimbaud R, Bécouarn Y, Adenis A, Raoul JL, Gourgou-Bourgade S, de la Fouchardière C, Bachet JB, Khemissa-Akouz F, Péré-Vergé D, Delbaldo C, Assenat E, Chauffert B, Michel P, Montoto-Grillot C, Ducreux M, Groupe Tumeurs Digestives of Unicancer, PRODIGE Intergroup. FOLFIRINOX versus gemcitabine for metastatic pancreatic cancer. N Engl J Med. 2011;364:1817–25.
6. Frese KK, Neesse A, Cook N, Bapiro TE, Lolkema MP, Jodrell DI, Tuveson DA. nab-Paclitaxel potentiates gemcitabine activity by reducing cytidine deaminase levels in a mouse model of pancreatic cancer. Cancer Discov. 2012;2:260–9.
7. Von Hoff DD, Ervin T, Arena FP, Chiorean EG, Infante J, Moore M, Seay T, Tjulandin SA, Ma WW, Saleh MN, Harris M, Reni M, Dowden S, Laheru D, Bahary N, Ramanathan RK, Tabernero J, Hidalgo M, Goldstein D, Van Cutsem E, Wei X, Iglesias J, Renschler MF. Increased survival in pancreatic cancer with nab-paclitaxel plus gemcitabine. N Engl J Med. 2013;369:1691–703.
8. Von Hoff DD, Ervin T, Arena FP, Chiorean EG, Infante JR, Moore MJ, Seay TE, Tjulandin S, Ma WW, Saleh MN, Harris M, Reni M, Ramanathan RK, Tabernero J, Hidalgo M, Van Cutsem E, Goldstein D, Wei X, Iglesias JL, Renschler MF. Randomized phase III study of weekly nab-paclitaxel plus gemcitabine versus gemcitabine alone in patients with metastatic adenocarcinoma of the pancreas (MPACT) [ASCO abstract LBA148]. J Clin Oncol. 2013;31 Suppl 4:LBA148.
9. McNeely S, Beckmann R, Bence Lin AK. CHEK again: revisiting the development of CHK1 inhibitors for cancer therapy. Pharmacol Ther. 2014; 142:1–10.
10. Azorsa DO, Gonzales IM, Basu GD, Choudhary A, Arora S, Bisanz KM, Kiefer JA, Henderson MC, Trent JM, Von Hoff DD, Mousses S. Synthetic lethal RNAi screening identifies sensitizing targets for gemcitabine therapy in pancreatic cancer. J Transl Med. 2009;7:43.
11. King C, Diaz H, Barnard D, Barda D, Clawson D, Blosser W, Cox K, Guo S, Marshall M. Characterization and preclinical development of LY2603618: a selective and potent Chk1 inhibitor. Invest New Drugs. 2014;32:213–26.
12. Calvo E, Chen VJ, Marshall M, Ohnmacht U, Hynes SM, Kumm E, Diaz HB, Barnard D, Merzoug FF, Huber L, Kays L, Iversen P, Calles A, Voss B, Lin AB, Dickgreber N, Wehler T, Sebastian M. Preclinical analyses and phase I evaluation of LY2603618 administered in combination with pemetrexed and cisplatin in patients with advanced cancer. Invest New Drugs. 2014;32: 955–68.
13. Calvo E, Braiteh F, Von Hoff DD, McWilliams R, Becerra C, Galsky MD, Jameson G, Lin J, McKane S, Wickremsinhe ER, Hynes SM, Bence Lin AK, Hurt K, Richards D. Phase I study of CHK1 inhibitor LY2603618 in combination with gemcitabine in patients with solid tumors. Oncology. 2016;91:251–60.
14. Congdon P. Applied bayesian modeling. 2nd ed. Hoboken: Wiley; 2003.
15. Ibrahim J, Chen M-H, Sinha D. Bayesian survival analysis. New York: Springer; 2001.
16. Oettle H, Richards D, Ramanathan RK, van Laethem JL, Peeters M, Fuchs M, Zimmermann A, John W, Von Hoff D, Arning M, Kindler HL. A phase III trial of pemetrexed plus gemcitabine versus gemcitabine in patients with unresectable or metastatic pancreatic cancer. Ann Oncol. 2005;16:1639–45.

Dancey J, Arbuck S, Gwyther S, Mooney M, Rubinstein L, Shankar L, Dodd L, Kaplan R, Lacombe D, Verweij J. New response evaluation criteria in solid tumours: revised RECIST guideline (version 1.1). Eur J Cancer. 2009;45:228–47.

19. Wickremsinhe ER, Lutzke B, Jones B, Schultz GA, Freeman AB, Pratt SE, Bones AM, Ackermann BL. Quantification of gemcitabine incorporation into human DNA by LC/MS/MS as a surrogate measure for target engagement. Anal Chem. 2010;82:6576–83.

20. Daud AI, Ashworth MT, Strosberg J, Goldman JW, Mendelson D, Springett G, Venook AP, Loechner S, Rosen LS, Shanahan F, Parry D, Shumway S, Grabowsky JA, Freshwater T, Sorge C, Kang SP, Isaacs R, Munster PN. Phase I dose-escalation trial of checkpoint kinase 1 inhibitor MK-8776 as monotherapy and in combination with gemcitabine in patients with advanced solid tumors. J Clin Oncol. 2015;33:1060–6.

21. Sausville E, LoRusso P, Carducci M, Carter J, Quinn MF, Malburg L, Azad N, Cosgrove D, Knight R, Barker P, Zabludoff S, Agbo F, Oakes P, Senderowicz A. Phase I dose-escalation study of AZD7762, a checkpoint kinase inhibitor, in combination with gemcitabine in US patients with advanced solid tumors. Cancer Chemother Pharmacol. 2014;73:539–49.

22. Infante J, Hollebecque A, Postel-Vinay S, Bauer T, Blackwood B, Evangelista M, Mahrus S, Peale F, Lu X, Sahasranaman S, Zhu R, Chen Y, Ding X, Murray E, Schutzman J, Lauchle J, Soria J-C, LoRusso P. Phase I study of GDC-0425, a checkpoint kinase 1 inhibitor, in combination with gemcitabine in patients with refractory solid tumors [AACR abstract CT139]. Cancer Res. 2015;75: CT139.

23. Weiss GJ, Donehower R, Iyengar T, Ramanathan RK, Lewandowski K, Westin E, Hurt K, Hynes SM, Anthony SP, McKane S. Phase I dose-escalation study to examine the safety and tolerability of LY2603618, a checkpoint 1 kinase inhibitor, administered 1 day after pemetrexed 500 mg/m(2) every 21 days in patients with cancer. Invest New Drugs. 2013;31:136–44.

24. Collins DC, Morris PG. Systemic therapy for advanced pancreatic cancer: individualising cytotoxic therapy. Expert Opin Pharmacother. 2015;16: 851–61.

25. Heinemann V, Boeck S, Hinke A, Labianca R, Louvet C. Meta-analysis of randomized trials: evaluation of benefit from gemcitabine-based combination chemotherapy applied in advanced pancreatic cancer. BMC Cancer. 2008;8:82.

Nanoliposomal irinotecan with fluorouracil for the treatment of advanced pancreatic cancer, a single institution experience

Danielle C. Glassman[1], Randze L. Palmaira[1], Christina M. Covington[1], Avni M. Desai[1], Geoffrey Y. Ku[1], Jia Li[1], James J. Harding[1], Anna M. Varghese[1], Eileen M. O'Reilly[1] and Kenneth H. Yu[1,2]*

Abstract

Background: Effective treatment options for advanced pancreatic cancer are finite. NAPOLI-1, a phase III randomized trial, demonstrated the efficacy of nanoliposomal irinotecan with fluorouracil/leucovorin (nal-IRI + 5-FU/LV) for the treatment of advanced pancreatic cancer following progression on gemcitabine-based chemotherapy. There are limited additional data on the safety and efficacy of nal-IRI + 5-FU/LV following FDA approval in October 2015. We examined the post-approval safety and effectiveness of nal-IRI + 5-FU/LV in advanced pancreatic cancer patients receiving treatment at Memorial Sloan Kettering Cancer Center.

Methods: A retrospective chart review was conducted of all patients beginning treatment with nal-IRI + 5-FU/LV from October 2015 through June 2017. Using the electronic medical record and institutional database, information was extracted pertaining to demographics, performance status (ECOG), prior therapies, dose, duration of treatment, adverse events, progression free survival (PFS), overall survival (OS) and treatment response.

Results: Fifty six patients were identified. Median progression free survival (PFS) was 2.9 months and median overall survival (OS) was 5.3 months. Patients with prior disease progression on irinotecan experienced PFS and OS of 2.2 and 3.9 mo, respectively. Patients without prior irinotecan exposure experienced significantly longer PFS (4.8 mo, $p = 0.02$) and OS (7.7 mo, $p = 0.002$), as did patients who received prior irinotecan without disease progression (PFS, 5.7 mo, $p = 0.04$; OS, 9.0 mo, $p = .04$). Progression on prior irinotecan was associated with greater lines of prior advanced disease chemotherapy (2 vs 1). Dose reductions (DR) were most frequently due to fatigue (42%) and diarrhea (37%), but were not associated with worse outcomes. In fact, patients with ≥1 DR experienced longer PFS (5.4 v 2.6 mo, $p = 0.035$). Sequential therapy with nab-paclitaxel + gemcitabine (nab-P + Gem) followed by nal-IRI + 5-FU/LV ($n = 25$) resulted in OS of 23.0 mo. Mutations in TP53 were associated with shorter PFS.

Conclusions: These data support the safety and efficacy of nal-IRI + 5-FU/LV, reinforcing results of NAPOLI-1. Patients without disease progression on prior irinotecan fared significantly better than patients with progression, when treated with nal-IRI + 5-FU/LV. Sequential therapy with nab-P + Gem followed by nal-IRI + 5-FU/LV demonstrates encouraging median OS. These findings provide guidance for patients most likely to benefit from nal-IRI + 5-FU/LV.

Keywords: Pancreatic cancer, Nanoliposomal irinotecan, MM-398, Nal-IRI, 5-fluorouracil

* Correspondence: yuk1@mskcc.org
[1]David M. Rubenstein Center for Pancreatic Cancer Research, Memorial Sloan Kettering Cancer Center, Weil Cornell Medical College, New York, NY, USA
[2]Gastrointestinal Oncology Service, Memorial Sloan Kettering Cancer Center, 300 East 66th Street, New York, NY 10065, USA

Background

Pancreatic ductal adenocarcinoma (PDAC) remains an intractable illness due to late stage of presentation, a propensity to metastasize, relative resistance to cytotoxic treatment and the lack of effective targeted agents. In 2017, an estimated 53,670 new cases of pancreatic cancer were diagnosed [1]. The majority of patients have either regional (11.5%) or distant (52%) spread at presentation. With a low 5-year survival rate of only 8.2%, PDAC ranks as the 3rd leading cause of cancer deaths, with an estimated 43,090 patient deaths in 2017. It is estimated that PDAC will rise to the second leading cause of cancer mortality by 2030 [2].

The treatment landscape for advanced PDAC has significantly changed since 2010. Randomized phase III trials have demonstrated significant survival benefits of FOLFIRINOX (folinic acid, 5-fluorouracil, irinotecan and oxaliplatin) [3] or nab-paclitaxel + gemcitabine (nab-P + Gem) [4] compared with the prior standard of care, single agent gemcitabine, for frontline treatment. Nanoliposomal irinotecan (nal-IRI) is a novel formulation of irinotecan, encapsulating drug molecules within long-circulating liposome-based nanoparticles with resulting favorable pharmacokinetic and biodistribution properties [5]. Recently, the randomized phase III NAPOLI-1 trial demonstrated significant survival benefit of nal-IRI with fluorouracil/leucovorin (nal-IRI + 5-FU/LV) compared with 5-FU alone after disease-progression on gemcitabine-based chemotherapy, progression-free survival (PFS) of 3.1 vs 1.5 months, respectively ($p = 0.0001$) and overall survival (OS) of 6.1 vs 4.2 months ($p = 0.012$). Nal-IRI received FDA approval on October 22nd, 2015.

Due to the aggressiveness of this disease, and, until recently, the dearth of effective therapies, the majority of patients receive only a single line of chemotherapy [6, 7]. With the current availability of several lines of active combination therapy, studies describing outcomes of sequential therapy are greatly needed. In particular, evidence for how to best integrate nal-IRI + 5-FU/LV into the treatment algorithm is needed and to understand the dosing schedule of the regimen. This retrospective, single institution analysis was conducted to address these questions.

Methods

Patients

A retrospective review was conducted of all consecutive patients with advanced PDAC who began receiving treatment with nal-IRI + 5-FU/LV at Memorial Sloan Kettering Cancer Center (MSKCC) and its regional care network between October 2015 and June 2017. The electronic medical record (EMR) was interrogated for patient demographics, performance status (ECOG), date of diagnosis, date of advanced disease diagnosis and carbohydrate antigen 19–9 (CA 19–9) level at baseline, tumor and germline genomic results, prior treatment details and duration, nal-IRI + 5-FU/LV starting dose, nal-IRI + 5-FU/LV dose reductions, nal-IRI + 5-FU/LV treatment duration, adverse events and survival. Tumor and germline genomics were performed under an IRB approved protocol (NCT01775072). The MSK-IMPACT somatic analysis utilizes targeted next generation sequencing (NGS) of pancreatic tumor tissue to interrogate a panel of 410–481 genes. Germline analysis on DNA obtained from normal peripheral blood utilizes NGS to interrogate a panel of 76 genes associated with hereditary cancer predisposition. This retrospective analysis was granted a research waiver by the MSKCC Institutional Review Board.

Outcome measures

All treatment related adverse events (AEs) that occurred while patients were treated with nal-IRI + 5-FU/LV were collected. All AEs and SAEs were graded per National Cancer Institute Common Terminology Criteria for Adverse Events (NCI-CTCAE V4.0).

Patients were assessed every 8–12 weeks by computed tomography (CT). Disease response was assessed using RECIST version 1.1 criteria. Response by change in CA 19–9 level was recorded. Date of disease progression on nal-IRI + 5-FU/LV treatment and date of death were recorded.

Statistical analysis

Descriptive statistics were calculated as mean, median or percentages as appropriate. PFS was calculated from the time of first nal-IRI + 5-FU/LV administration to disease progression or death, whichever occurred first. Nal-IRI + 5-FU/LV OS was calculated from time of first nal-IRI + 5-FU/LV administration to death. Advanced disease OS was calculated from time of advanced disease diagnosis to death.

Patients without progression or death were censored at the last follow-up date as of November 2nd, 2017. Survival curves and median survival were estimated using the Kaplan–Meier method. Survival curves were compared using Log-rank (Mantel-Cox) test or Log-rank test for trend. Hazard ratios were calculated using Log-rank test with 95% confidence intervals.

Results

Patient and tumor characteristics

During the accrual period, $N = 56$ patients with advanced PDAC received treatment with nal-IRI + 5-FU/LV at MSKCC. All patients who received one or more administrations of nal-IRI + 5-FU/LV were included in the analysis. The patient characteristics are listed in Table 1. The median age was 68 years, range 42 to 88 years. The significant majority of patients had metastatic disease at the time of treatment onset, with only two patients with locally advanced

Table 1 Characteristics of patients and tumors

	N = 56 (%)
Median Age (years, range)	68 (42–88)
Gender	
Male	29 (52)
Female	27 (48)
ECOG Performance Status	
0	3 (5)
1	41 (73)
2	12 (21)
Primary tumor location	
Head	28 (50)
Body	11 (20)
Tail	12 (21)
Body and tail	5 (9)
Stage at start of treatment	
III	2 (4)
IV	54 (96)
Metastatic sites	
Liver	41 (73)
Peritoneum	16 (29)
Lung	15 (27)
Distant lymph nodes	18 (32)
Other	10 (18)
Number of metastatic sites	
1	29 (52)
2	8 (14)
3 or more	16 (29)
Prior lines of advanced disease therapy	
0	4 (7)
1	20 (36)
2	21 (38)
3 or more	11 (20)

disease. The majority (79%) of patients had an Eastern Cooperative Oncology Group (ECOG) performance status of 0 or 1, the remainder (20%) had an ECOG performance status of 2. Nineteen patients had prior surgery and nine patients received prior radiation therapy. Although the majority of patients received at least one (36%) or more (58%) lines of chemotherapy prior to receiving nal-IRI + 5-FU/LV, 4 (7%) patients were treated with nal-IRI + 5-FU/LV in the frontline, metastatic setting after failure of gemcitabine-based chemotherapy in the adjuvant setting.

Dosing and drug delivery

The majority of patients (70%) started nal-IRI + 5-FU/LV treatment with a dose of nal-IRI below the

recommended 70 mg/m^2 dose level, see Table 2. The median starting dose was 55 mg/m^2. The choice of a lower starting dose at our institution is based on physician preference. Line of therapy and ECOG performance status were not factors associated with lower starting dose. The only statistically significant factor identified was age; the median age of patients starting at full dose was 63 versus 70 ($p = 0.01$). The majority of patients never experienced a dose reduction of nal-IRI, with 15 (27%) experiencing a single dose reduction and only 3 (5%) experiencing two dose reductions. Examining the sequence of chemotherapy regimens prior to nal-IRI + 5-FU/LV treatment, the vast majority followed one of two patterns. The most common sequence was treatment with either 5-FU based chemotherapy, typically FOLFIRINOX or FOLFOX, followed by gemcitabine-based chemotherapy, typically single agent gemcitabine or nab-P + Gem, or the inverse (referred to going forward as **Sequence 1**). Twenty-six (46%) experienced this pattern of treatment, followed by nal-IRI + 5-FU/LV treatment in the 3rd line or later. The second most common sequence, received by 25 (45%) patients, was treatment with gemcitabine-based chemotherapy, typically either gemcitabine alone or nab-P + Gem in the frontline or adjuvant setting followed by nal-IRI + 5-FU/LV treatment in the 2nd line (referred to going forward as **Sequence 2**). A small number of patients, 3 (5%), received nab-P + Gem followed by Gem/capecitabine (Cap), followed by nal-IRI + 5-FU/LV in the 3rd line. Two (4%) patients received sequential treatment that did not fit any of these patterns due to participation in clinical trials.

Table 2 Dosing, dose reductions and sequencing of nal-IRI + 5-FU/LV

	N = 56 (%)
Starting nal-IRI dose (mg/m2)	
< 50	23 (41)
55	9 (16)
60	7 (13)
70	17 (30)
Dose reductions (#)	
0	38 (68)
1	15 (27)
2	3 (5)
Treatment sequencing	
FOLF (IRIN) OX ← → (nab-P) + Gem → nal-IRI + 5-FU/LV	26 (46)
nab-P + Gem → nal-IRI + 5-FU/LV	25 (45)
nab-P + Gem → Gem/Cap → nal-IRI + 5-FU/LV	3 (5)
other	2 (4)

Efficacy

For the entire cohort of $N = 56$ the median PFS was 2.9 months and the median OS was 5.3 months (Table 3). Three patients had a PR (5%) and 23 (41%) had SD per RECIST. Ten patients (18%) experienced > 50% reduction of CA 19–9 at maximal response compared to baseline. Patients were classified based on whether they received irinotecan ($N = 33$, 59%) in prior lines of chemotherapy, or not ($N = 23$, 41%). Of patients receiving prior irinotecan, patients were further divided into those whose disease progressed on prior irinotecan-based chemotherapy ($N = 27$, 48%), or not ($N = 6$, 11%). The latter generally were patients who presented initially with locally advanced disease who completed a course of FOLFIRINOX chemotherapy in the neoadjuvant setting without disease progression before moving on to surgery or radiation therapy. By contrast, patients whose disease progressed on prior irinotecan-based chemotherapy typically received FOLFIRINOX as front-line therapy for metastatic disease. Patients receiving nal-IRI + 5-FU/LV after progressing on prior irinotecan-based chemotherapy experienced significantly shorter PFS and OS compared with patients not previously treated with irinotecan (PFS, 2.2 v 4.6 mo, $p = 0.022$; OS, 3.9 v 7.7 mo, $p = 0.0021$), and also when compared with patients previously treated with irinotecan without progression (PFS, 2.2 v 5.7 mo, $p = 0.041$; OS, 3.9 v 9.0 mo, $p = 0.035$) (Fig. 1). Importantly, patients

Table 3 Overall efficacy and response to treatment with nal-IRI + 5-FU/LV

	N = 56 (%)
PFS (median, mo)	2.9
OS (median, mo)	5.3
Response rate	
Partial response	3 (5)
Stable disease	23 (41)
Progressive disease	23 (41)
Not evaluabe	7 (13)
CA 19–9 response (maximal response/baseline)	
> 1	19 (34)
0.5 to 1	15 (27)
< 0.5	10 (18)
not evaluable	10 (18)
not measurable	2 (4)
Advanced disease, OS (median, mo)	
All	24.2
Sequence 1	25.5
Sequence 2	23.0
nab-P + Gem → Gem/Cap → nal-IRI + 5-FU/LV	28.6
other	23.0

with progression on prior irinotecan-based chemotherapy typically received nal-IRI + 5-FU/LV in a later line of therapy (median, 3rd-line) compared with the other sub-groups. Looking specifically at line of advanced disease therapy, there was a significant trend to longer PFS ($p = 0.0031$) and OS ($p = 0.0002$) for patients receiving nal-IRI + 5-FU/LV in earlier lines of therapy, compared with later (Fig. 2).

ECOG performance status at start of nal-IRI + 5-FU/LV treatment was not significantly associated with PFS or OS. Twenty percent of patients in our cohort began treatment with an ECOG performance status of 2. This contrasts with patients treated with nal-IRI + 5-FU/LV in the NAPOLI-1 trial, where only 8.5% of patients began treatment with equivalent Karnofsky performance status of 70 or worse [8]. Starting dose of nal-IRI was also not significantly associated with survival, however, dose-reduction of nal-IRI was. Increasing numbers of dose reductions were associated with increased PFS ($p = 0.016$). There was also a trend to increased OS, though this did not meet statistical significance ($p = 0.073$). Comparing patients with or without any dose reductions, PFS was 5.4 v 2.6 mo ($p = 0.035$), OS was 7.1 v 4.5 mo (not significant, $p = 0.1226$).

Treatment sequences were significantly associated with survival (Fig. 3). Patients receiving Sequence 1 experienced significantly shorter PFS (2.2 v 4.8 mo, $p = 0.0094$) and OS (4.1 v 9.0 mo, $p = 0.0006$) compared with Sequence 2. OS from the time of advanced disease diagnosis was analyzed. Median OS from time of documentation of stage III or IV disease was 24.2 mo for all patients receiving nal-IRI + 5-FU/LV. OS was similar across all sequences of treatment (Table 3). A sequence of particular interest was Sequence 2, with patients receiving frontline Gem with or without nab-P, followed by nal-IRI + 5-FU/LV. Median OS was 23.0 mo.

Safety

Patients were evaluated for toxicity through history and physical exam, complete blood count, and comprehensive metabolic panel. Treatment was discontinued at the discretion of treating physician due to toxicity or progression of disease. The number of dose reductions and attributed reasons for dose reductions are detailed in Table 4. Of the 20 total dose reductions, the most common reasons were for fatigue and diarrhea. Some dose reductions were attributed to multiple reasons. Adverse and serious adverse events are detailed in Table 5. Compared to the pivotal NAPOLI-1 trial, overall toxicity was comparable. There were lower rates of grade 3 or 4 toxicities seen in the MSKCC patient cohort across all of the most common toxicities observed, likely due in part to the lower median starting dose administered.

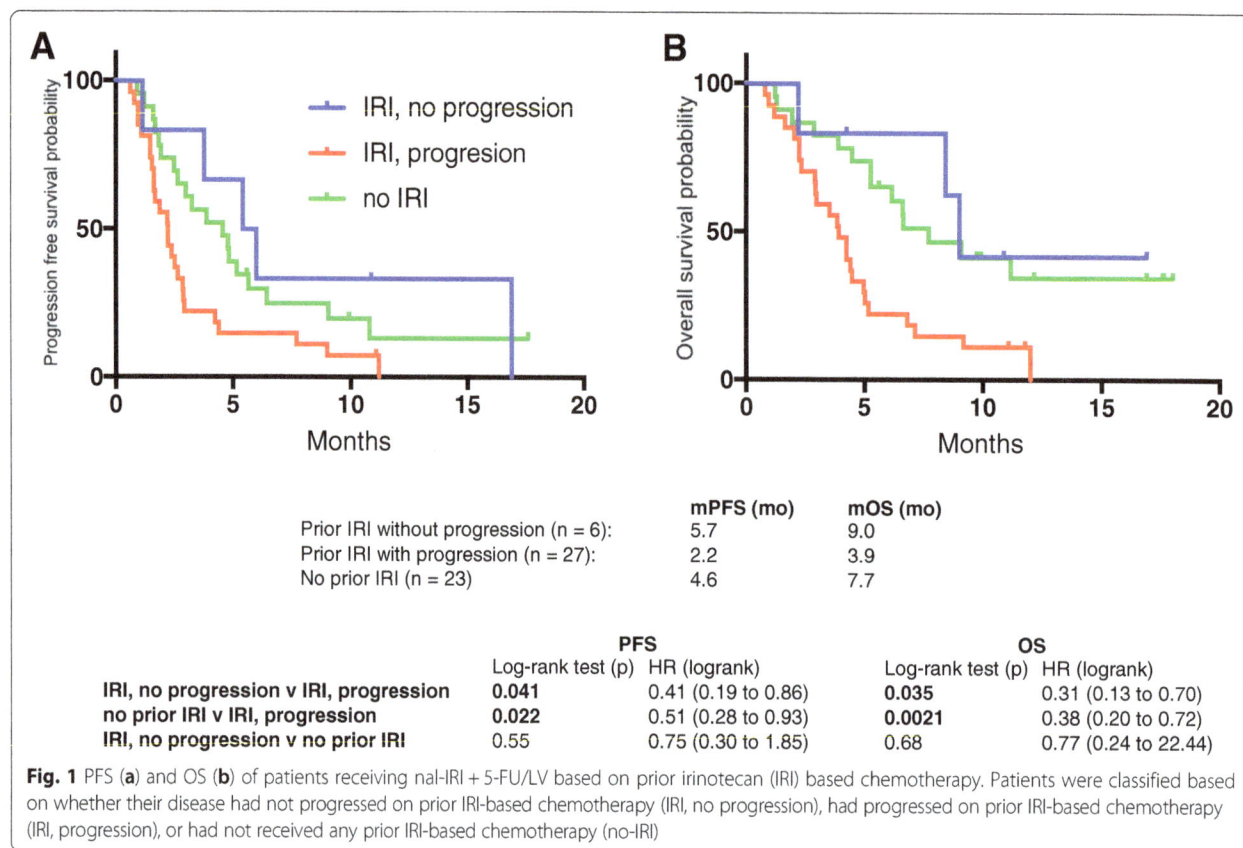

	mPFS (mo)	mOS (mo)
Prior IRI without progression (n = 6):	5.7	9.0
Prior IRI with progression (n = 27):	2.2	3.9
No prior IRI (n = 23):	4.6	7.7

	PFS		OS	
	Log-rank test (p)	HR (logrank)	Log-rank test (p)	HR (logrank)
IRI, no progression v IRI, progression	**0.041**	0.41 (0.19 to 0.86)	**0.035**	0.31 (0.13 to 0.70)
no prior IRI v IRI, progression	**0.022**	0.51 (0.28 to 0.93)	**0.0021**	0.38 (0.20 to 0.72)
IRI, no progression v no prior IRI	0.55	0.75 (0.30 to 1.85)	0.68	0.77 (0.24 to 22.44)

Fig. 1 PFS (**a**) and OS (**b**) of patients receiving nal-IRI + 5-FU/LV based on prior irinotecan (IRI) based chemotherapy. Patients were classified based on whether their disease had not progressed on prior IRI-based chemotherapy (IRI, no progression), had progressed on prior IRI-based chemotherapy (IRI, progression), or had not received any prior IRI-based chemotherapy (no-IRI)

Tumor and germline genomics

Somatic with or without germline genomic results were available for 41 (73%) patients. The most commonly somatic gene mutations identified in the present study are similar to those identified in previously conducted, large genomic studies, and in similar proportions [9–13]. Activating mutations in KRAS were the most commonly identified, found in 83% of patients, followed by inactivating mutations in TP53 (66%), CDKN2A (29%) and SMAD4 (27%) (Additional file 1: Table S1). Germline mutations associated with cancer susceptibility were identified in 21% of patients, a frequency in-line with what our group has recently published in a large patient cohort. [14] BRCA2 was mutated in 3 patients. Although KRAS mutation status was not associated with PFS, TP53 mutation status was associated with significantly shorter PFS (2.2 v 6.0 mo, $p = 0.039$) (Additional file 1: Figure S1). There was a trend to shorter PFS in patients with mutations in SMAD4 and CDKN2A, however, neither of these differences reached statistical significance. Mutations in the four most common somatic genes were not associated with overall survival from the time of advanced disease diagnosis in this cohort. Germline mutations, including those in BRCA1 and BRCA2, were also not associated with differences in PFS or advanced disease overall survival, although

the numbers of patients in these cohorts were exceedingly small.

Discussion

Treatment options for advanced PDAC are expanding but nonetheless finite. Although PDAC remains a challenging disease, the last decade has seen the development of three new and effective combination chemotherapy regimens. The current study is the first report of post-approval, real-world analysis of nal-IRI + 5-FU/LV for the treatment of patients with advanced PDAC. This is also the first study reporting outcomes for patients in an era where two active, combination chemotherapy regimens, FOLFIRINOX and nab-P + Gem, are available for treating patients in the frontline/neoadjuvant settings, and an active, combination chemotherapy regimen, nal-IRI + 5-FU/LV, is available in the second-line setting.

The optimal sequencing of therapy remains undefined, and in practice, is largely defined by patient performance status, age, patient and physician preference. Molecular biomarkers, such as mutations in BRCA1/2 or microsatellite instability, to guide therapy are found in only a small minority of our patients [15]. For patients receiving FOLFIRINOX in the frontline setting, treatment with nab-P + Gem has been studied in a number of cohort studies. One of the largest was performed by the

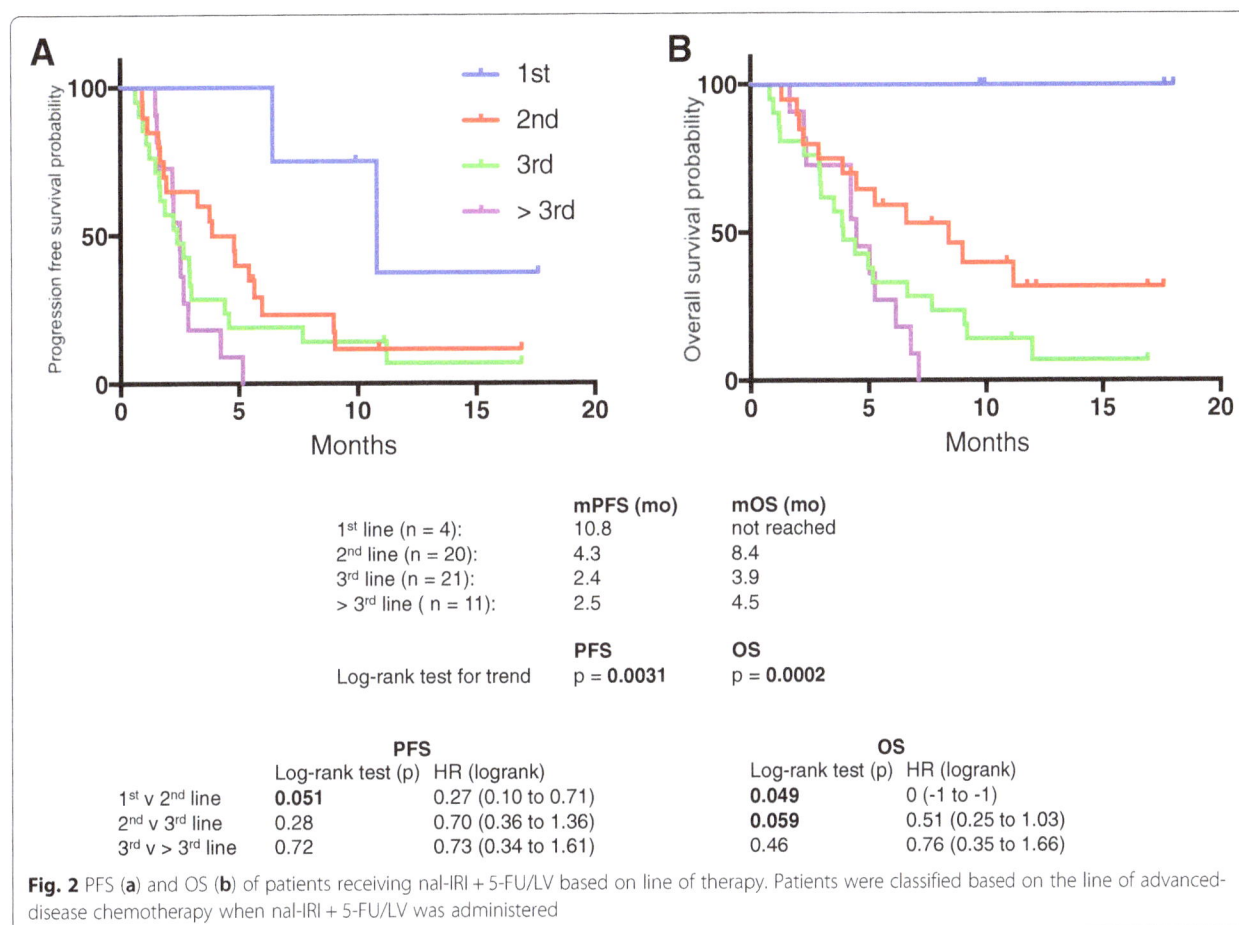

	mPFS (mo)	mOS (mo)
1st line (n = 4):	10.8	not reached
2nd line (n = 20):	4.3	8.4
3rd line (n = 21):	2.4	3.9
> 3rd line (n = 11):	2.5	4.5
	PFS	**OS**
Log-rank test for trend	p = **0.0031**	p = **0.0002**

	PFS		**OS**	
	Log-rank test (p)	HR (logrank)	Log-rank test (p)	HR (logrank)
1st v 2nd line	**0.051**	0.27 (0.10 to 0.71)	**0.049**	0 (-1 to -1)
2nd v 3rd line	0.28	0.70 (0.36 to 1.36)	**0.059**	0.51 (0.25 to 1.03)
3rd v > 3rd line	0.72	0.73 (0.34 to 1.61)	0.46	0.76 (0.35 to 1.66)

Fig. 2 PFS (**a**) and OS (**b**) of patients receiving nal-IRI + 5-FU/LV based on line of therapy. Patients were classified based on the line of advanced-disease chemotherapy when nal-IRI + 5-FU/LV was administered

French AGEO (Association des Gastro-Entérologues Oncologues), [16] which studied a similarly sized cohort (N = 57) as our current study. Portal and colleagues found reasonable PFS (5.1 mo), OS (8.8 mo) and an encouraging median OS of 18 months from the beginning of advanced disease therapy. For patients receiving nab-P + Gem chemotherapy in the frontline setting, a number of 5-FU-based chemotherapy regimens have been studied. Chiorean and colleagues performed a retrospective analysis of patients enrolled in the pivotal MPACT study to evaluate 2nd therapy received [6]. In patients who received 2nd-line therapy, primarily 5-FU-based, after frontline nab-P + Gem, overall survival was 12.8 mo. The most common 5-FU-based regimens administered contained oxaliplatin. Irinotecan-based chemotherapy was uncommon, and none of these individuals received nal-IRI + 5-FU/LV.

Before the approval of nal-IRI + 5-FU/LV, the most common regimens for treatment after failure of gemcitabine-based chemotherapy were FOLFIRI and FOLFOX. The activity of FOLFIRI has been studied in a number of single arm studies. In one of the largest such studies, Zaniboni and colleagues found PFS and OS of 3.2 and 5 mo, respectively [17]. No randomized studies

have been performed to support the efficacy of FOLFIRI in the 2nd line. Two randomized studies investigating the activity of 5-FU and oxaliplatin combinations report conflicting results. The randomized phase III CONKO-003 trial demonstrated a benefit of OFF, a 5-FU and oxaliplatin regimen commonly administered in Europe, compared to 5-FU alone, with PFS of 2.9 v 2.0 mo (p = 0.019), respectively, and OS of 5.9 v 3.3 mo (p = 0.010), respectively [18]. By contrast, the PANCREOX trial demonstrated no benefit of mFOLFOX6 compared with 5-FU, with PFS of 3.1 v 2.9 mo, and surprisingly a detriment in OS, 6.1 v 9.9 mo (p = 0.02) [19]. A single randomized phase II study has compared second line therapy with FOLFIRI to FOLFOX [20]. Both regimens performed similarly, with PFS of 1.9 and 1.4 mo, respectively, and OS of 3.8 and 3.4 mo, respectively. Overall survival from beginning of frontline therapy was 10.8 mo for both groups. A recent meta-analysis performed by Sonbol and colleagues comparing second-line therapies concluded that although both oxaliplatin and irinotecan improved PFS compared with 5-FU alone, only irinotecan appeared to improve OS [21].

Nal-IRI is a liposomal encapsulated formulation of irinotecan with favorable pharmacokinetic properties as

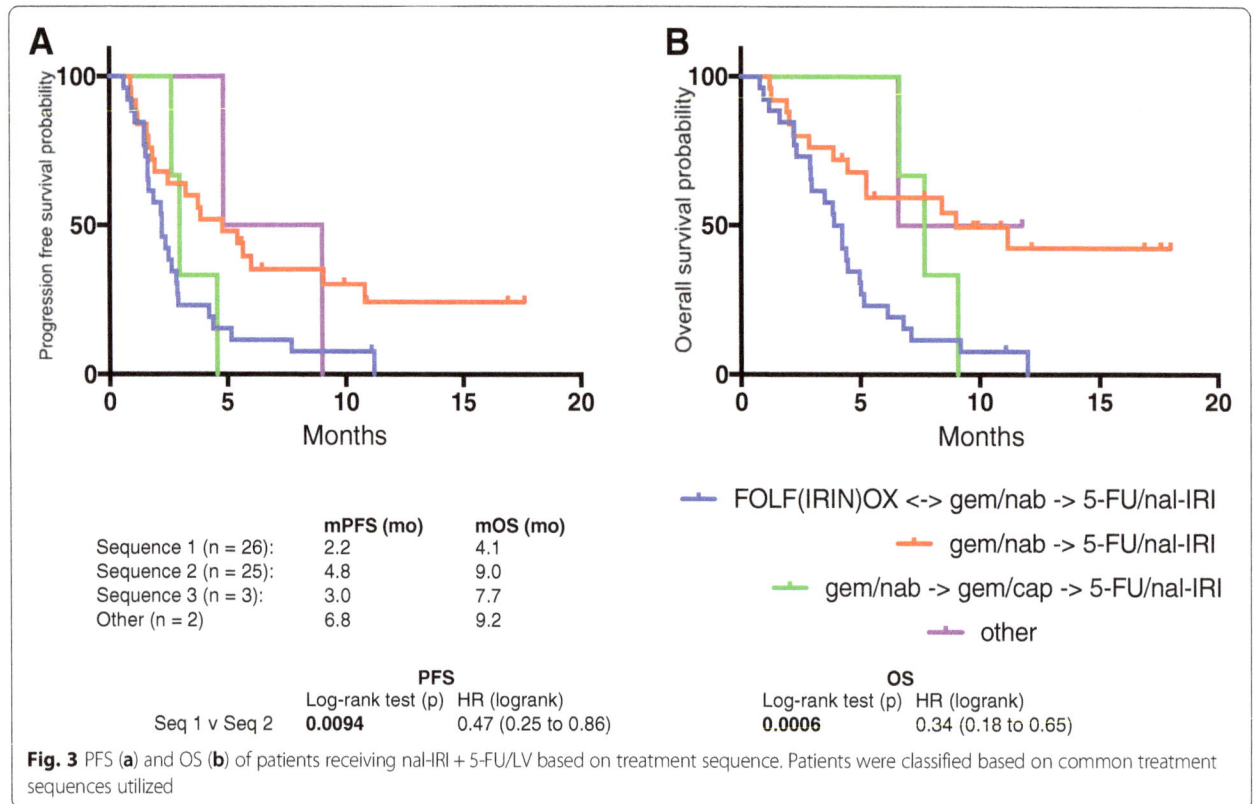

	mPFS (mo)	mOS (mo)
Sequence 1 (n = 26):	2.2	4.1
Sequence 2 (n = 25):	4.8	9.0
Sequence 3 (n = 3):	3.0	7.7
Other (n = 2)	6.8	9.2

	PFS		OS	
	Log-rank test (p)	HR (logrank)	Log-rank test (p)	HR (logrank)
Seq 1 v Seq 2	**0.0094**	0.47 (0.25 to 0.86)	**0.0006**	0.34 (0.18 to 0.65)

Fig. 3 PFS (**a**) and OS (**b**) of patients receiving nal-IRI + 5-FU/LV based on treatment sequence. Patients were classified based on common treatment sequences utilized

demonstrated in preclinical [5] and preliminary clinical studies [22]. These results led to a phase II trial, [23] then the randomized phase III NAPOLI-1 trial. [8] NAPOLI-1 was a global study which enrolled 417 patients who previously received Gem-based chemotherapy. Patients were initially randomized to receive either nal-IRI monotherapy dosed at 120 mg/m^2 every 3 weeks or 5-FU/LV monotherapy dosed at 2000 mg/m^2/continuous infusion over 24 h weekly for 4 out of every

6-week cycle. A third arm, nal-IRI + 5-FU/LV, dosed at nal-IRI (70 mg/m^2) with 5-FU/LV (2400 mg/m^2/continuous infusion over 46 h), was added once the phase II dose of the combination was established. As previously discussed, NAPOLI-1 demonstrated both PFS (3.1 vs 1.5 mo, *p = 0.0001*) and OS benefit (6.1 vs 4.2 mo, *p = 0.012*) of nal-IRI + 5-FU/LV compared with 5-FU. In our current study, PFS (2.88 mo) for all patients treated with similar to that seen in the NAPOLI-1 study. A number of key factors were significantly associated with longer survival, including

Table 4 Dose reductions and attributed reasons for dose reductions of nal-IRI + 5-FU/LV

Number of dose reductions	N = 18 (%)
1	15 (83)
2	3 (17)
Reason attributed for dose	
Fatigue	8 (44)
Diarrhea	8 (44)
Nausea	2 (11)
Neutropenia	2 (11)
Anorexia	2 (11)
Abdominal cramping	1 (6)
Ageusia	1 (6)
Not defined	1 (6)

Table 5 Adverse events and serious (grade 3 or 4) adverse events reported

	MSKCC	
Treatment	nal-IRI + 5-FU/LV	
Patients	56	
toxicities	any grade (%)	grade 3/4 (%)
Nausea	33 (59)	2 (4)
Vomiting	18 (32)	2 (4)
Diarrhea	35 (63)	1 (2)
Fatigue	45 (80)	1 (2)
Anorexia	32 (57)	0 (0)
Neutropenia	16 (29)	1 (2)
Anemia	50 (89)	10 (18)

earlier line of therapy, non-progression on prior irinotecan-based chemotherapy, and dose-reductions while on treatment. In this real-world study, safety was comparable to that seen in the NAPOLI-1 study. The main toxicities seen were fatigue, gastrointestinal toxicities and cytopenias. The incidence of grade 3 or 4 toxicities was low. As part of the NAPOLI-1 study, patients found to be homozygous for the UGT1A1*28 allele were dosed at 50 mg/m^2, then dose escalated to 70 mg/m^2 in the absence of toxicity. Reassuringly, a separate safety analysis of the NAPOLI-1 study found that patients homozygous for the UGT1A1*28 allele (7/117) experienced similar treatment toxicity compared to those without [24]. Patients treated at our institution are not routinely tested for UGT1A1 genotype. Of note, the median starting dose administered of 55 mg/m^2 is below that used in the NAPOLI-1 trial. This pre-emptive dose reduction represents real-world practice patterns and likely played a major role in the low rate of serious adverse events seen. Neither starting dose, nor dose reductions were associated with worse outcomes with regards to PFS or OS. This observation has been made in other regimens used for the treatment of advanced PDAC. For example, Ahn and colleagues found improved safety and promising efficacy when nab-P + Gem was administered at a lower, every other week, frequency [25]. Similarly, FOLFIRINOX with a variety of dose modifications is currently being studied. Two studies have found that dose reductions result in improved safety and similar [26] if not improved [27] efficacy. Lee and colleagues have developed a tool to optimize dose intensity for both toxicity and efficacy and applied their approach to FOLFIRINOX. [28] Studies to systematically examine this and other strategies to improve patient tolerance and outcomes should be undertaken.

With the increased prevalence of tumor somatic and patient germline sequencing, our ability to study the relationship between genomics and treatment response and survival will grow. A number of prior studies have studied gene mutations in KRAS, CDKN2A, TP53 and SMAD4 with regards to survival with mixed results. Hayashi and colleagues found that fewer numbers of mutations in these 4 key genes were associated with better prognosis [29]. Other studies have similarly found low p53 expression, [30] mutations in p16 and TP53, [31] and SMAD4 [32] as predictive of poor prognosis. While mutations in these genes did not correlate with overall survival from advanced stage disease in our patient cohort, there was a correlation between TP53 mutation status and PFS on nal-IRI + 5-FU/LV treatment, with a trend seen for CDKN2A and SMAD4. One preclinical study has previously demonstrated a relationship between TP53 mutation status and irinotecan sensitivity

[33]. While no definitive conclusions can be drawn from a study of this size, our results suggest an interesting pharmacogenomic signal that merits further study and validation in larger, controlled patient cohorts.

The overall survival seen across all sequences of treatment was encouraging. In particular, patients receiving frontline nab-P + Gem followed by 2nd line nal-IRI + 5-FU/LV (*Sequence 2*) experienced an OS of 23.0 mo from the time of advanced disease diagnosis. Patients treated with FOLFIRINOX and nab-P + Gem prior to nal-IRI + 5-FU/LV (*Sequence 1*) also experienced excellent OS (25.5 mo), however, this was not significantly longer. This study represents the first published experience documenting survival in a patient population receiving treatment with access to all modern, FDA-approved chemotherapeutic agents. Given the toxicities experienced by some patients receiving FOLFIRINOX, the excellent survival seen in patients who did not receive FOLFIRINOX (*Sequence 2*) is encouraging and further studies to explore optimal sequencing are warranted. Overall advanced disease survival seen in our study compares favorably to OS reported with sequential nab-P + Gem then 5-FU-based chemotherapy (13.5 mo) [6] and sequential FOLFIRINOX and nab-P + Gem (18 mo). [16] Patient selection is likely a critical issue. Further studies are warranted to confirm the prolonged OS outcomes seen in this study. Patients who received nal-IRI + 5-FU/LV in the frontline metastatic setting experienced prolonged mPFS (10.82 mo) and mOS (not reached), however, the number of patients was very small. The use of nal-IRI for the frontline treatment of patients deserves further evaluation, and an ongoing study (ClinicalTrials.gov Identifier NCT02551991) will hopefully provide a definitive answer to this question.

As a single institution, retrospective analysis, the current study has limitations. Only patients without significant deterioration after prior gemcitabine-based chemotherapy and remained eligible for nal-IRI + 5-FU/LV chemotherapy were included. Patients treated at our tertiary referral center may not experience the same outcomes as patients treated in the community. Nevertheless, our results are encouraging and support continued utilization and study of the nal-IRI + 5-FU/LV regimen to treat patients with advanced pancreatic cancer, and to further optimize selection of patients most likely to benefit.

Conclusions

This real-world study supports the findings of NAPOLI-1, demonstrating the safety and efficacy of nal-IRI + 5-FU/LV for the treatment of advanced PDAC following gemcitabine-based chemotherapy. Patients receiving nal-IRI + 5-FU/LV in earlier lines of therapy, and without irinotecan-refractory disease, experienced significantly longer PFS. Dose reductions were not associated with worse outcomes. Exploratory genetic predictors of response identified candidates which warrant validation. Promising OS was seen integrating nal-IRI + 5-FU/LV sequentially with active combination chemotherapy.

Abbreviations
AE: adverse event; CA 19–9: carbohydrate antigen 19–9; CT: computed tomography; DR: dose reductions; ECOG: Eastern Cooperative Oncology Group; EMR: electronic medical record; FOLFIRINOX: folinic acid, 5-fluorouracil, irinotecan and oxaliplatin; MSKCC: Memorial Sloan Kettering Cancer Center; nab-P + Gem: nab-paclitaxel + gemcitabine; nal-IRI + 5-FU/LV: nanoliposomal irinotecan with fluorouracil/leucovorin; NCI-CTCAE: National Cancer Institute Common Terminology Criteria for Adverse Events; NGS: next generation sequencing; OS: overall survival; PDAC: pancreatic ductal adenocarcinoma; PFS: performance status, progression free survival; SAE: serious adverse event

Acknowledgements
The study has been presented in part at the 2018 Gastrointestinal Cancers Symposium.

Funding
KHY (Research reported in this manuscript was supported by National Cancer Institute of the National Institutes of Health under award number R01CA202762).

Authors' contributions
DCG and KHY conceived and designed the study, DCG, KHY and EOR analyzed and interpreted the data, DCG, RLP, CMC and KHY acquired data, AMD, GYK, JL, JJH, AMV, EOR and KHY enrolled patients and collected patient information and data. DCG, RLP, CMC, AMD, GYK, JL, JJH, AMV, EOR and KHY were involved in drafting and revising the manuscript, gave final approval and agree to be accountable for all aspects of the work regarding accuracy or integrity.

Competing interests
KHY (consultant or advisory role, Ipsen), EOR (consultant or advisory role, Ipsen).

References
1. Siegel RL, Miller KD, Jemal A. Cancer statistics, 2017. CA Cancer J Clin. 2017; 67(1):7–30. https://doi.org/10.3322/caac.21387.
2. Rahib L, Smith BD, Aizenberg R, Rosenzweig AB, Fleshman JM, Matrisian LM. Projecting cancer incidence and deaths to 2030: the unexpected burden of thyroid, liver, and pancreas cancers in the United States. Cancer Res. 2014; 74(11):2913–21. https://doi.org/10.1158/0008-5472.CAN-14-0155.
3. Conroy T, Desseigne F, Ychou M, Bouche O, Guimbaud R, Becouarn Y, et al. FOLFIRINOX versus gemcitabine for metastatic pancreatic cancer. N Engl J Med. 2011;364(19):1817–25. https://doi.org/10.1056/NEJMoa1011923.
4. Von Hoff DD, Ervin T, Arena FP, Chiorean EG, Infante J, Moore M, et al. Increased survival in pancreatic cancer with nab-paclitaxel plus gemcitabine. N Engl J Med. 2013;369(18):1691–703. https://doi.org/10.1056/NEJMoa1304369.
5. Drummond DC, Noble CO, Guo Z, Hong K, Park JW, Kirpotin DB. Development of a highly active nanoliposomal irinotecan using a novel intraliposomal stabilization strategy. Cancer Res. 2006;66(6):3271–7. https://doi.org/10.1158/0008-5472.CAN-05-4007

6. Chiorean EG, Von Hoff DD, Tabernero J, El-Maraghi R, Wee Ma W, Reni M, et al. Second-line therapy after nab-paclitaxel plus gemcitabine or after gemcitabine for patients with metastatic pancreatic cancer. Br J Cancer. 2016;115(9):e13. https://doi.org/10.1038/bjc.2016.306.
7. Abrams TA, Meyer G, Meyerhardt JA, Wolpin BM, Schrag D, Fuchs CS. Patterns of chemotherapy use in a U.S.-based cohort of patients with metastatic pancreatic Cancer. Oncologist. 2017;22(8):925–33. https://doi.org/10.1634/theoncologist.2016-0447.
8. Wang-Gillam A, Li CP, Bodoky G, Dean A, Shan YS, Jameson G, et al. Nanoliposomal irinotecan with fluorouracil and folinic acid in metastatic pancreatic cancer after previous gemcitabine-based therapy (NAPOLI-1): a global, randomised, open-label, phase 3 trial. Lancet. 2016;387(10018):545–57. https://doi.org/10.1016/S0140-6736(15)00986-1.
9. Jones S, Zhang X, Parsons DW, Lin JC, Leary RJ, Angenendt P, et al. Core signaling pathways in human pancreatic cancers revealed by global genomic analyses. Science. 2008;321(5897):1801–6.
10. Yachida S, Jones S, Bozic I, Antal T, Leary R, Fu B, et al. Distant metastasis occurs late during the genetic evolution of pancreatic cancer. Nature. 2010; 467(7319):1114–7.
11. Biankin AV, Waddell N, Kassahn KS, Gingras MC, Muthuswamy LB, Johns AL, et al. Pancreatic cancer genomes reveal aberrations in axon guidance pathway genes. Nature. 2012;491(7424):399–405. https://doi.org/10.1038/nature11547.
12. Waddell N, Pajic M, Patch AM, Chang DK, Kassahn KS, Bailey P, et al. Whole genomes redefine the mutational landscape of pancreatic cancer. Nature. 2015;518(7540):495–501. https://doi.org/10.1038/nature14169.
13. Bailey P, Chang DK, Nones K, Johns AL, Patch AM, Gingras MC, et al. Genomic analyses identify molecular subtypes of pancreatic cancer. Nature. 2016;531(7592):47–52. https://doi.org/10.1038/nature16965.
14. Mandelker D, Zhang L, Kemel Y, Stadler ZK, Joseph V, Zehir A, et al. Mutation detection in patients with advanced Cancer by universal sequencing of Cancer-related genes in tumor and normal DNA vs guideline-based germline testing. JAMA. 2017;318(9):825–35. https://doi.org/10.1001/jama.2017.11137.
15. Lowery MA, Jordan EJ, Basturk O, Ptashkin RN, Zehir A, Berger MF, et al. Real-time genomic profiling of pancreatic ductal adenocarcinoma: potential Actionability and correlation with clinical phenotype. Clin Cancer Res. 2017; 23(20):6094–100. https://doi.org/10.1158/1078-0432.CCR-17-0899.
16. Portal A, Pernot S, Tougeron D, Arbaud C, Bidault AT, de la Fouchardiere C, et al. Nab-paclitaxel plus gemcitabine for metastatic pancreatic adenocarcinoma after Folfirinox failure: an AGEO prospective multicentre cohort. Br J Cancer. 2015;113(7):989–95. https://doi.org/10.1038/bjc.2015.328.
17. Zaniboni A, Aitini E, Barni S, Ferrari D, Cascinu S, Catalano V, et al. FOLFIRI as second-line chemotherapy for advanced pancreatic cancer: a GISCAD multicenter phase II study. Cancer Chemother Pharmacol. 2012;69(6):1641–5. https://doi.org/10.1007/s00280-012-1875-1.
18. Oettle H, Riess H, Stieler JM, Heil G, Schwaner I, Seraphin J, et al. Second-line oxaliplatin, folinic acid, and fluorouracil versus folinic acid and fluorouracil alone for gemcitabine-refractory pancreatic cancer: outcomes from the CONKO-003 trial. J Clin Oncol. 2014;32(23):2423–9. https://doi.org/10.1200/JCO.2013.53.6995.
19. Gill S, Ko YJ, Cripps C, Beaudoin A, Dhesy-Thind S, Zulfiqar M, et al. PANCREOX: a randomized phase III study of fluorouracil/Leucovorin with or without Oxaliplatin for second-line advanced pancreatic Cancer in patients who have received gemcitabine-based chemotherapy. J Clin Oncol. 2016; 34(32):3914–20. https://doi.org/10.1200/JCO.2016.68.5776.
20. Yoo C, Hwang JY, Kim JE, Kim TW, Lee JS, Park DH, et al. A randomised phase II study of modified FOLFIRI.3 vs modified FOLFOX as second-line therapy in patients with gemcitabine-refractory advanced pancreatic cancer. Br J Cancer. 2009;101(10):1658–63. https://doi.org/10.1038/sj.bjc.6605374.
21. Sonbol MB, Firwana B, Wang Z, Almader-Douglas D, Borad MJ, Makhoul I, et al. Second-line treatment in patients with pancreatic ductal adenocarcinoma: a meta-analysis. Cancer. 2017;123(23):4680–6. https://doi.org/10.1002/cncr.30927.
22. Chang TC, Shiah HS, Yang CH, Yeh KH, Cheng AL, Shen BN, et al. Phase I study of nanoliposomal irinotecan (PEP02) in advanced solid tumor patients. Cancer Chemother Pharmacol. 2015;75(3):579–86. https://doi.org/10.1007/s00280-014-2671-x
23. Ko AH, Tempero MA, Shan YS, Su WC, Lin YL, Dito E, et al. A multinational phase 2 study of nanoliposomal irinotecan sucrosofate (PEP02, MM-398) for

patients with gemcitabine-refractory metastatic pancreatic cancer. Br J Cancer. 2013;109(4):920–5. https://doi.org/10.1038/bjc.2013.408.

24. Chen LT, Siveke J, Wang-Gillam A, Hubner R, Pant S, Dragovich T, et al. PD-023Safety across subgroups in NAPOLI-1: a phase 3 study of nal-IRI (MM-398) ± 5-fluorouracil and leucovorin (5-FU/LV) versus 5-FU/LV in metastatic pancreatic cancer (mPAC) previously treated with gemcitabine-based therapy. Ann Oncol. 2016;27(Suppl 2):ii110-ii. https://doi.org/10.1093/annonc/mdw200.23.

25. Ahn DH, Krishna K, Blazer M, Reardon J, Wei L, Wu C, et al. A modified regimen of biweekly gemcitabine and nab-paclitaxel in patients with metastatic pancreatic cancer is both tolerable and effective: a retrospective analysis. Ther Adv Med Oncol. 2017;9(2):75–82. https://doi.org/10.1177/1758834016676011.

26. Li X, Ma T, Zhang Q, Chen YG, Guo CX, Shen YN, et al. Modified-FOLFIRINOX in metastatic pancreatic cancer: a prospective study in Chinese population. Cancer Lett. 2017;406:22–6. https://doi.org/10.1016/j.canlet.2017.07.012.

27. Ohba A, Ueno H, Sakamoto Y, Kondo S, Morizane C, Okusaka T. Retrospective comparison of modified FOLFIRINOX with full-dose FOLFIRINOX for advanced pancreatic cancer: A Japanese cancer center experience. J Clin Oncol. 2018;36(4_suppl):469. https://doi.org/10.1200/JCO.2018.36.4_suppl.469.

28. Lee JC, Kim JW, Ahn S, Kim HW, Lee J, Kim YH, et al. Optimal dose reduction of FOLFIRINOX for preserving tumour response in advanced pancreatic cancer: using cumulative relative dose intensity. Eur J Cancer. 2017;76:125–33. https://doi.org/10.1016/j.ejca.2017.02.010.

29. Hayashi H, Kohno T, Ueno H, Hiraoka N, Kondo S, Saito M, et al. Utility of assessing the number of mutated KRAS, CDKN2A, TP53, and SMAD4 genes using a targeted deep sequencing assay as a prognostic biomarker for pancreatic Cancer. Pancreas. 2017;46(3):335–40. https://doi.org/10.1097/MPA.0000000000000760.

30. Grochola LF, Taubert H, Greither T, Bhanot U, Udelnow A, Wurl P. Elevated transcript levels from the MDM2 P1 promoter and low p53 transcript levels are associated with poor prognosis in human pancreatic ductal adenocarcinoma. Pancreas. 2011;40(2):265–70.

31. Luo Y, Tian L, Feng Y, Yi M, Chen X, Huang Q. The predictive role of p16 deletion, p53 deletion, and polysomy 9 and 17 in pancreatic ductal adenocarcinoma. Pathol Oncol Res. 2013;19(1):35–40. https://doi.org/10.1007/s12253-012-9555-3.

32. Blackford A, Serrano OK, Wolfgang CL, Parmigiani G, Jones S, Zhang X, et al. SMAD4 gene mutations are associated with poor prognosis in pancreatic cancer. Clin Cancer Res. 2009;15(14):4674–9. https://doi.org/10.1158/1078-0432.CCR-09-0227.

33. Abal M, Bras-Goncalves R, Judde JG, Fsihi H, De Cremoux P, Louvard D, et al. Enhanced sensitivity to irinotecan by Cdk1 inhibition in the p53-deficient HT29 human colon cancer cell line. Oncogene. 2004;23(9):1737–44. https://doi.org/10.1038/sj.onc.1207299.

The Warburg effect in human pancreatic cancer cells triggers cachexia in athymic mice carrying the cancer cells

Feng Wang[1*†], Hongyi Liu[2†], Lijuan Hu[1], Yunfei Liu[1], Yijie Duan[1,3], Rui Cui[1] and Wencong Tian[1]

Abstract

Background: Cancer cachexia is a cancer-induced metabolic disorder and a major cause of cancer-induced death. The constituents of cancer cachexia include an increase in energy expenditure, hepatic gluconeogenesis, fat lipolysis, and skeletal-muscle proteolysis and a decrease in body weight. The aetiology of cancer cachexia is unclear and may involve cancer-cell metabolism and secretion. In this study, we investigated whether the high glycolysis in cancer cells (the Warburg effect) triggers cachexia in athymic mice carrying pancreatic cancer cells.

Methods: First, we examined five human pancreatic cancer cell lines for glycolysis and cachectic-cytokine secretion. Consequently, MiaPaCa2 and AsPC1 cells were selected for the present study, because the glycolysis in MiaPaCa2 cells was typically high and that in AsPC1 cells was exceptionally low. In addition, both MiaPaCa2 and AsPC1 cells were competent in the secretion of examined cytokines. Next, we transplanted MiaPaCa2 and AsPC1 cells subcutaneously in different athymic mice for 8 weeks, using intact athymic mice for control. In another experiment, we treated normal mice with the supernatants of MiaPaCa2 or AsPC1 cells for 7 days, using vehicle-treated mice for control. In both models, we measured food intake and body weight, assayed plasma glucose, triglycerides, and TNF-α and used Western blot to determine the proteins that regulated hepatic gluconeogenesis, fat lipolysis, and skeletal-muscle proteolysis in the corresponding tissues. We also studied the effect of MiaPaCa2-cell supernatants on the proteolysis of C2C12 skeletal-muscle cells in vitro.

Results: The athymic mice carrying high-glycolytic MiaPaCa2 cells had anorexia and also showed evidence for cachexia, including increased hepatic gluconeogenesis, fat lipolysis and skeletal-muscle proteolysis and decreased body weight. The athymic mice carrying low-glycolytic AsPC1 cells had anorexia but did not show the above-mentioned evidence for cachexia. When normal mice were treated with the supernatants of MiaPaCa2 or AsPC1 cells, their energy homeostasis was largely normal. Thus, the cachexia in the athymic mice carrying MiaPaCa2 cells may not result from humeral factors released by the cancer cells. In vitro, MiaPaCa2-cell supernatants did not induce proteolysis in C2C12 cells.

Conclusion: The Warburg effect in pancreatic cancer cells is an independent aetiological factor for pancreatic cancer-induced cachexia.

Keywords: Cancer cachexia, The Warburg effect, Pancreatic cancer, Cytokines, Mouse

* Correspondence: fengwangpi@163.com
†Equal contributors
[1]The Institute of Integrative Medicine for Acute Abdominal Diseases, Nankai Hospital, No. 6, Changjiang Road, Nankai, Tianjin 300100, China
Full list of author information is available at the end of the article

Background

Cancer cachexia is a metabolic syndrome present in 50% of all cancer patients and more frequent in the patients with pancreatic cancer [1–4]. The components of cancer cachexia include increased energy expenditure, augmented hepatic gluconeogenesis, uncontrolled fat lipolysis, unrestrained skeletal-muscle proteolysis, and decreased body weight [1, 2]. How these pathologies are initiated to induce cachexia is unclear, but several hypotheses are proposed. For instance, cachectic cytokines such as tumour necrosis factor-α (TNF-α), interferon-γ (IFN-γ), and different interleukins (ILs., e.g. IL-1β and IL-6) may be increased in the peripheral circulation of cancer patients and induce cancer cachexia [1, 2, 5]. In addition to regular cytokines, cancer cells may release cachectic proteins that are not available in normal subjects, such as lipid mobilizing factor (LMF) and proteolysis inducing factor (PIF) [6–9]. Further, the endocrine pancreas may be impaired in cancer patients and, thereafter, involved in cancer cachexia [3, 4, 10–12]. Last but not least, cancer cachexia may be triggered by cancer-cell glycolysis [13–17].

Mammalian cells produce energy primarily by oxidative phosphorylation (36 ATP/glucose). However, cancer cells switch their major way of energy production from oxidative phosphorylation to glycolysis (2 ATP/glucose). The aberrant way of energy production in cancer cells is known as the Warburg effect [18]. To get enough energy by glycolysis, cancer cells over-express key regulators of glycolysis, such as glucose transporters and glycolytic enzymes. Cancer-induced hypoxia-inducible factor-1α (HIF-1α) plays a key role in the over-expression of glucose transporters and glycolytic enzymes [19]. After

HIF-1α is decreased in cancer cells, the Warburg effect in the same cells is decreased as well [13].

The Warburg effect in cancer cells increases total expenditure of glucose and in the meantime produces lactate as waste. In the liver, the lactate is recycled to glucose at cost of energy (Fig. 1a). When the glucose is released into the circulation, cancer cell may take it for glycolysis again (Fig. 1a). The futile glucose-lactate shuttle is called Cori cycle that increases energy expenditure and hepatic gluconeogenesis (Fig. 1b) [20]. Consequently, fat and skeletal muscle undergoes catabolic metabolisms to mobilize more glucose precursors for gluconeogenesis. When such conditions persist, body weight decreases. In this light, the Warburg effect in cancer cells hypothetically triggers cancer cachexia (Fig. 1b). In keeping with this hypothesis were the results from one of our previous studies: When wild-type human pancreatic cancer cells were transplanted in growing athymic mice, the mice showed decreased body-weight gain; when the HIF-1α gene was silenced to inhibit the Warburg effect in the cancer cells, the tumour carrier's body weight was improved [13].

So far, it is unclear whether the Warburg effect in cancer cells induces cachexia independent of other cachexia-inducing abilities the cancer cells possess. It is also unclear whether the levels of cancer-cell glycolysis determine the levels of hepatic gluconeogenesis, fat lipolysis, and skeletal-muscle proteolysis in cancer cachexia. In the present study, we sought to address these questions. However, when cancer cells grow in vivo, they may exercise all cachexia-inducing capabilities to induce the disease, so it is difficult to single out the

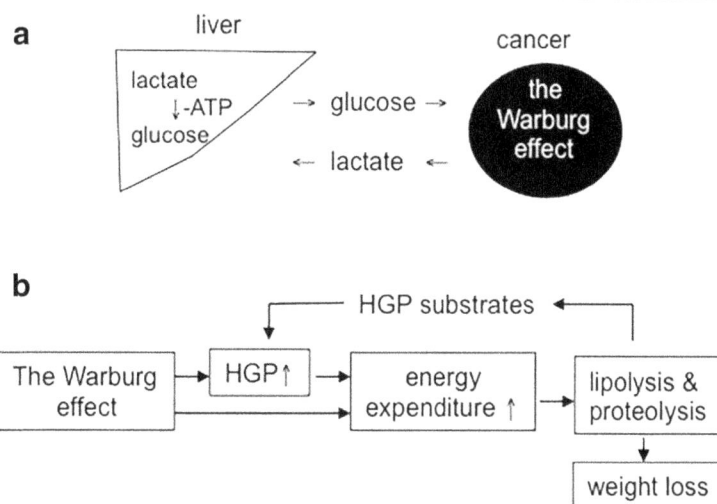

Fig. 1 The Warburg effect and cancer cachexia **a**. The Warburg effect in cancer cells increases glucose expenditure and lactate production in the tumour carrier. The cancer-produced lactate is recycled to glucose in the liver. When the glucose is put back in the blood, cancer cells may take it for glycolysis again. **b** The Warburg effect increases both energy expenditure and hepatic glucose production (HGP). Thus, fat lipolysis and skeletal-muscle proteolysis increase to mobilize more glucose precursors. Consequently, body weight decreases

contribution made by the Warburg effect to the genesis of cancer cachexia.

To overcome this obstacle, we examined five human pancreatic cancer cells for their glycolysis and secretion of TNF-α, IL-1β, and IFN-γ. As a result, we selected for the present study two cell lines namely MiaPaCa2 and AsPC1. The glycolysis levels were typically high in MiaPaCa2 cells and exceptionally low in AsPC1 cells. In addition, both MiaPaCa2 and AsPC1 cells were competent in the secretion of TNF-α, IL-1β, and IFN-γ. In one experiment, these cell lines were implanted in different athymic mice, so the cancer cells may exert all capabilities to induce cachexia. In another experiment, we used the supernatants of these cell lines to treat normal mice to see whether soluble factors from these cells induced cachexia. When data from these models were compared with each other, the role of the Warburg effect in the induction of cancer cachexia was revealed.

Methods
Animals and cancer cells
Normal and athymic Balb/c mice (male) were bought from Hua-Fu-Kang Bioscience (Beijing, China). When mice arrived, they were 4 or 5 weeks old and weighed 17–23 g. After acclimation, they were randomly designated to experimental groups. Throughout experiment, they lived in a room with 12 h/12 h light/dark cycle and had free access to chow and water.

We bought from the Cell Bank of Chinese Academy of Science (Shanghai, China) five human pancreatic

cancer cell lines, i.e. AsPC1 (#CC2404), BxPC3 (#CC2405), HPAF-2 (#CC2407), MiaPaCa2 (#CC2408), and Panc-1 (#CC2401), as well as C2C12 mouse myoblasts (#CC9003). Unless indicated otherwise, all cells were cultured at 37°C in normoxia (95% air and 5% CO_2), using RPMI-1640 media and Dulbecco modified Eagle's media (DMEM) supplemented with foetal bovine serum (FBS, 10%), glutamine (2 mM), penicillin (100 U/ml), and streptomycin (100 μg/ml). Culture media and supplements were bought from the distributor of Gibco Thermo Fisher Scientific in Beijing (China).

Pancreatic cancer cells' Warburg effect and cytokine secretion in vitro
AsPC1, BxPC3, HPAF-2, MiaPaCa2, and Panc-1 cells were cultured till 90% confluence. After rinsing with phosphate buffered saline, these cells were cultured in serum-free media for 6 h in normoxia or hypoxia (1% O_2, 5% CO_2, 94% N_2) [13]. After whole-cell proteins were extracted, glucose transporter-1 (Glut1), hexokinase-2 (HK-II), and phosphofructokinase-1 (PFK-1) were determined by Western blot. Glucose, lactate, TNF-α, IL-1β, and IFN-γ were assayed in removed media. Rongsheng Life Pharmacological (Shanghai, China) and Jiancheng Bio-engineering (Nanjing, China) produced the kits for the glucose and lactate assays. Human TNF-α, IL-1β, and IFN-γ were determined, using ELISA kits from Four-A Biotech (Beijing, China).

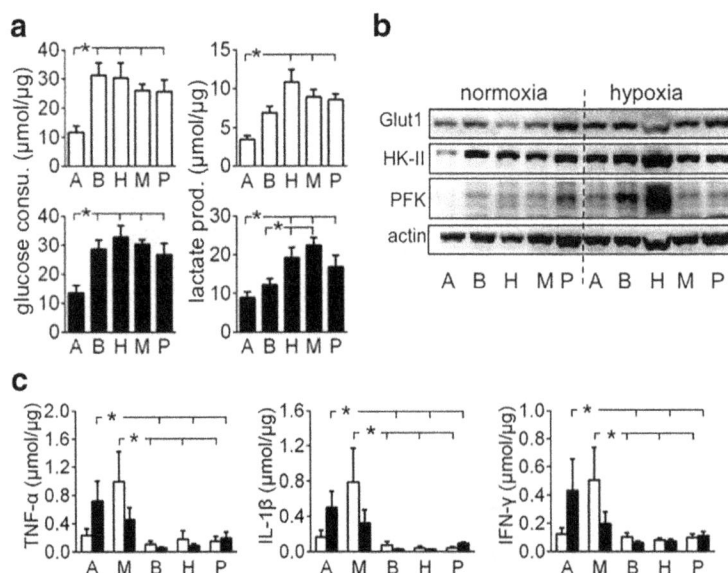

Fig. 2 Pancreatic cancer cell's Warburg effect and cytokine secretion AsPC1 (a), BxPC3 (b), HPAF-2 (H), MiaPaCa2 (M), and Panc-1 (P) pancreatic cancer cells were incubated for 6 h in normoxia or hypoxia. a Glucose and lactate were determined in removed media to assess glucose consumption and lactate production by the cells. Original data were normalized with cellular protein. White bars = normoxia, black bars = hypoxia, n = 12, *P < 0.05. b Glucose transporter-1 (Glut1), hexokinase-2 (HK-II), and phosphofructokinase-1 (PFK-1) were determined by Western blot. c TNF-α, IL-1β, and IFN-γ were determined in removed media. Data were normalized by cellular protein. White bars = normoxia, black bars = hypoxia, n = 6, * P < 0.05

Transplantation of MiaPaCa2 and AsPC1 cells in athymic mice

MiaPaCa2 and AsPC1 cells were suspended in RPMI-1640 media and transplanted subcutaneously in athymic mice (3×10^6 cells/mouse), giving a group of MiaPaCa2-cell carriers ($n = 10$) and a group of AsPC1-cell carriers ($n = 13$). Intact athymic mice were used as normal controls ($n = 14$). In the next 8 weeks, food intake and body weight were recorded on a weekly basis. In the end of week 8, all mice were anesthetized, using 5% chloral hydrate. Blood was collected from the orbital sinus and centrifuged (1500 x g, 10 min, 4°C) to obtain plasma. After mice were killed by cervical dislocation, subcutaneous tumour and inguinal fat pads were removed and weighed. Skeletal muscle was removed from hind legs. The abdominal cavity was opened, epididymal fat pads were removed and weighed, and the liver was sampled. Plasma and tissue samples were kept at – 80°C.

Treating normal mice with the supernatants of MiaPaCa2 or AsPC1 cells

MiaPaCa2 and AsPC1 cells were cultured in different Petri dishes (diameter = 10 cm) till 90% confluence. Then, the cells were incubated in 15 ml serum-free RPMI-1640 medium for 24 h under normoxic conditions. The media that were conditioned by MiaPaCa2 and AsPC1 cells, respectively, were collected. The media were centrifuged to remove debris and then were saved for experiment.

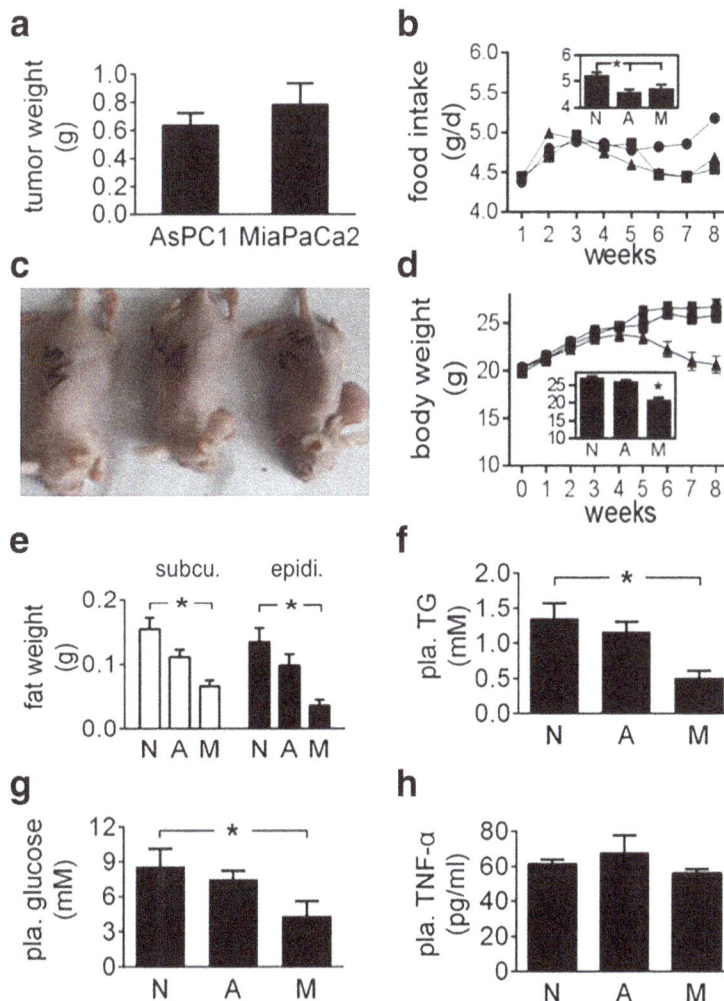

Fig. 3 Energy homeostasis in athymic mice carrying pancreatic cancer cells MiaPaCa2 and AsPC1 cells were transplanted subcutaneously in different athymic mice for 8 weeks, giving group M ($n = 10$) and group A ($n = 13$), respectively. Normal athymic mice were used for control (group N, $n = 14$). **a** Tumour weight. **b** Weekly food intake was plotted. The data of 8 individual weeks were averaged and the results are shown in the inset. **c** Nutritional states in 3 mice representative of groups N (left), A (central), and M (right), respectively. **d** Body weight was plotted for the 8 weeks. The final body weight is shown in the inset. **e** The weight of subcutaneous and epididymal fat. **f-h** Plasma triglyceride (TG), glucose, and TNF-α levels. Data are mean ± SEM (See n in the parentheses). *$P < 0.05$

Normal Balb/c mice were divided in three groups (6 mice per group). Then, they were subjected to subcutaneous injection (0.5 ml, twice a day) of normal control medium or the media that were conditioned by MiaPaCa2 and AsPC1 cells, respectively. After 7 days, all mice were sacrificed as in the preceding experiment.

In a follow-up experiment, normal Balb/c mice were divided in three groups. Mice in two groups (10 mice per group) were subjected to subcutaneous injection of normal control medium or the MiaPaCa2-cell conditioned medium as in the preceding experiment (0.5 ml, twice a day). The mice in the third group ($n = 11$) were subjected to subcutaneous injection of an increased amount of the MiaPaCa2-cell conditioned medium (1.0 ml, twice a day). After 7 days, all mice were sacrificed as described before.

Incubating skeletal-muscle cells with media conditioned by MiaPaCa2 cells

C2C12 mouse myoblasts were cultured in 6-well plates, using DMEM containing 10% FBS. When cells were 95% confluent, they were cultured for 48 h in DMEM with 2% horse serum so as to differentiate to skeletal-muscle cells. Then, the cells were incubated for 4 h in normal control medium or in the medium that was conditioned by MiaPaCa2 cells. Intracellular atrogin-1 and myosin (heavy chain) were determined by Western blotting.

Western blots

We performed Western blots to determine Glut1, HK-II, PFK-1, pyruvate carboxylase (PCB), glucose-6-phosphatase (G-6-Pase), LMF, PIF, atrogin-1, muscle ring finger-1 (MURF1) protein, myosin (heavy chain), insulin-like growth factor binding protein (IGFBP)-3, and adipose triglyceride lipase (ATGL). β-Actin and β-tubulin were used as loading controls. Santa Cruz Biotechnology (Santa Cruz, CA) produced the antibodies for HK-II (#6521), PFK-1 (#377346), LMF (#11238), G-6-Pase (#27196), PCB (#43228), and β-actin (#47778). Abcam (Cambridge, UK) produced the antibodies for Glut1 (#115730) PIF (#52138), MURF1 (#172479), myosin (#124205), and ATGL (#3370–1). ECM Biosciences (Versailles, KY), R&D Systems (Minneapolis, MN), and Proteintech (Chicago, IL) produced the antibodies for atrogin-1 (#AP2041), IGFBP3 (#MAB305), and β-tubulin (#66240–1), respectively.

Tissue samples were homogenized with a mechanical homogenizer, and whole-cell proteins were extracted using RIPA lysis buffer. When proteins were extracted from cultured cells, the lysis buffer was used in the first place. Protein samples were separated in polyacrylamide gel, transferred to polyvinylidene difluoride membrane, and incubated with a primary antibody at 4°C overnight. After rinsing, the membrane was incubated with a secondary antibody at room temperature for 1 h. Specific

blotting was visualized, using an enhanced ECL detection kit.

Other assays

Plasma glucose and lactate were determined, using aforementioned kits. Plasma triglycerides were determined, using a kit produced by Jiancheng Bioengineering (Nanjing,

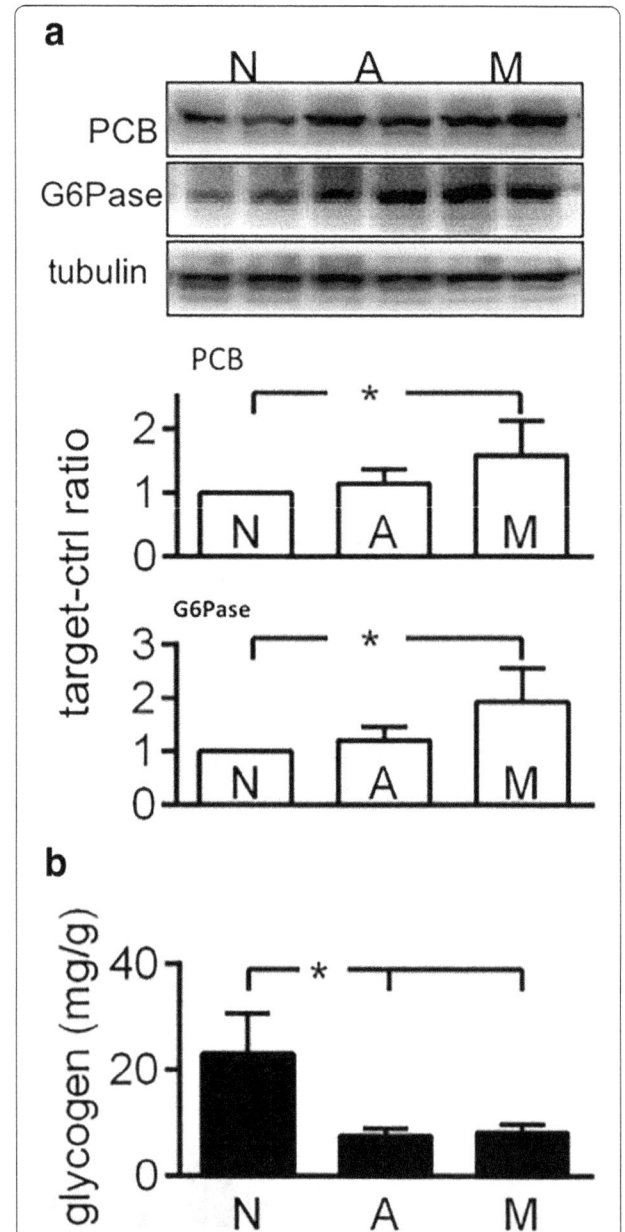

Fig. 4 The effect of tumour carriage on liver metabolism Liver tissues were obtained from normal athymic mice (group N, $n = 14$) and from those that carried MiaPaCa2 (group M, $n = 10$) or AsPC1 cells (group A, $n = 13$). **a** Western blots were performed to determine pyruvate carboxylase (PCB) and glucose-6-phosphatase (G6Pase), using β-tubulin as a loading control. The blots are representative data. The histograms show the results of all mice. **b** Glycogen was determined. Data are mean ± SEM (See n in the parentheses). *$P < 0.05$

China). To determine plasma TNF-α and IL-6, we used an ELISA kit for mouse TNF-α (#E02T0008, Bluegene Biotech, Shanghai, China) and an ELISA kit for mouse IL-6 (DKW12–2060, Dakewei Biotech, Shenzhen, China). When insulin-like growth factor-1 (IGF-1) was determined in skeletal muscle, we used an ELISA kit produced by Elabscience Biotechnology (Wuhan, China). Hepatic glycogen was determined using a kit produced by Jiancheng Bioengineering (Nanjing, China).

Statistics

Data are mean ± SEM. To evaluate difference in groups, we employed the analysis of variance followed with Bonferroni or student-Newman-Keuls post-hoc test. The computer programs of Statistical Product and Service Solutions (version 17.0) and Graph-Pad Prism (version 5.01) were used. $P < 0.05$ was considered statistically significant.

Results

Pancreatic cancer cell lines' Warburg effect and cytokine secretion

Five pancreatic cancer cell lines were incubated for 6 h in normoxia or hypoxia. Glucose and lactate were determined in removed media, and the resulting data were used to assess the Warburg effect. In both normoxia and hypoxia, BxPC3, HPAF-2, MiaPaCa2, and Panc-1 cells had similar levels of Warburg effect, but AsPC1 cells had lower levels of Warburg effect (Fig. 2a). Generally speaking, Glut1, HK-II, and PFK-1 expression were less in AsPC1 cells, than in the other cell lines (Fig. 2b). Further, MiaPaCa2 and AsPC1 cells secreted more TNF-α, IFN-γ, and IL-1β, than the remaining cell lines (Fig. 2c).

Energy homeostasis in athymic mice carrying MiaPaCa2 or AsPC1 cells

The subcutaneous tumours made of MiaPaCa2 and AsPC1 cells had similar weight (Fig. 3a). Both groups of tumour carriers had anorexia, compared to intact mice (Fig. 3b). The body weight of the mice that carried Mia-PaCa2 cells was decreased, as compared to the control value (Fig. 3c and d). No significant decrease was seen in the body weight of the mice that carried AsPC1 cells.

The weight of inguinal and epididymal fat was decreased significantly in the carriers of MiaPaCa2 cells but not AsPC1 cells, as compared to normal values (Fig. 3e), which suggests that lipolysis increased in the former group of tumour carriers but not the latter. Plasma triglycerides were decreased in the carriers of MiaPaCa2 cells, compared to normal value (Fig. 3f), which may a result of increased triglyceride consumption by the tumour carriers [21, 22]. Plasma glucose was decreased in the mice carrying MiaPaCa2 cells, compared to normal value (Fig. 3g). This result was essentially identical to that demonstrated before [23]. Plasma triglyceride and glucose levels were normal in the carriers of AsPC1 cells (Fig. 3f and g). Plasma levels of lactate were normal in both groups of tumour carriers, compared to the control value in the intact mice (data not shown).

Cachectic cytokines in cancer patients are derived from both neoplastic and non-neoplastic cells [1, 2, 5]. In the athymic mouse experiment, we determined plasma level of mouse TNF-α and used it as an index of cachectic cytokines. TNF-α levels in two groups of tumour carriers were not significantly different from those seen in the intact mice (Fig. 3h). This result may be due to the fact that the immune system in athymic mice is incompetent, so the mice in the present study did not release TNF-α in response to the cancer cells. PIF and LMF are cancer-induced cachectic factors [6–8]. We used Western blot to determine PIF and LMF in the plasma of athymic mice. As a result, we found neither of them therein, no matter the mice carried tumours or not (data not shown).

To assess the effect of tumour carriage on hepatic gluconeogenesis, we checked PCB and G-6-Pase expression

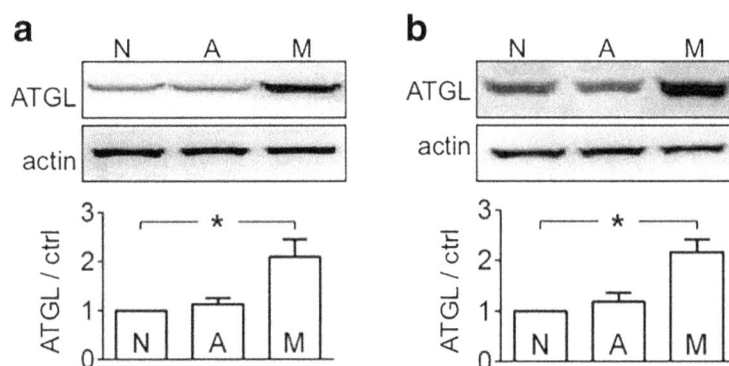

Fig. 5 The effect of tumour carriage on fat lipolysis Inguinal (**a**) and epididymal (**b**) fat were obtained from normal athymic mice (group N, $n = 14$) and from those that carried MiaPaCa2 (group M, $n = 10$) or AsPC1 cells (group A, $n = 13$). Western blots were performed to determine adipose triglyceride lipase (ATGL), using β-actin as a loading control. The blots are representative data. The histograms show the results of all mice (See n in the parentheses). *$P < 0.05$

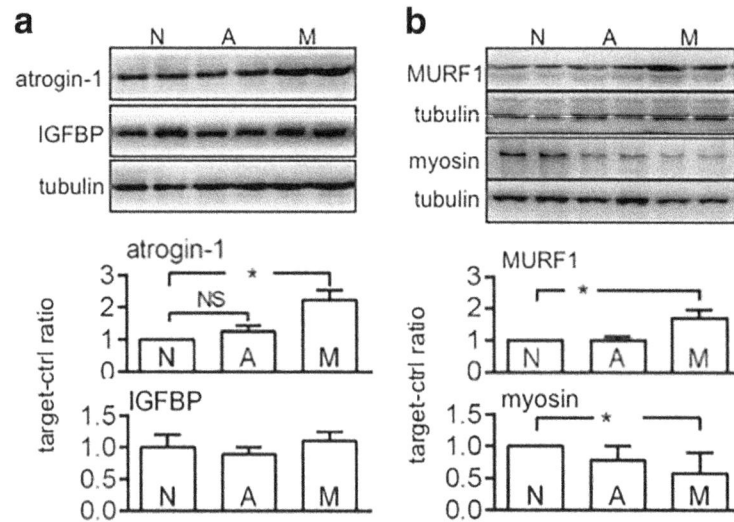

Fig. 6 The effect of tumour carriage on skeletal muscle Skeletal-muscle samples were obtained from normal athymic mice (group N, $n = 14$) and from those that carried MiaPaCa2 (group M, $n = 10$) or AsPC1 cells (group A, $n = 13$). Western blots were performed to determine atrogin-1 (**a**), IGFBP-3 (**a**), myosin (**b**), and MURF1 (**b**), using β-tubulin as a loading control. The blots are representative data. The histograms show the results of all mice (See n in the parentheses). *$P < 0.05$, NS: not significant

in the liver. PCB and G-6-Pase expression were increased significantly when athymic mice carried MiaPaCa2 cells, as compared to reference values seen in intact mice (Fig. 4a). This result suggests that hepatic gluconeogenesis was increased in the mice carrying MiaPaCa2 cells. No significant changes in PCB and G-6-Pase expression were seen when athymic mice carried AsPC1 cells (Fig. 4a). However, hepatic glycogen was decreased significantly in both groups of tumour carriers (Fig. 4b), compared to reference value in intact mice. ATGL regulates cancer-induced lipolysis [24]. When athymic mice carried MiaPaCa2 cells, ATGL

expression was increased in both inguinal and epididymal fat pads, compared to reference values in intact mice (Fig. 5). This result suggests that adipose tissues in these tumour carriers underwent increased lipolysis. No significant increase was seen in ATGL expression when athymic mice carried AsPC1 cells (Fig. 5).

Skeletal-muscle proteolysis is regulated by atrogin-1 and MURF1, and skeletal-muscle protein biosynthesis is regulated by IGF-1 [25–27]. In addition, the amount of free (active) IGF-1 is regulated by IGFBPs [28, 29]. In the present study, the athymic mice carrying MiaPaCa2 cells

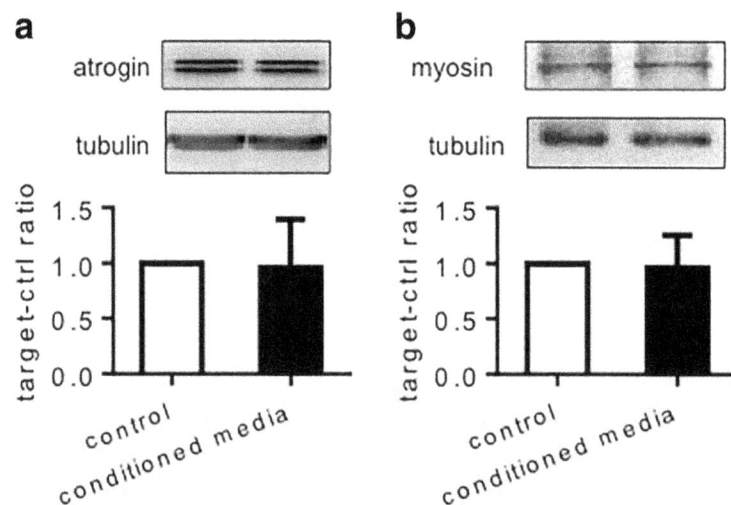

Fig. 7 Atrogin-1 and myosin expression by C2C12 cells in vitro C2C12 cells were incubated for 4 h in normal control medium or MiaPaCa2 cell-conditioned medium. Atrogin-1 and myosin were determined by Western blot, using β-tubulin as a loading control. The blots are representative data. The histograms summarize data from 6 experiments

showed increased atrogin-1 and MURF1 expression, normal IGFBP-3 expression, and decreased myosin expression in skeletal muscle, compared to reference values in intact mice (Fig. 6). However, IGF-1 contents in the same skeletal-muscle samples were similar to the normal value in intact mice (data not shown). Thus, the skeletal muscle in the carriers of MiaPaCa2 cells had an increased proteolysis without compensation in protein biosynthesis. When the same parameters were checked in the athymic mice that carried AsPC1 cells, no significant changes were seen (Figs. 6a–c). When we incubated C2C12 skeletal-muscle cells in the medium conditioned by MiaPaCa2 cells, the cells showed normal atrogin-1 and myosin expression, compared to reference data seen in the C2C12 cells that were incubated in normal medium (Fig. 7). Thus, the supernatants of MiaPaCa2 cells may not induce proteolysis in skeletal-muscle cells.

Energy homeostasis in mice treated with the supernatants of MiaPaCa2 or AsPC1 cells

When athymic mice carried MiaPaCa2 cells, the expression of PCB, G-6-Pase, ATGL, atrogin-1, MURF1, and myosin were changed in the liver, fat, and skeletal muscle, respectively. If these changes were induced by humoral factors that were released by MiaPaCa2 cells, the same results may be seen again when normal mice were subjected to the supernatants of MiaPaCa2 cells. After we treated normal mice with the supernatants of MiaPaCa2 and AsPC1 cells, we did not see any significant changes in the expression of PCB, G-6-Pase, ATGL, atrogin-1, and IGFBP-3, as compared to reference values seen in the mice that were treated with vehicle (Fig. 8).

After normal mice were treated with MiaPaCa2- or AsPC1-cell supernatants, food intake, body weight, and plasma levels of glucose and lactate were not changed

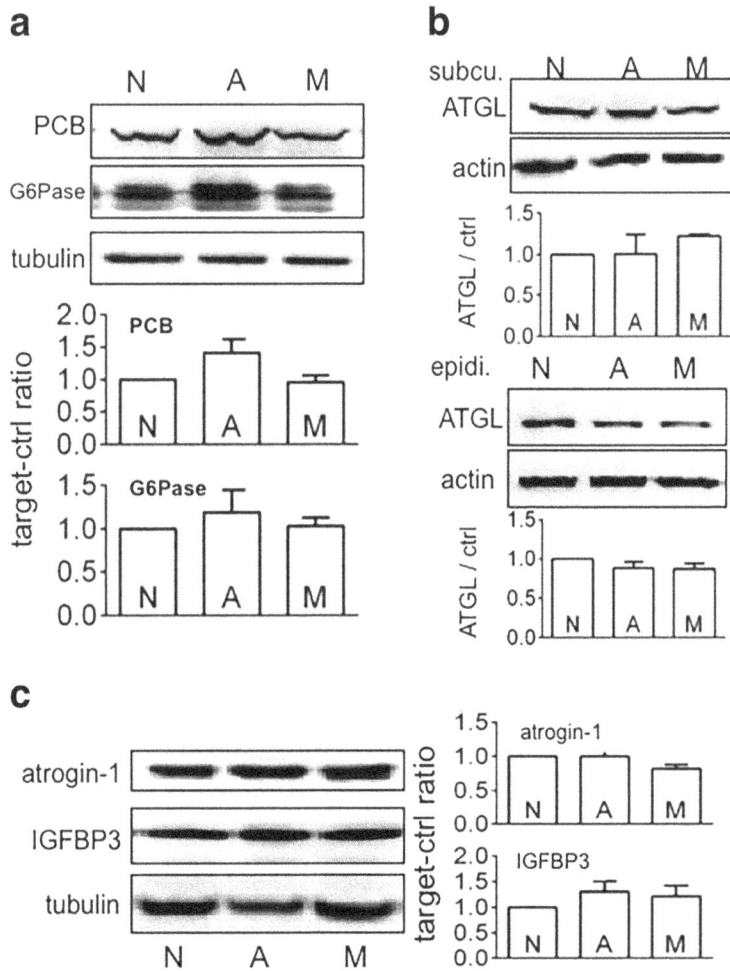

Fig. 8 The effects of MiaPaCa2 or AsPC1-cell supernatants on hepatic, fat, and skeletal-muscle metabolisms Normal mice in 3 groups (6 mice/group) were subjected to subcutaneous injection (0.5 ml, twice a day) of normal control medium (group N) or the media that were conditioned by MiaPaCa2 cells (group M) or by AsPC1 cells (group A). After 7 days, all mice were sacrificed. Their liver, fat, and skeletal muscle were obtained. Western blots were performed, using β-tubulin and β-actin as loading controls. a PCB and G6Pase expression in the liver. b ATGL expression in subcutaneous and epididymal fat. c Atrogin-1 and IGFBP-3 expression in skeletal muscle. Blots are representative results. The histograms show the results of all mice

significantly, as compared to reference values seen in the mice treated with vehicle (Fig. 9a–d). Plasma triglycerides were decreased when mice were treated with the supernatants of MiaPaCa2 cells but not AsPC1 cells, compared to reference value seen in the mice treated with vehicle (Fig. 9e). Of note, the decrease in plasma triglycerides was comparable to that seen when athymic mice carried MiaPaCa2 cells (Fig. 3f). Taken together, MiaPaCa2 cells may secrete something that increased the utilization of triglycerides in these mice. When mouse TNF-α was determined in plasma, a significant increase was seen in the mice that were treated with the supernatants of MiaPaCa2 cells but not AsPC1 cells, as compared to reference value seen in the mice treated with vehicle (Fig. 9f). In the follow-up experiment, we treated normal mice with two doses of MiaPaCa2-cell supernatants, one being as in the preceding experiment and the other being twice as much. The increase in MiaPaCa2-cell supernatants did not change food intake and body weight, but it did induce a significant increase in plasma glucose (Fig. 10a-c). IL-6 may be a key regulator of cancer cachexia [30]. However, MiaPaCa2 cells did not release IL-6 [31]. When we determined mouse IL-6 in the plasma, no significant difference was found in the different groups of mice (Fig. 10d).

Discussion

In recent years, a big progress has been made in the research for cancer cachexia [32]. For instance, there is an international consensus on both definition and classification of cancer cachexia [33]. In addition, ketone-body metabolism is known to play a role in cancer cachexia [34]. The mechanism by which cancer cachexia suppresses anti-tumour immunity is defined [30, 35]. So is the mechanism by which malignant tumours trigger white adipose tissue browning [36–38].

Several lines of evidence have supported the hypothesis that the Warburg effect in cancer cells triggers cancer cachexia [13–17]. However, this hypothesis has not been tested systemically. In the present study, high-glycolytic MiaPaCa2 cells increased hepatic gluconeogenesis, fat lipolysis, and skeletal-muscle proteolysis in the athymic mice carrying the cancer cells. On the other hand, energy homeostasis in the athymic mice carrying low-glycolytic AsPC1 cells was largely normal with the exception of anorexia and decreased hepatic glycogen. Anorexia is usually induced by anorectic cytokines (e.g. TNF-α, IFN-γ, and IL-1β) and neuropeptides [1, 39]. When these factors are increased in cancer patients, they attack the part of hypothalamus that regulates appetite to induce anorexia [1].

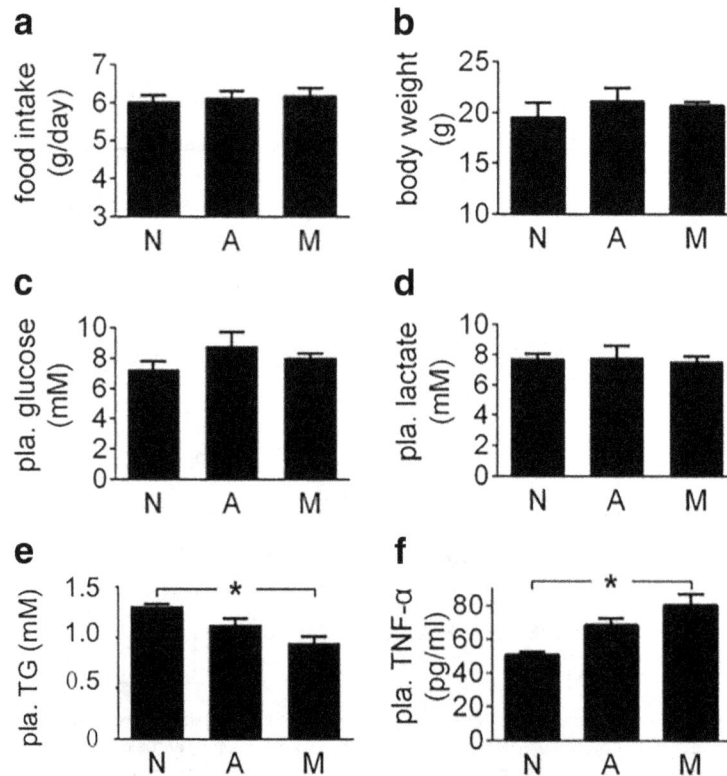

Fig. 9 The effects of MiaPaCa2 or AsPC1-cell supernatants on energy homeostasis See the legend of Fig. 8 for study design. **a** Daily food intake was averaged for the 7-day experiment. **b** Final body weight. **c-f** Plasma levels of glucose, lactate, triglycerides (TG), and TNF-α; *P < 0.05

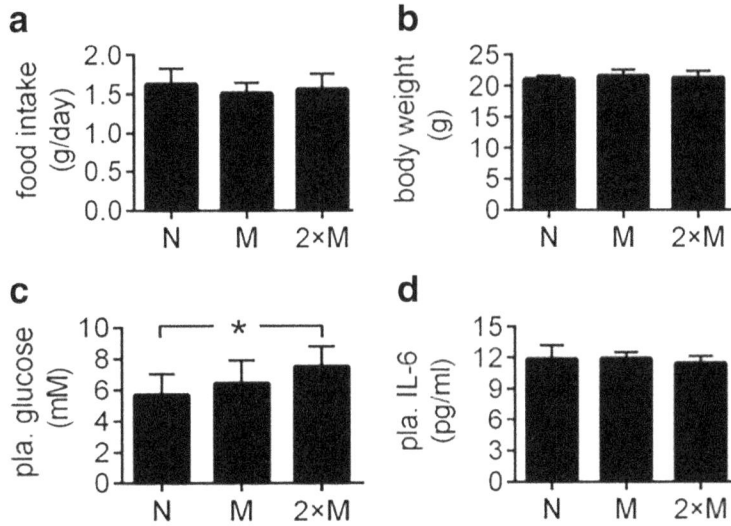

Fig. 10 The effects of different amounts of MiaPaCa2-cell supernatants on energy homeostasis Mice in 2 groups (10 mice/group) were injected (s.c.) with 0.5 ml of MiaPaCa2-cell supernatants (group M) or vehicle (group N) for 7 days. In the meantime, mice in a third group (n = 11) were injected with 1.0 ml of the MiaPaCa2-cell supernatants (group 2×M). **a** Daily food intake was averaged for the 7 days. **b** Final body weight. **c** Plasma levels of glucose. **d** Plasma levels of IL-6. *$P < 0.05$

Numerous studies have shown evidence that glucose, lipid, and protein turnover are increased in cancer patients [14–17]. Radioactive tracers are usually used to demonstrate the increase in nutrient turnover [14–16]. Sometimes, cancer-induced increase in glucose turnover is seen as a decrease in circulating glucose [23]. In keeping with this notion, plasma glucose was decreased when athymic mice carried high-glycolytic MiaPaCa2 cells.

Cancer cells may induce cachexia by secreting cachectic cytokines [1, 2]. In addition to cancer cells, macrophages and other non-cancer cells may release cachectic cytokines in the presence of cancer [1, 5]. When cachectic cytokines are increased in peripheral circulation, they may target liver, skeletal muscle, and fat to induce cachexia. In the present study, both MiaPaCa2 and AsPC1 cells secreted cachectic TNF-α, IL-1β, and IFN-γ in vitro. However, energy homeostasis was largely undisturbed when normal mice were treated with the supernatants of MiaPaCa2 and AsPC1 cells. Thus, the cachexia seen in the athymic mice carrying MiaPaCa2 cells may not be induced by humoral factors released by these cells.

In the present study, MiaPaCa2 and AsPC1 cells did not release PIF and LMF. Using immunohistochemical methods, Kamoshida and co-workers looked for PIF and LMF in five human pancreatic cancer cell lines (including MiaPaCa2) carried by athymic mice. Three cell lines (including MiaPaCa2) had neither PIF nor LMF, and two cell lines showed weak expression of PIF or LMF, respectively [9].

Orthotopic and subcutaneous transplantation of human pancreatic cancer cells in athymic mice are two models that are frequently used in pancreatic-cancer research. When pancreatic cancer cells are transplanted orthotopically, they may cause ascetic fluid, jaundice, and liver metastasis, and these intra-abdominal complications may induce cachectic states directly [40]. This being the case, we chose the subcutaneous model for the present study. Unfortunately, the subcutaneous model cannot be used to study how the endocrine pancreas is involved in pancreatic cancer-induced cachexia. However, previous studies have showed that the endocrine pancreas is impaired in pancreatic cancer, and the impairment in turn contributes to the pathogenesis of pancreatic cancer-induced cachexia [3, 4, 10–12, 41, 42]. For instance, when pancreatic cancer was induced in hamsters, the endocrine pancreas showed a decrease in insulin-producing cells and an increase in other hormonal cells [41]. In addition, the circulating profiles of pancreatic hormones were changed in the hamsters with pancreatic cancer [42]. Similar abnormalities in the anatomy and function of the endocrine pancreas are also seen in pancreatic cancer patients [3, 4, 10–12].

Data from the present study suggest that the Warburg effect in pancreatic cancer cells drives the pathogenesis of pancreatic cancer-induced cachexia. Inhibiting the Warburg effect in pancreatic cancer cells may attenuate the cachexia induced by pancreatic cancer [13, 43, 44].

Conclusion

The Warburg effect in pancreatic cancer cells triggers metabolic abnormalities in liver, fat, and skeletal muscle and thus induces cachexia. Inhibiting the Warburg effect in pancreatic cancer cells may help the tumour carrier restore energy homeostasis.

Abbreviations

ATGL: Adipose triglyceride lipase; ELISA: Enzyme-linked immunosorbent assay; G-6-Pase: Glucose-6-phosphatase; Glut1: Glucose transporter-1; HGP: Hepatic glucose production; HK-II: Hexokinase-2; IFN-γ: Interferon-γ; IGF-1: Insulin-like growth factor-1; IGFBP: IGF binding protein; IL: Interleukin; LMF: Lipid mobilizing factor; MURF1: Muscle ring finger-1; PCB: Pyruvate carboxylase; PFK-1: Phosphofructokinase-1; PIF: Proteolysis inducing factor; TNF-α: Tumour necrosis factor-α

Acknowledgements

Not applicable.

Funding

Natural Science Foundation of China supported the work [No. 81572318]. The foundation played no role in the study design and collection, analysis, and interpretation of data.

Authors' contributions

FW conceived, designed, and described the study. YD screened five cell lines to find appropriate ones for mouse experiments. HL, LH and YL were involved in different experiments, with LH being mainly in the experiment of cancer supernatants and YL in the experiment of athymic mice. RC and WT performed the experiment regarding LMF and PIF. All authors have read and approved the manuscript.

Authors' information

No special information.

Competing interests

The authors declare that they have no competing interests.

Author details

[1]The Institute of Integrative Medicine for Acute Abdominal Diseases, Nankai Hospital, No. 6, Changjiang Road, Nankai, Tianjin 300100, China. [2]The Post-doctoral Working Station, Tianjin Medical University, Tianjin 300070, China. [3]Present Address: The Centre of Disease Control, Dagang, Tianjin 300270, China.

References

1. Tisdale MJ. Mechanisms of cancer cachexia. Physiol Rev. 2009;89:381–410.
2. Tayek JA. A review of cancer cachexia and abnormal glucose metabolism in humans with cancer. J Am Coll Nutr. 1992;11:445–56.
3. Schwarts SS, Zeidler A, Moossa AR, Kuku SF, Rubenstein AH. A prospective study of glucose tolerance, insulin, C-peptide, and glucagon responses in patients with pancreatic carcinoma. Am J Dig Dis. 1978;23:1107–14.
4. Permert J, Ihse I, Jorfeldt L, von Schenck H, Arnqvist HJ, Larsson J. Pancreatic cancer is associated with impaired glucose metabolism. Eur J Surg. 1993;159:101–7.
5. Martignoni ME, Kunze P, Hildebrandt W, Künzli B, Berberat P, Giese T, et al. Role of mononuclear cells and inflammatory cytokines in pancreatic cancer-related cachexia. Clin Cancer Res. 2005;11:5802–8.
6. Todorov P, Cariuk P, McDevitt T, Coles B, Fearon K, Tisdale M. Characterization of a cancer cachectic factor. Nature. 1996;379:739–42.
7. Todorov PT, Field WN, Tisdale MJ. Role of a proteolysis-inducing factor (PIF) in cachexia induced by a human melanoma (G361). Br J Cancer. 1999;80:1734–7.
8. Todorov PT, McDevitt TM, Meyer DJ, Ueyama H, Ohkubo I, Tisdale MJ. Purification and characterization of a tumor lipid-mobilizing factor. Cancer Res. 1998;58:2353–8.
9. Kamoshida S, Watanabe K, Suzuki M, Mizutani Y, Sakamoto K, Sugimoto Y, et al. Expression of cancer cachexia-related factors in human cancer xenografts: an immunohistochemical analysis. Biomed Res. 2006;27:275–81.
10. Pour PM, Permert J, Mogaki M, Fujii H, Kazakoff K. Endocrine aspects of exocrine cancer of the pancreas. Their patterns and suggested biologic significance. Am J Clin Pathol. 1993;100:223–30.
11. Permert J, Larsson J, Westermark GT, Herrington MK, Christmanson L, Pour PM, et al. Islet amyloid polypeptide in patients with pancreatic cancer and diabetes. N Engl J Med. 1994;330:313–8.
12. Cersosimo E, Pisters PW, Pesola G, McDermott K, Bajorunas D, Brennan MF. Insulin secretion and action in patients with pancreatic cancer. Cancer. 1991;67:486–93.
13. Wang F, Li SS, Segersvärd R, Strömmer L, Sundqvist KG, Holgersson J, et al. Hypoxia inducible factor-1 mediates effects of insulin on pancreatic cancer cells and disturbs host energy homeostasis. Am J Pathol. 2007;170:469–77.
14. Burt ME, Lowry SF, Gorschboth C, Brennan MF. Metabolic alterations in a noncachectic animal tumor system. Cancer. 1981;47:2138–46.
15. Lundholm K, Edström S, Karlberg I, Ekman L, Scherstén T. Glucose turnover, gluconeogenesis from glycerol, and estimation of net glucose cycling in cancer patients. Cancer. 1982;50:1142–50.
16. Torosian MH, Bartlett DL, Chatzidakis C, Stein TP. Effect of tumor burden on futile glucose and lipid cycling in tumor-bearing animals. J Surg Res. 1993;55:68–73.
17. Edén E, Edström S, Bennegård K, Scherstén T, Lundholm K. Glucose flux in relation to energy expenditure in malnourished patients with and without cancer during periods of fasting and feeding. Cancer Res. 1984;44:1718–24.
18. Warburg O, Wind F, Negelein E. The metabolism of tumours in the body. J Gen Physiol. 1927;8:519–30.
19. Semenza GL, Wang GL. A nuclear factor induced by hypoxia via de novo protein synthesis binds to the human erythropoietin gene enhancer at a site required for transcriptional activation. Mol Cell Biol. 1992;12:5447–54.
20. Waterhouse C, Keilson J. Cori cycle activity in man. J Clin Invest. 1969;48:2359–66.
21. Wang F, Kumagai-Braesch M, Herrington MK, Larsson J, Permert J. Increased lipid metabolism and cell turnover of MiaPaCa2 cells induced by high-fat diet in an orthotopic system. Metabolism. 2009;58:1131–6.
22. Shaw JH, Wolfe RR. Fatty acid and glycerol kinetics in septic patients and in patients with gastrointestinal cancer. The response to glucose infusion and parenteral feeding. Ann Surg. 1987;205:368–76.
23. Zhang D, Cui L, Li SS, Wang F. Insulin and hypoxia-inducible factor-1 cooperate in pancreatic cancer cells to increase cell viability. Oncol Lett. 2015;10:1545–50.
24. Das SK, Eder S, Schauer S, Diwoky C, Temmel H, Guertl B, et al. Adipose triglyceride lipase contributes to cancer-associated cachexia. Science. 2011;333:233–8.
25. Eley HL, Tisdale MJ. Skeletal muscle atrophy, a link between depression of protein synthesis and increase in degradation. J Biol Chem. 2007;282:7087–97.
26. Schwarzkopf M, Coletti D, Sassoon D, Marazzi G. Muscle cachexia is regulated by a p53-PW1/Peg3-dependent pathway. Genes Dev. 2006;20:3440–52.
27. Saini A, Nasser AL, Stewart CEH. Waste management - cytokines, growth factors and cachexia. Cytokine Growth Factor Rev. 2006;17:475–86.
28. Foulstone EJ, Savage PB, Crown AL, Holly JM, Stewart CE. Adaptations of the IGF system during malignancy: human skeletal muscle versus the systemic environment. Horm Metab Res. 2003;35:667–74.
29. Huang XY, Huang ZL, Yang JH, Xu YH, Sun JS, Zheng Q, et al. Pancreatic cancer cell-derived IGFBP-3 contributes to muscle wasting. J Exp Clin Cancer Res. 2016;35:46.
30. Flint TR, Janowitz T, Connell CM, Roberts EW, Denton AE, Coll AP, et al. Tumor-induced IL-6 reprograms host metabolism to suppress anti-tumor immunity. Cell Metab. 2016;24:672–84.
31. Block KM, Hanke NT, Maine EA, Baker AF. IL-6 stimulates STAT3 and Pim-1 kinase in pancreatic cancer cell lines. Pancreas. 2012;41:773–81.
32. Petruzzelli M, Wagner EF. Mechanisms of metabolic dysfunction in cancer-associated cachexia. Genes Dev. 2016;30:489–501.
33. Fearon K, Strasser F, Anker SD, Bosaeus I, Bruera E, Fainsinger RL, et al. Definition and classification of cancer cachexia: an international consensus. Lancet Oncol. 2011;12:489–95.
34. Shukla SK, Gebregiworgis T, Purohit V, Chaika NV, Gunda V, Radhakrishnan P, et al. Metabolic reprogramming induced by ketone bodies diminishes pancreatic cancer cachexia. Cancer Metab. 2014;2:18.

35. Flint TR, Fearon DT, Janowitz T. Connecting the Metabolic and Immune Responses to Cancer. Trends Mol Med. 2017;23:451–64.

36. Kir S, White JP, Kleiner S, Kazak L, Cohen P, Baracos VE, et al. Tumour-derived PTH-related protein triggers adipose tissue browning and cancer cachexia. Nature. 2014;513:100–4.

37. Petruzzelli M, Schweiger M, Schreiber R, Campos-Olivas R, Tsoli M, Allen J, et al. A switch from white to brown fat increases energy expenditure in cancer-associated cachexia. Cell Metab. 2014;20:433–47.

38. Abdullahi A, Jeschke MG. Taming the flames: targeting white adipose tissue browning in hypermetabolic conditions. Endocr Rev. 2017;38:538–49.

39. Matthys P, Dijkmans R, Proost P, Van Damme J, Heremans H, Sobis H, et al. Severe cachexia in mice inoculated with interferon-gamma-producing tumor cells. Int J Cancer. 1991;49:77–82.

40. Hotz HG, Reber HA, Hotz B, Yu T, Foitzik T, Buhr HJ, et al. An orthotopic nude mouse model for evaluating pathophysiology and therapy of pancreatic cancer. Pancreas. 2003;26:e89–98.

41. Asano N, Manabe T, Imanishi K, Tobe T. Changes of A, B and D cells in Langerhans islets in pancreatic cancers of hamsters. Nihon Geka Hokan. 1991;60:233–42.

42. Permert J, Herrington M, Kazakoff K, Pour PM, Adrian TE. Early changes in islet hormone secretion in the hamster pancreatic cancer model. Teratog Carcinog Mutagen. 2001;21:59–67.

43. Xiao H, Li S, Zhang D, Liu T, Yu M, Wang F. Separate and concurrent use of 2-deoxy-D-glucose and 3-bromopyruvate in pancreatic cancer cells. Oncol Rep. 2013;29:329–34.

44. Hu L, Cui R, Liu H, Wang F. Emodin and rhein decrease hypoxia-inducible factor-1α in human pancreatic cancer cells and attenuate cancer cachexia in athymic mice carrying the cancer cells. Oncotarget. 2017;8:88008–20.

Trends in pancreatic adenocarcinoma incidence and mortality in the United States in the last four decades; a SEER-based study

Anas M. Saad[1†], Tarek Turk[2†], Muneer J. Al-Husseini[3†] and Omar Abdel-Rahman[4,5*] (iD)

Abstract

Background: Pancreatic cancer is the fourth-leading cause of cancer deaths in the United States. The silent nature of the disease and its poor prognosis, the need for further research, along with the need to assess the outcomes of current approaches necessitate an ongoing evaluation of the epidemiology and mortality-trends of this malignancy. Continuous monitoring of disease-patterns, on population-levels, may help scientists assess the quality of healthcare delivery, boost their understanding of diseases' characteristics and risk factors, and detect gaps whereby further research is needed. None of the previous reports shed light on pancreatic adenocarcinomas (PAC), the most common type of Pancreatic Cancer, as the primary outcome. In this study we aim to investigate PAC's incidence and mortality trends over the last four decades in the United States.

Methods: We used SEER 9 database to study PAC cases during 1974-2014. Incidence and mortality rates were calculated by sex, age, race, state and stage of PAC. Annual percent change (APC) was calculated using joinpoint regression software.

Results: We reviewed 67,878 PAC cases; most of these cases were in the head of pancreas. Overall PAC incidence rates increased 1.03% (95% CI, 0.86-1.21, p <.001) per year over the study period. Rates of adenocarcinoma of the head of pancreas increased 0.87% (95% CI, 0.68-1.07, p <.001), and rates of adenocarcinoma of the body and tail of pancreas increased 3.42% (95% CI, 3.06-3.79, p <.001) per year during 1973-2014. PAC incidence-based mortality increased 2.22% (95% CI, 1.93-2.51, p <.001) per year. However, during 2012-2014 there was a statistically significant decrease in PAC incidence-based mortality; APC, -24.70% (95% CI, -31.78 - -16.88, p <.001).

Conclusion: PAC's incidence and mortality rates have been increasing for decades. However, the last few years have shown a promising decrease in mortality. We believe that further advances in healthcare delivery and research can lead to a further mortality decrease. Future studies can use this paper as a baseline to keep monitoring the outcomes of PAC's therapy.

Keywords: Incidence, Mortality, Pancreatic adenocarcinoma, SEER

* Correspondence: omar.abdelrhman@med.asu.edu.eg
†Anas M. Saad, Tarek Turk and Muneer J. Al-Husseini contributed equally to this work.
[4]Clinical Oncology Department, Faculty of Medicine, Ain Shams University, Lofty Elsayed Street, Cairo 11566, Egypt
[5]Department of Oncology, University of Calgary and Tom Baker Cancer Center, Calgary, Alberta, Canada
Full list of author information is available at the end of the article

Background

Pancreatic cancer (PC) is an intractable malignancy, and the fourth-leading cause of cancer deaths in the United States, with an estimated of 55 440 new cases, and 44 330 deaths in 2018 [1]. It relatively constitutes a smaller percentage of all cancers' deaths around the globe (7.2%). However, it is one of the most fatal types of cancers with a five-year relative survival rate of 8% [1, 2]. The vast majority (85%) of pancreatic malignancies are adenocarcinomas arising in exocrine glands of the pancreas [3]. Other less common histologies include neuroendocrine tumors such as gastrinoma, insulinoma, somatostatinoma, glucagonoma and non-functional islet cells tumors. Pancreatic adenocarcinoma (PAC) is most commonly diagnosed in the head and neck of the pancreas [2].

At its early stages, pancreatic cancer is usually symptom-free [4]. Upon tumor progression, it manifests as a gradual onset of nonspecific symptoms including jaundice, light-colored stools, abdominal pain, weight loss and fatigue [1]. The available diagnostic tests can also be nonspecific and may miss patients with early stage disease [4]. Surgery, radiotherapy and chemotherapy are traditionally used to extend survival and/or relieve patients' symptoms. However, there is still no definite cure for advanced-stage cases [5]. The silent nature of the disease and its poor prognosis, the need for further research and new local and systemic therapies, along with the need to assess the outcomes of these approaches necessitate an ongoing evaluation of the epidemiology and mortality trends of this malignancy.

The Surveillance, Epidemiology, and End Results (SEER) program of the National Cancer Institute has been collecting data on cancer epidemiology for decades [3]. Such continuous monitoring of disease-patterns, on population-levels, may help scientists to assess the quality of healthcare delivery as well as boost their understanding of diseases' characteristics and risk factors, and detect gaps where further research and interventions are needed [3, 6, 7]. In pancreatic carcinomas, several reports described the trends of incidence and survival [8, 9]. However, these reports varied in conclusions. In addition, recent data show that PC new cases have been rising on average 0.5% each year over the past ten years [3]. Furthermore, none of the previous reports shed light on pancreatic adenocarcinomas as the primary outcome. Therefore, in this study, we aim to add a piece to the puzzle by investigating PAC's incidence and incidence-based mortality trends over the last four decades in the United States.

Methods

Data source

We used the SEER*stat software (version 8.3.4) to obtain data of PAC cases diagnosed during 1973-2014 from SEER nine registries [10]. "Incidence - SEER 9 Regs Research Data, Nov 2016 Sub (1973-2014) <Katrina/Rita Population Adjustment>"database covers approximately 9.4% of the US population (based on 2010 census) [11].

Study population

The study included patients with PAC diagnosed during 1973-2014; 'Site Recode ICD-O-3/WHO 2008 classification' and 'Histology recode - broad groupings' variables were used for this selection. We excluded cases whose diagnosis relied only on autopsy or death certificates. Within this population, we looked into the following variables: sex, age at diagnosis, race, state, stage at diagnosis (using SEER historic stage A) and site of the tumor within the pancreas (using the 'primary site' variable).

Outcomes

We calculated two main outcomes: incidence and incidence-based mortality rates. All rates were adjusted to the 2000 US standard population and expressed by 100 000 person-years. These rates were calculated during 1973-2014 according to demographic and tumor characteristics. Incidence-based mortality rates were calculated as the number of pancreatic cancer deaths among cases diagnosed over person-time at risk among people in the SEER areas [12]. Rates for Washington and Georgia were calculated starting from 1974 and 1975; respectively, as recording of cases started in these areas after these dates.

Then we calculated the Annual Percentage Changes (APCs) of incidence and incidence-based mortality rates over the study period according to baseline demographic and tumor characteristics.

Statistical analysis

The SEER*stat software (version 8.3.4) was used to calculate all incidence and incidence-based mortality rates. The National Cancer Institute's Joinpoint Regression program, version 4.5.0.1 was used to calculate APCs [13]. The Joinpoint Regression software used t tests to determine if APCs were statistically significant from zero; difference was considered statistically significant when $P < .05$. The software analyzed rates over time and detected significant changes in APCs, then selected the best model with the minimum number of joinpoints [14]. All statistical tests were two sided.

Results

Baseline characteristics

We reviewed 67 878 PAC cases that were diagnosed from 1973 - 2014 and met our inclusion criteria (Table 1). Most of these cases were white (55 222 patients [81.35%]), older than 60 years (51,573 patients [75.98%]), and had a metastatic cancer (38 852 patients [57.24%]). The most

Table 1 Pancreatic adenocarcinoma Incidence rates (1973-2014)

Characteristic	Incidence of pancreatic adenocarcinoma		Incidence of adenocarcinoma of the head of pancreas		Incidence of adenocarcinoma of the body and tail of pancreas	
	Cases, No (%)[a]	Rate (95% CI)[b]	Cases, No (%)[a]	Rate (95% CI)[b]	Cases, No (%)[a]	Rate (95% CI)[b]
Overall	67,878 (100)	6.95 (6.90 - 7.00)	33,728 (100)	3.46 (3.42 - 3.50)	14,321 (100)	1.46 (1.43 - 1.48)
Sex						
Male	35,062 (51.65)	8.16 (8.07 - 8.24)	17,033 (50.50)	3.98 (3.92 - 4.04)	7,666 (53.53)	1.76 (1.72 - 1.81)
Female	32,816 (48.35)	5.99 (5.93 - 6.06)	16,695 (49.50)	3.05 (3.00 - 3.09)	6,655 (46.47)	1.22 (1.19 - 1.25)
Race						
White	55,222 (81.35)	6.77 (6.71 - 6.83)	27,492 (81.51)	3.37 (3.33 - 3.42)	11,414 (79.70)	1.40 (1.37 - 1.42)
Black	7,797 (11.49)	9.85 (9.63 -10.08)	3,961 (11.74)	5.02 (4.86 - 5.19)	1,727 (12.06)	2.16 (2.05 - 2.27)
Others[c]	4,755 (7.01)	5.80 (5.63 - 5.97)	2,229 (6.61)	2.72 (2.61 - 2.84)	1,153 (8.05)	1.39 (1.31 - 1.48)
Unknown[d]	104 (0.15)	-	46 (0.14)	-	27 (0.19)	-
Age at diagnosis, y						
<60	16,305 (24.02)	1.93 (1.90 - 1.96)	7,729 (22.92)	0.92 (0.90- 0.94)	3,750 (26.19)	0.44 (0.43 - 0.46)
>60	51,573 (75.98)	32.28 (32.00 - 32.56)	25,999 (77.08)	16.30 (16.10 - 16.50)	10,571 (73.81)	6.58 (6.46 - 6.71)
State[e]						
California	10,960 (16.15)	7.06 (6.93 - 7.20)	5,563 (16.49)	3.60 (3.50 - 3.69)	2,347 (16.39)	1.50 (1.44-1.56)
Connecticut	10,906 (16.07)	7.41 (7.27 - 7.55)	5,363 (15.90)	3.64 (3.54 - 3.74)	2,306 (16.10)	1.57 (1.51-1.63)
Georgia	5,113 (7.53)	7.09 (6.89 - 7.29)	2,585 (7.66)	3.61 (3.46 - 3.75)	1,178 (8.22)	1.61 (1.52-1.71)
Hawaii	2,955 (4.35)	6.47 (6.23 - 6.71)	1,316 (3.90)	2.88 (2.73 - 3.04)	700 (4.89)	1.53 (1.41-1.64)
Iowa	9,079 (13.38)	6.75 (6.61 - 6.89)	4,631 (13.73)	3.42 (3.33 - 3.53)	1,941 (13.55)	1.46 (1.39-1.52)
Michigan	12,539 (18.47)	7.87 (7.73 - 8.01)	6,182 (18.33)	3.89 (3.79 - 3.99)	2,556 (17.85)	1.60 (1.53-1.66)
New Mexico	3,890 (5.73)	6.09 (5.89 - 6.28)	1,928 (5.72)	3.01 (2.87 - 3.15)	671 (4.69)	1.04 (0.96-1.12)
Utah	3,172 (04.67)	5.32 (5.13 - 5.51)	1,581 (4.69)	2.67 (2.54 - 2.81)	667 (4.66)	1.11 (1.02-1.19)
Washington	9,264 (13.65)	6.68 (6.55 - 6.82)	4,579 (13.58)	3.31 (3.22 - 3.41)	1,955 (13.65)	1.40 (1.34-1.47)
Stage at diagnosis[f]						
Localized	5,796 (8.54)	0.60 (0.58 - 0.62)	3,678 (10.90)	0.38 (0.37 - 0.40)	1,123 (7.84)	0.11 (0.11 - 0.12)
Regional	18,623 (27.43)	1.90 (1.88 - 1.93)	13,193 (39.12)	1.35 (1.33 - 1.37)	2,140 (14.94)	0.22 (0.21 - 0.23)
Distant	38,852 (57.24)	3.96 (3.92 - 3.998)	14,685 (43.54)	1.50 (1.47 - 1.52)	10,600 (74.02)	1.08 (1.06 - 1.10)
Unstaged	4,607 (6.79)	0.48 (0.47-0.50)	2,172 (6.44)	0.23 (0.22-0.24)	458 (3.20)	0.05 (0.04-0.05)

[a]Cases included first primary tumors that matched the selection criteria, were microscopically confirmed, and were not identified only from autopsy records or death certificates
[b]Rates were calculated as number of cases per 100,000 person-years and age adjusted to the 2000 US standard population
[c]Includes American Indian/Alaskan Native and Asian/Pacific Islander
[d]Rates for patients with unknown race could not be calculated, as 'race' is a population variable and must be known to calculate rates
[e]Rates were calculated between 1973-2014 for all states except Georgia; 1975-2014, and Washington; 1974-2014
[f]Using SEER historic stage A

common sub-site for PAC was the head (33 728 patients [49.69%]), followed by the body and tail (14 321 patients [21.1%]). Additional file 1, shows 2014 incidence rates according to demographic and tumor factors. Additional file 2 shows pancreatic adenocarcinoma incidence rates in each individual year from 1973 to 2014.

During the study period, 63 426 eligible cases died of pancreatic cancer and were included in the incidence-based mortality analysis (Table 2). Most of these deaths occurred in whites (51 742 [81.58%]), people older than 60 years (49 994 [78.82%]), and had a metastatic cancer (37 327 [58.85%]). Additional file 3

shows 2014 incidence-based mortality rates according to demographic and tumor factors. Additional file 4 shows pancreatic adenocarcinoma incidence-based mortality rates in each individual year from 1973 to 2014.

Incidence rates and trends over time

PAC incidence rates were highest among males (8.16 [95% CI, 8.07 - 8.24]), blacks (9.85 [95% CI, 9.63 -10.08]), and people older than 60 years (32.28 [95% CI, 32.00 - 32.56]) (Table 1).

PAC incidence rates increased 1.03% (95% CI, 0.86-1.21, $p<.001$) per year over the study period. Rates

Table 2 Pancreatic adenocarcinoma Incidence-based mortality rates (1973-2014)

characteristic	Incidence-based mortality of pancreatic adenocarcinoma		Incidence-based mortality of adenocarcinoma of the head of pancreas		Incidence-based mortality of adenocarcinoma of the body and tail of pancreas	
	Cases, No (%)[a,b]	Rate (95% CI)[c]	Cases, No (%)[a,b]	Rate (95% CI) [c]	Cases, No (%)[a,b]	Rate (95% CI) [c]
Overall	63,426 (100)	6.52 (6.47 - 6.57)	31,609 (100)	3.26 (3.22 - 3.30)	12,859 (100)	1.32 (1.29 - 1.39)
Sex						
Male	32,771 (51.67)	7.73 (7.65 - 7.82)	15,975 (50.54)	3.79 (3.73 - 3.86)	6,903 (53.68)	1.61 (1.57 - 1.65)
Female	30,655 (48.33)	5.58 (5.52 - 5.64)	15,634 (49.46)	2.84 (2.79 - 2.89)	5,956 (46.32)	1.09 (1.06 - 1.11)
Race						
White	51,742 (81.58)	6.36 (6.30 - 6.41)	25,815 (81.67)	3.18 (3.14 - 3.22)	10,289 (80.01)	1.26 (1.24 - 1.28)
Black	7,309 (11.52)	9.42 (9.19 - 9.64)	3,736 (11.82)	4.84 (4.68 – 5.00)	1,557 (12.11)	1.99 (1.89 - 2.09)
Others[d]	4,313 (6.80)	5.34 (5.18 - 5.50)	2,030 (6.42)	2.52 (2.41 - 2.64)	997 (7.75)	1.22 (1.15 - 1.30)
Unknown[e]	62 (0.10)	-	28 (0.09)	-	16 (0.13)	-
Age at death, y						
<60	13,432 (21.18)	1.59 (1.56 - 1.62)	6,358 (20.11)	0.75 (0.73 - 0.77)	2,869 (22.31)	0.34 (0.33 - 0.35)
>60	49,994 (78.82)	31.45 (31.16 - 31.73)	25,251 (79.89)	15.93 (15.73 - 16.13)	9,990 (77.69)	6.25 (6.13 - 6.38)
State[f]						
California	10,192 (16.07)	6.60 (6.47 - 6.73)	5,196 (16.44)	3.38 (3.29 - 3.47)	2,092 (16.27)	1.35 (1.29 - 1.41)
Connecticut	10,146 (16.00)	6.90 (6.76 - 7.03)	4,991 (15.79)	3.39 (3.30 - 3.49)	2,077 (16.15)	1.41 (1.35 - 1.47)
Georgia	4,635 (7.30)	6.57 (6.38 - 6.77)	2,362 (7.47)	3.38 (3.24 - 3.52)	1,012 (7.87)	1.41 (1.33 - 1.51)
Hawaii	2,776 (4.38)	6.11 (5.88 - 6.34)	1,245 (3.94)	2.75 (2.60 - 2.91)	631 (4.91)	1.38 (1.27 - 1.49)
Iowa	8,556 (13.49)	6.31 (6.17 - 6.44)	4,383 (13.87)	3.22 (3.12 - 3.32)	1,767 (13.74)	1.31 (1.25-1.37)
Michigan	11,916 (18.79)	7.52 (7.38 - 7.66)	5,882 (18.61)	3.73 (3.63 - 3.82)	2,350 (18.27)	1.48 (1.42 -1.54)
New Mexico	3,660 (5.77)	5.77 (5.59 - 5.97)	1,817 (5.75)	2.86 (2.73 - 3.00)	613 (4.77)	0.96 (0.88 - 1.04)
Utah	2,948 (4.65)	4.99 (4.81 - 5.17)	1,471 (4.65)	2.51 (2.38 - 2.64)	591 (4.60)	0.99 (0.91 -1.07)
Washington	8,597 (13.55)	6.25 (6.12 - 6.38)	4,262 (13.48)	3.11 (3.02 - 3.21)	1,726 (13.42)	1.25 (1.19-1.31)
Stage at diagnosis[g]						
Localized	4,656 (7.34)	0.49 (0.47 - 0.50)	3,250 (10.28)	0.34 (0.33 - 0.35)	610 (4.74)	0.06 (0.06 - 0.07)
Regional	16,977 (26.77)	1.75 (1.72- 1.78)	12,083 (38.23)	1.25 (1.22 - 1.27)	1,878 (14.60)	0.19 (0.18 - 0.20)
Distant	37,327 (58.85)	3.81 (3.78 - 3.85)	14,170 (44.83)	1.45 (1.42 - 1.47)	9,929 (77.21)	1.01 (0.99 - 1.03)
Unstaged	4,466 (7.04)	0.47 (0.46-0.48)	2,106 (6.66)	0.22 (0.21-0.23)	442 (3.45)	0.05 (0.04-0.05)

[a]Cases included first primary tumors that matched the selection criteria, were microscopically confirmed, and were not identified only from autopsy records or death certificates
[b]No. (%) of deaths were based on cases diagnosed during 1973-2014
[c]Rates were calculated as number of deaths per 100 000 person-years and age adjusted to the 2000 US standard population
[d]Includes American Indian/Alaskan Native and Asian/Pacific Islander
[e]Rates for patients with unknown race could not be calculated, as 'race' is a population variable and must be known to calculate rates
[f]Rates were calculated between 1973-2014 for all states except Georgia; 1975-2014, and Washington; 1974-2014
[g]Using SEER historic stage A

did not increase significantly during 1983-1999; APC, -0.18% (95% CI,-0.56 - 0.20, p = .35), but increased 2.43% (95% CI, 2.11-2.74, p <.001) per year during 1999-2014. PAC incidence rates increased for all sex, race, age, state and stage sub-groups. Table 3 describes PAC incidence trends during 1973-2014 by sex, race, age at diagnosis and stage. Additional file 5 summarizes PAC incidence trends by geographical distribution.

Rates of adenocarcinoma of the head of pancreas increased 0.87% (95% CI, 0.68-1.07, p <.001), and rates of adenocarcinoma of the body and tail of pancreas

increased 3.42% (95% CI, 3.06-3.79, p <.001) per year during 1973-2014. Adenocarcinoma of the head of pancreas increased during 1973-2014 for sex, race, age and stage sub-groups except for blacks group and localized stage group, which did not increase significantly. Adenocarcinoma of the body and tail of pancreas increased during 1973-2014 for all sex, race, age and stage sub-groups. Figure 1 shows incidence trends for selected characteristics. Additional file 6 summarizes adenocarcinoma of the head of pancreas, and adenocarcinoma of the body and tail of pancreas incidence trends by sex, race, age at diagnosis and stage.

Table 3 Trends in Pancreatic adenocarcinoma Incidence Rates (1973-2014)

| | Overall (1973-2014) | | Trends | | | | | | | | |
| | | | 1 | | | 2 | | | 3 | | |
	APC[a] (95% CI)	P value[b]	year	APC[a] (95% CI)	P value[b]	year	APC[a] (95% CI)	P value[b]	year	APC[a] (95% CI)	P value[b]
Overall	1.03 (0.86-1.21)	<.001	1973-1983	1.84 (0.97-2.71)	<.001	1983-1999	-0.18 (-0.56-0.20)	.35	1999-2014	2.43 (2.11-2.74)	<.001
Sex											
Male	0.88 (0.69-1.06)	<.001	1973-1983	1.10 (0.11-2.09)	.03	1983-1999	-0.25 (-0.69-0.20)	0.27	1999-2014	2.33 (1.97-2.69)	<.001
Female	1.16 (0.97-1.36)	<.001	1973-1984	2.49 (1.40-3.59)	<.001	1984-1999	-0.27 (-0.87-0.34)	.37	1999-2014	2.54 (2.09-3.00)	<.001
Race											
White	1.09 (0.91-1.28)	<.001	1973-1983	1.77 (0.84-2.70)	<.001	1983-1999	-0.14 (-0.55-0.28)	0.50	1999-2014	2.59 (2.24-2.95)	<.001
Black	0.65 (0.43-0.87)	<.001	1973-1986	1.85 (0.31-3.40)	.02	1986-1998	-0.73 (-2.20-0.76)	.32	1998-2014	1.47 (0.76-2.18)	<.001
Others[c]	0.89 (0.61-1.18)	<.001	1973-2006	0.26 (-0.09-0.62)	.14	2006-2009	8.41 (-7.86-27.55)	.32	2009-2014	-1.21 (-4.41-2.10)	.46
Age at diagnosis, y											
<60	0.38 (0.18-0.59)	<.001	1973-1984	0.91 (-0.16-1.98)	0.09	1984-1993	-2.14 (-3.76- -0.50)	0.01	1993-2014	1.48 (1.16-1.80)	<.001
>60	1.23 (1.05-1.40)	<.001	1973-1984	2.11 (1.32-2.90)	<.001	1984-1999	-0.07 (-0.50-0.36)	.74	1999-2014	2.58 (2.26-2.91)	<.001
Stage at diagnosis[d]											
Localized	1.67 (1.03-2.32)	<.001	1973-1981	6.05 (1.61-10.69)	.01	1981-2001	-2.11 (-3.06- -1.16)	<.001	2001-2014	7.98 (6.63-9.35)	<.001
Regional	1.84 (1.63-2.04)	<.001	1973-2014	1.84 (1.63-2.04)	<.001						
Distant	0.95 (0.73-1.18)	<.001	1973-1976	7.56 (-0.44-16.41)	.06	1976-1995	-0.55 (-0.96- -0.14)	0.01	1995-2014	2.20 (1.90-2.50)	<.001

[a]Annual Percentage Changes, calculated using Joinpoint regression software
[b]Two-sided P value was calculated using t test to determine the significance of APC change
[c]Includes American Indian/Alaskan Native and Asian/Pacific Islander
[d]Using SEER historic stage A

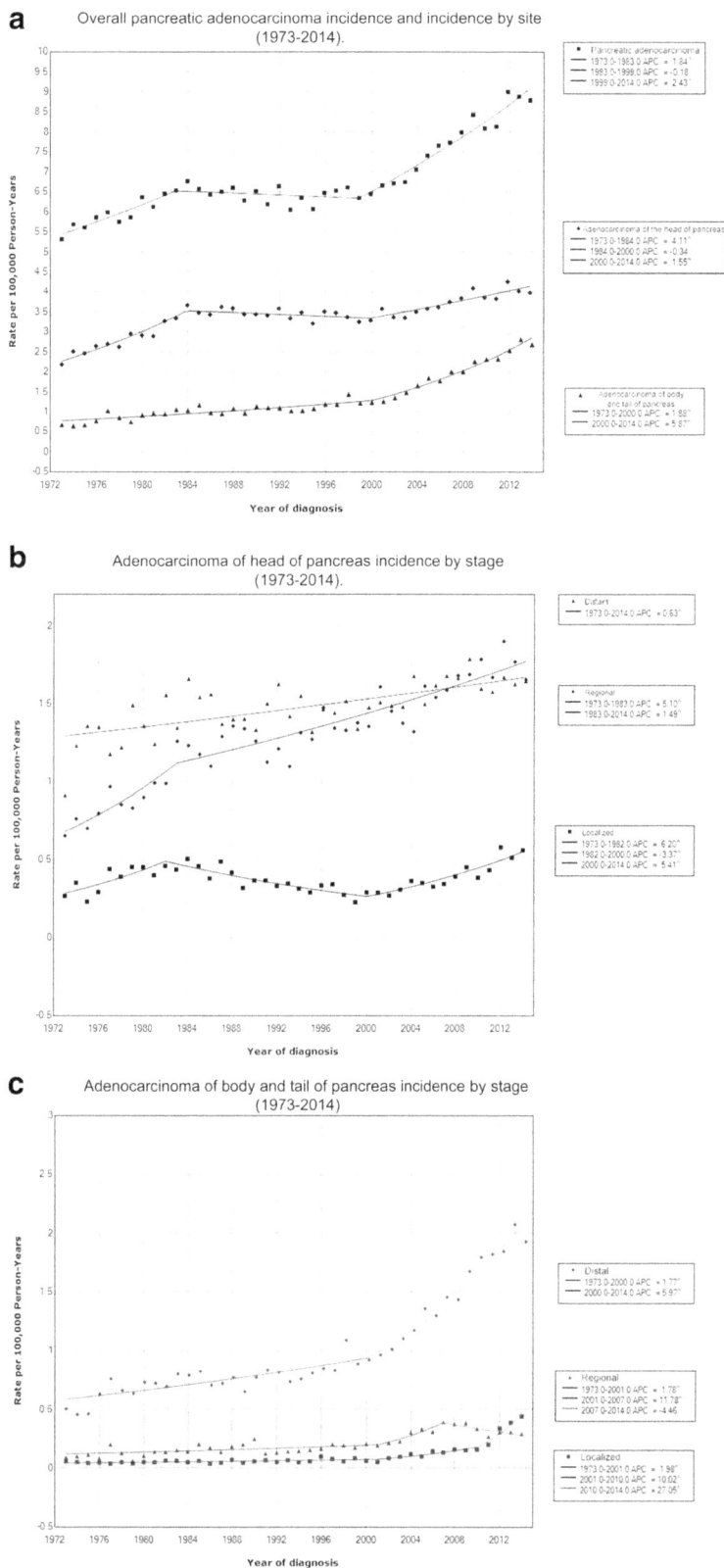

Fig. 1 Trends in annual pancreatic adenocarcinoma incidence; **a** according to subsite; **b** according to stage among pancreatic head tumors; **c** according to stage among pancreatic body and tail tumors

Incidence-based mortality rates and trends over times

PAC incidence-based mortality rates were highest among males (7.73 [95% CI, 7.65 - 7.82]), blacks (9.42 [95% CI, 9.19 - 9.64]), and people older than 60 years (31.45 [95% CI, 31.16 - 31.73]) (Table 2).

PAC incidence-based mortality increased 2.22% (95% CI, 1.93-2.51, p <.001) per year over the study period. However, during 2012-2014 there was a statistically significant decrease in PAC incidence-based mortality; APC, -24.70% (95% CI, -31.78 - -16.88, p <.001). PAC incidence-based mortality rates increased for all sex, race, age, state and stage sub-groups during the study period. Interestingly, incidence based-mortality rates decreased between 2012 and 2014 in all states except Georgia, Hawaii and Utah. Table 4 describes PAC incidence-based mortality trends during 1973-2014 by sex, race, age at death and stage. Additional file 7 summarizes PAC incidence-based mortality trends by geographical distribution.

During 1973-2014 there was a statistically significant increase in mortality rates of adenocarcinoma of the head of pancreas; APC, 2.11% (95% CI, 1.73-2.50, p <.001), and adenocarcinoma of body and tail of pancreas; APC, 4.31% (95% CI, 3.88-4.74, p <.001). Incidence-based mortality rates of both adenocarcinoma of head of pancreas, and adenocarcinoma of body and tail increased in all sex, race, age, and stage sub-groups during 1973-2014. Figure 2 shows incidence-based mortality trends for selected characteristics. Additional file 6 summarizes adenocarcinoma of the head of pancreas, and adenocarcinoma of the body and tail of pancreas incidence trends by sex, race, age at diagnosis and stage.

Discussion

To our knowledge, this is the first study to outline the trends of PAC during the past four decades. Our results revealed an overall increase in incidence and incidence-based mortality rates of PAC during the study period.

Being a rapidly fatal malignancy, PAC represents a challenge for clinicians in terms of early detection and management [15]. Such a poor prognosis can be attributed to the relatively silent progression of pancreatic tumors at early stages; the tumor usually invades locally and/or spreads before diagnosis [15]. Consequently, this tumor's mortality rates are notably close to its incidence rates [9]. Few studies have investigated the temporal trends of pancreatic cancer with its incidence and mortality [8, 9, 16–18]. Besides few variations, results from these studies have almost always showed an increase in all types of pancreatic cancer incidence and mortality, which is consistent with our results on PAC. This continuous increase draws attention to the need for more research and efforts on preventive measures to battle

PCs. Besides smoking cessation, several lifestyle changes were recommended as preventive measures including controlled alcohol consumption, weight loss and consuming more fruit and whole grains [19]. However, there is still no level I evidence supporting the efficacy of these recommendations.

Calculating incidence based-mortality (IBM) using population-based registries allows partitioning of mortality by variables associated with the cancer onset [12, 13]. In addition, it can reflect the effectiveness of present treatment modalities. For PAC, surgery is the mainstay treatment in resectable tumors (+/- perioperative treatment). A recent review demonstrated significant advances in pancreatic cancer treatment on different levels including surgical technology, imaging technology and systemic therapy regimens [5]. These advances could explain the significant decrease in incidence based-mortality (IBM) rates between 2012 and 2014 that was reported in our study. These results, along with the promising research on targeted therapy, highlight the importance of continuous monitoring and updating of PAC IBM rates to assess the implication of clinical approaches. This result could also be, potentially, attributed to the recent introduction of the FOLFIRINOX regimen, which is a combination of several chemotherapy agents (Fluorouracil 5-FU; Leucovorin; Irinotecan; Oxaliplatin) that was presented at the 2010 American Society of Clinical Oncology (ASCO) meeting [20]. However, there is still not hard evidence to support this claim, and further research is required in this context.

Despite the recent advances in molecular understanding of PAC, scientists still lack a full picture on its etiology. However, several risk factors were linked to a higher risk of pancreatic neoplasia [21]. Tobacco smoking represents the most well-established risk factor, with an estimated two-fold risk of pancreatic malignancy in smokers compared to nonsmokers [22, 23]. However, researchers argue that smoking alone does not sufficiently explain the variation in pancreatic cancer's incidence around the globe, and that more attention should be paid to other risk factors such as diet and hormonal influences in addition to certain strain types of H. Pylori [9, 21, 24, 25]. Generally, a more in-depth understanding of the trends of PAC can play role in assessing and investigating these risk agents, for instance, although Risch et al found that H.Pylori CagA Strain type might increase the incidence of PC, other researchers like Schulte et al in their meta-analysis concluded that there was no overall relationship between H. Pylori and pancreatic cancer [25, 26]. Unfortunately, as reported in previous SEER-based studies on pancreatic cancer, we could not evaluate the effect of these factors due to the lack of such data in the available registries [9].

Table 4 Trends in Pancreatic Cancer Incidence-based mortality Rates (1973-2014)

| | Overall (1973-2014) | | Trend | | | | | | | | | | | | |
	APC[a] (95% CI)	P value[b]	1 Year	APC[a] (95% CI)	P value[b]	2 Year	APC[a] (95% CI)	P value[b]	3 Year	APC[a] (95% CI)	P value[b]	4 Year	APC[a] (95% CI)	P value[b]
Overall	2.22 (1.93-2.51)	<.001	1973-1982	4.58 (3.38-5.79)	<.001	1982-2000	1.45 (1.08-1.83)	<.001	2000-2012	3.83 (3.21-4.45)	<.001	2012-2014	-24.70 (-31.78 - -16.88)	<.001
Sex														
Male	2.31 (2.03-2.59)	<.001	1973-1975	15.14 (0.57-31.82)	.04	1975-2000	1.83 (1.59-2.06)	<.001	2000-2012	4.03 (3.40-4.67)	<.001	2012-2014	-24.52 (-31.71 - -16.57)	<.001
Female	2.17 (1.85-2.49)	<.001	1973-1983	5.34 (3.99-6.71)	<.001	1983-2000	1.20 (0.68-1.73)	<.001	2000-2012	3.66 (2.85-4.47)	<.001	2012-2014	-24.79 (-33.89 - -14.44)	<.001
Race														
White	1.92 (1.64-2.21)	<.001	1973-1976	12.10 (4.45-20.30)	<.001	1976-2001	1.53 (1.29-1.78)	<.001	2001-2012	3.50 (2.73-4.28)	<.001	2012-2014	-24.89 (-32.58 - -16.32)	<.001
Black	2.91 (2.54-3.27)	<.001	1973-1980	8.93 (4.65-13.38)	<.001	1980-2001	2.19 (1.55-2.82)	<.001	2001-2012	4.46 (3.00-5.94)	<.001	2012-2014	-24.30 (-37.98 - -7.60)	.01
Others[c]	4.86 (4.40-5.31)	<.001	1973-2012	5.23 (4.92-5.53)	<.001	2012-2014	-22.08 (-37.33 - -3.13)	.03						
Age at death, y														
<60	1.50 (1.10-1.91)	<.001	1973-1993	0.19 (-0.34-0.73)	.46	1993-2005	4.03 (2.84-5.24)	<.001	2005-2012	0.44 (-2.06-3.00)	.72	2012-2014	-33.46 (-45.65 - -18.53)	<.001
>60	2.40 (2.10-2.70)	<.001	1973-1983	5.42 (4.30-6.55)	<.001	1983-2002	1.46 (1.11-1.82)	<.001	2002-2012	4.57 (3.69-5.46)	<.001	2012-2014	-22.92 (-30.31 - -14.75)	<.001
Stage at diagnosis[d]														
Localized	1.39 (0.92-1.87)	<.001	1973-1981	9.30 (5.75-12.97)	<.001	1981-1999	-0.94 (-1.83 - -0.04)	.04	1999-2012	4.57 (3.09-6.07)	<.001	2012-2014	-27.92 (-44.80 - -5.87)	.02
Regional	2.94 (2.47-3.41)	<.001	1973-1977	12.80 (2.50-24.14)	.02	1977-2012	3.13 (2.88-3.38)	<.001	2012-2014	-36.81 (-49.61 - -20.77)	<.001			
Distant	2.35 (2.07-2.63)	<.001	1973-1975	25.14 (6.66-46.83)	.01	1975-1995	1.10 (0.72-1.49)	<.001	1995-2012	3.83 (3.42-4.25)	<.001	2012-2014	-17.61 (-25.68 - -8.66)	<.001

[a] Annual Percentage Changes, calculated using Joinpoint regression software
[b] Two-sided P value was calculated using t test to determine the significance of APC change
[c] Includes American Indian/Alaskan Native and Asian/Pacific Islander
[d] Using SEER historic stage A

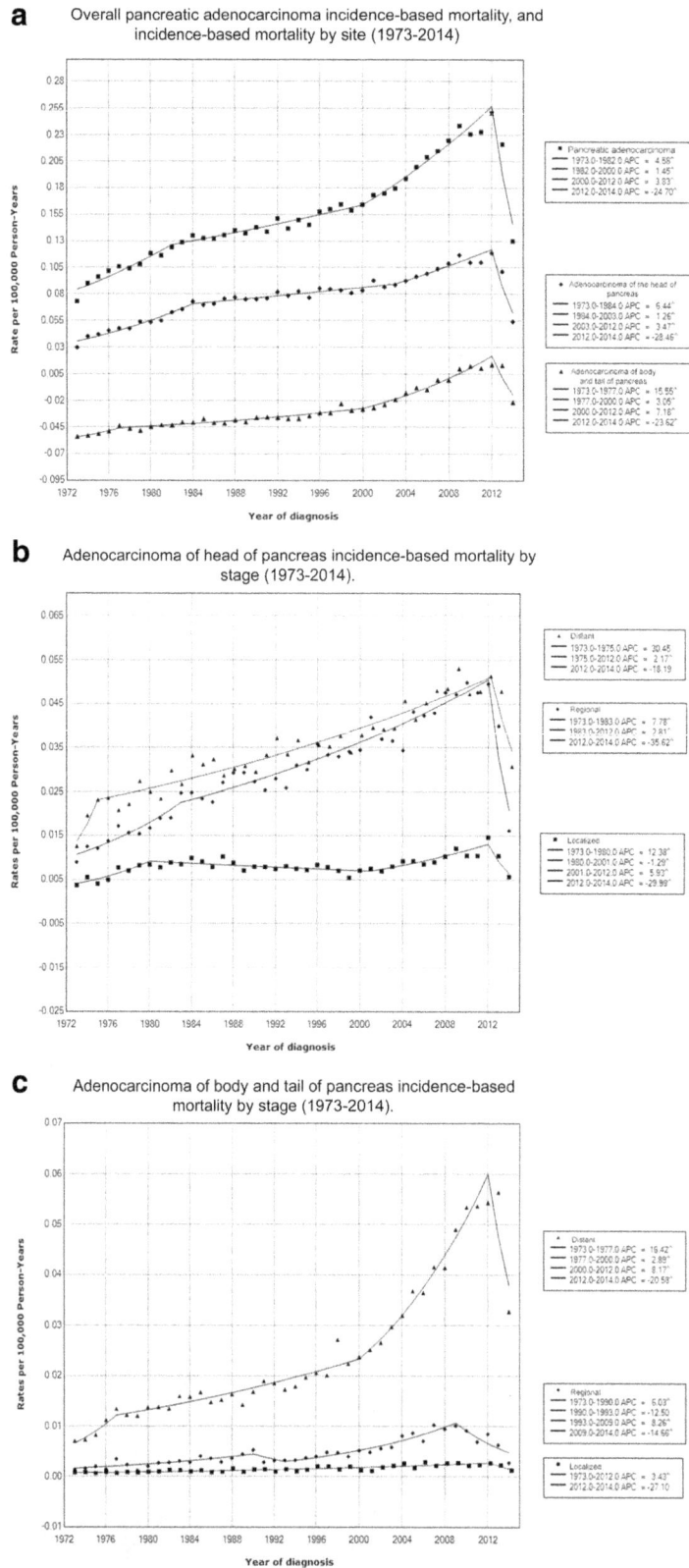

Fig. 2 Trends in annual pancreatic adenocarcinoma incidence-based mortality; **a** according to subsite; **b** according to stage among pancreatic head tumors; **c** according to stage amog pancreatic body and tail tumors

Although pancreatic masses in any site must trigger a red alarm, the primary location of a tumor can be a valuable indicator of a tumor's prognosis [27]. It is also pivotal to plan any surgical and non-surgical approach. Previous reports on pancreatic malignancies have shown the head of pancreas to be the most common site; our results in PAC are consistent with these results [8, 9]. However, the increase in body and tail tumors over the past four decades is statistically higher than in-head tumors, which was also found by Lau *et al* in their study over the period from 1973 till 2002 [8]. The latest finding could be one of the interpretations to the increased IBM since body and tail tumors are usually associated with poor prognosis due to their late presentation [28].

Like risk factors and tumor locations, geographic distribution of incidence and mortality rates adds valuable information to the epidemiological characteristics of diseases. Our results showed that Georgia, Hawaii and Utah were the only states where incidence-based mortality rates did not decrease in 2012-2014. The reason behind this finding is yet to be investigated. It can be due to fewer cases in these states that hindered the detection of a significant decrease in incidence based-mortality (IBM), to different quality of healthcare delivery, or can even be related to the characteristics of patients in these states and their health-awareness and lifestyle.

This study, like other SEER-based studies, is limited by the availability of data in the registries. For instance, some analyses and comparisons may not be feasible due to the unavailability or incompleteness of certain variables. In addition, the course of treatment and the factors that lead to a certain approach may also be missing. All details related to SEER-related limitations are demonstrated in separate reports [29, 30].

Conclusion

In summary, PAC's incidence and mortality rates have been increasing for decades, and it is expected to become the second leading cause of cancer-related death in the US by 2030 [31]. However, the past few years have shown a promising decrease in mortality. Further advances in healthcare delivery and research can lead to a further mortality decrease. Healthcare professionals and policy-makers can also make more efforts to control the associated risk factors, especially smoking. These efforts could range from awareness campaigns and advocating for lifestyle changes to imposing more strict smoking-related laws. All these attempts, along with persistent monitoring of the outcomes, can help to tackle the burden of PAC on a global scale.

Additional files

Additional file 1: Pancreatic adenocarcinoma Incidence rates (2014).

Additional file 2: Pancreatic adenocarcinoma Incidence rates for each individual year (1973-2014).

Additional file 3: Pancreatic adenocarcinoma Incidence-based mortality rates (2014).

Additional file 4: Pancreatic adenocarcinoma Incidence-based mortality rates for each individual year (1973-2014).

Additional file 5: Trends in Pancreatic adenocarcinoma Incidence Rates by state (1973-2014)

Additional file 6: Trends in Adenocarcinoma of head of pancreas and Adenocarcinoma of body and tail of pancreas Incidence and incidence-based mortality rates (1973-2014).

Additional file 7: Trends in Pancreatic adenocarcinoma Incidence-based mortality Rates by state (1973-2014).

Abbreviations
APC: Annual percent change; IBM: Incidence based-mortality; PAC: Pancreatic adenocarcinomas; PC: Pancreatic cancer; SEER: The Surveillance, Epidemiology, and End Results

Acknowledgements
We would like to thank Obai Alsalhani and Qosai Omar for their help in tables and figures preparation.

Funding
This research did not receive any specific grant from funding agencies in the public, commercial, or not-for-profit sectors.

Authors' contributions
All authors participated in designing the concept of the paper. All authors have contributed to study design and analysis of the data and had the access to it. All authors have contributed to data interpretation and writing the paper. All authors have revised and agreed to the content of the paper. OA supervised the whole project scientifically and had final responsibility for the decision to submit for publication. AS Managed and coordinated the research activity planning and execution. AS, MA, and TT contributed equally to this manuscript. All authors agreed to be accountable for all aspects of the work in ensuring that questions related to the accuracy or integrity of any part of the work are appropriately investigated and resolved.

Competing interests
The authors declare that they have no competing interests.

Author details
[1]Faculty of Medicine, Damascus University, Damascus, Syria. [2]Faculty of Medicine, Damascus University, Damascus, Syria. [3]Faculty of Medicine, Ain Shams University, Cairo, Egypt. [4]Clinical Oncology Department, Faculty of Medicine, Ain Shams University, Lofty Elsayed Street, Cairo 11566, Egypt. [5]Department of Oncology, University of Calgary and Tom Baker Cancer Center, Calgary, Alberta, Canada.

References

1. Siegel RL, Miller KD, Jemal A. Cancer statistics, 2018. CA Cancer J Clin. 2018;68(1):7–30. https://doi.org/10.3322/caac.21442.
2. Siegel RL, Miller KD, Jemal A. Cancer statistics, 2016. CA: a cancer journal for clinicians. 2016;66(1):7–30.
3. National Cancer Institute. Estimated new cancer cases and deaths for 2013. SEER (Surveillance Epidemiology and End Results) cancer statistics review. Available from: http://www.seer.cancer.gov.
4. De La Cruz M, Young AP, Ruffin MT. Diagnosis and management of pancreatic cancer. *Am Fam Physician*. 2014;89(8):626–32.
5. Mohammed S, George Van Buren I, Fisher WE. Pancreatic cancer: advances in treatment. World Journal of Gastroenterology: WJG. 2014;20(28):9354.
6. National Research Council (US) Committee on Future Directions for Behavioral and Social Sciences Research at the National Institutes of Health; Singer BH, Ryff CD, editors. New Horizons in Health: An Integrative Approach. Washington (DC): National Academies Press (US); 2001. 8, Population Perspectives: Understanding Health Trends and Evaluating the Health Care System. Available from: https://www.ncbi.nlm.nih.gov/books/NBK43784/.
7. Pearce N. Epidemiology as a population science. Int J Epidemiol. 1999;28(5):S1015.
8. Lau MK, Davila JA, Shaib YH. Incidence and survival of pancreatic head and body and tail cancers: a population-based study in the United States. Pancreas. 2010;39(4):458–62.
9. Zhang J, Dhakal I, Yan H, et al. Trends in pancreatic cancer incidence in nine SEER Cancer Registries, 1973–2002. Annals of oncology. 2007;18(7):1268–79.
10. Surveillance Research Program, National Cancer Institute SEER*Stat software (www.seer.cancer.gov/seerstat) version 8.3.4.
11. Surveillance, Epidemiology, and End Results (SEER) Program (www.seer.cancer.gov) SEER*Stat Database: Incidence - SEER 9 Regs Research Data, Nov 2016 Sub (1973-2014) <Katrina/Rita Population Adjustment> - Linked To County Attributes - Total U.S., 1969-2015 Counties, National Cancer Institute, DCCPS, Surveillance Research Program, released April 2017, based on the November 2016 submission.
12. Chu KC, Miller BA, Feuer EJ, et al. A method for partitioning cancer mortality trends by factors associated with diagnosis: An application to female breat cancer. J Clin Epidemiol. 1994;47(12):1451–61.
13. Joinpoint Regression Program, Version 4.5.0.1. June, 2017; Statistical Research and Applications Branch, National Cancer Institute. https://surveillance.cancer.gov/joinpoint/. Last Accessed on 26/7/2017.
14. Kim H-J, Fay MP, Feuer EJ, et al. Permutation tests for joinpoint regression with applications to cancer rates. Statistics in medicine. 2000;19(3):335–51.
15. Ryan DP, Hong TS, Bardeesy N. Pancreatic adenocarcinoma. N Engl J Med. 2014;371(11):1039–49.
16. Zheng T, Holford TR, Ward BA, et al. Time trend in pancreatic cancer incidence in Connecticut, 1935–1990. Int J Can. 1995;61(5):622–7.
17. Wood H, Gupta S, Kang J, et al. Pancreatic cancer in England and Wales 1975–2000: patterns and trends in incidence, survival and mortality. Aliment Pharmacol Ther. 2006;23(8):1205–14.
18. Levi F, Lucchini F, Negri E, et al. Pancreatic cancer mortality in Europe: the leveling of an epidemic. Pancreas. 2003;27(2):139–42.
19. Pericleous M, Rossi RE, Mandair D, et al. Nutrition and pancreatic cancer. Anticancer Res. 2014;34(1):9–21.
20. Conroy T, Desseigne F, Ychou M, et al. Randomized phase III trial comparing FOLFIRINOX (F: 5FU/leucovorin [LV], irinotecan [I], and oxaliplatin [O]) versus gemcitabine (G) as first-line treatment for metastatic pancreatic adenocarcinoma (MPA): preplanned interim analysis results of the PRODIGE 4/ACCORD 11 trial. J Clin Oncol. 2010;28(15_suppl):4010-4010.

21. Lowenfels AB, Maisonneuve P. Epidemiology and risk factors for pancreatic cancer. Best Pract Res Clin Gastroenterol. 2006;20(2):197–209.
22. Lin Y, Tamakoshi A, Kawamura T, et al. A prospective cohort study of cigarette smoking and pancreatic cancer in Japan. Cancer Causes and Control. 2002;13(3):249–54.
23. Iodice S, Gandini S, Maisonneuve P, et al. Tobacco and the risk of pancreatic cancer: a review and meta-analysis. Langenbeck's Archives of Surgery. 2008;393(4):535–45.
24. de Gonzalez AB, Sweetland S, Spencer E. A meta-analysis of obesity and the risk of pancreatic cancer. Br J Cancer Suppl. 2003;89(3):519.
25. Risch HA, Lu L, Kidd MS, Wang J, Zhang W, Ni Q, Gao YT, Yu H. Helicobacter pylori seropositivities and risk of pancreatic carcinoma. Biomarkers & Prevention: Cancer Epidemiology; 2014. https://doi.org/10.1158/1055-9965.
26. Schulte A, Pandeya N, Fawcett J, Fritschi L, Risch HA, Webb PM, Whiteman DC, Neale RE. Association between Helicobacter pylori and pancreatic cancer risk: a meta-analysis. Cancer Causes & Control. 2015; https://doi.org/10.1007/s10552-015-0595-3.
27. Artinyan A, Soriano PA, Prendergast C, et al. The anatomic location of pancreatic cancer is a prognostic factor for survival. HPB. 2008;10(5):371–6.
28. Barreto SG, Shukla PJ, Shrikhande SV. Tumors of the Pancreatic Body and Tail. World J Oncol. 2010; https://doi.org/10.4021/wjon2010.04.200w.
29. James BYM, Gross CP, Wilson LD, et al. NCI SEER public-use data: applications and limitations in oncology research. Oncology. 2009;23(3):288.
30. Noone A-M, Lund JL, Mariotto A, et al. Comparison of SEER treatment data with Medicare claims. Medical care. 2016;54(9):e55.
31. Rahib L, Smith BD, Aizenberg R, et al. Projecting cancer incidence and deaths to 2030: the unexpected burden of thyroid, liver, and pancreas cancers in the United States. Cancer research. 2014;74(11):2913–21.

Programmed cell death ligand 1 cut-point is associated with reduced disease specific survival in resected pancreatic ductal adenocarcinoma

Basile Tessier-Cloutier[1,2], Steve E. Kalloger[2,5,7,9*] ⓘ, Mohammad Al-Kandari[1], Katy Milne[6], Dongxia Gao[3], Brad H. Nelson[6,8], Daniel J. Renouf[3,5,7], Brandon S. Sheffield[9] and David F. Schaeffer[1,2,4,5]

Abstract

Background: Programmed cell death 1 (PD1) inhibitors have recently shown promising anti-cancer effects in a number of solid tumor types. A predictive biomarker to this class of drugs has not been clearly identified; however, overexpression of the PD1 ligand (PD-L1) has shown particular promise in lung adenocarcinoma. In this study, we explore the staining characteristics, prevalence, and clinico-molecular correlates of PD-L1 overexpression in pancreatic ductal adenocarcinoma (PDAC).

Methods: A tissue microarray (TMA) was constructed from cases of resected PDAC. PD-L1 immunohistochemistry (IHC) was performed using the SP142 primary antibody. Immunohistochemical assessment for deficient mismatch repair status (MMRd), CD3 and CD8 were performed. All biomarkers were assessed independently by two anatomical pathologists and consensus achieved on all cases. Survival analysis was performed using three thresholds ($> = 1\%$, $>5\%$ and $>10\%$) for tumor cell membrane staining.

Results: Two-hundred fifty-two cases were included in the TMA and evaluable by IHC. Thirty-one (12%), 17 (7%), 12(5%) cases were positive at percentage cut offs of >0, >5, and >10% respectively. Increased PD-L1 expression was associated with inferior prognosis ($p = 0.0367$). No statistically significant association was identified between PD-L1 status and MMR status or tumor infiltrating lymphocytes.

Conclusions: This data suggests that there is an inverse relationship between PD-L1 expression and disease specific survival times in resected PDAC. Consequently, this association may represent a phenotype where increased PD-L1 expression has an effect on tumor biology and could therefore identify a subgroup where PD1 blockade could have enhanced effectiveness.

Keywords: Pancreatic cancer, Programmed cell death 1 ligand, DNA mismatch repair, Tumor-infiltrating lymphocytes, Biomarkers, Immuno-oncology

* Correspondence: skalloger@mac.com
Daniel J. Renouf and David F. Schaeffer co-supervised this work.
Basile Tessier-Cloutier and Steve E Kalloger contributed equally to this work.
[2]Department of Pathology & Laboratory Medicine, University of British Columbia, Vancouver, British Columbia, Canada
[5]Pancreas Centre BC, Vancouver, British Columbia, Canada
Full list of author information is available at the end of the article

Background

Pancreatic ductal adenocarcinoma (PDAC) ranks fourth for overall cancer-related death with over forty-thousand estimated deaths in 2015 in the United States. The five-year survival rate is 26% in resectable disease and drops to 2% if unresectable. Surgical resection is only attempted in 20% of cases [1].

Inhibitors of the programmed cell death 1 (PD1) signalling axis have yielded improved survival benefits for a number of solid tumor types. Large randomized clinical trials have been successful in treating melanoma, non-small cell lung cancer, and renal cell carcinoma [2, 3]. Three phase 1/2 drug trials are ongoing involving treatment of PDACs with immunotherapy (NCT02583477, NCT02305186, NCT02452424). To date, no biomarker has been established to predict benefit from PD1-axis inhibition for this disease [4].

PD-1 is an inhibitory receptor expressed by T cells and other immune cell types. It plays an important role in immune suppression when activated by its ligand (PD-L1). The latter is physiologically expressed by normal tissue and can occasionally be aberrantly expressed by tumor cells as a means for evading immune destruction [4–8]. Blockade of the PD-1/PD-L1 interaction promotes T-cell response against tumor cells [3, 9].

The response to PD-1/PD-L1 inhibition has been mixed in various malignancies such as colorectal, prostatic and pancreatic adenocarcinomas and is exemplified in the results of a study by Brahmer et al. which failed to show an objective response to anti-PD-L1 therapy in 14 patients with pancreatic cancer [3, 10]. In those cases, the use of biomarkers may have been useful in the identification of patients who are more likely to respond to PD1-axis inhibition. Mismatch repair (MMR) status has been shown to be predictive in colorectal carcinoma [11] and PD-L1 expression by immunohistochemistry (IHC) may be useful in lung and bladder carcinomas [12, 13]. However, no cut-off has been uniformly defined for PD-L1 expression that would trigger the use of PD-L1 inhibitors in PDAC. Current clinical trials often use 1% [14] but evidence suggests that higher cut-points may optimize patient stratification for PD-L1 therapies [15]. PD-1 expression in tumor infiltrating immune cells, the direct target of nivolumab, has shown, unlike tumor PD-L1 expression, only borderline association with clinical outcome to PD-1 blockade [16]. Other methods to predict response to immune checkpoint inhibitors have also been investigated, including immune cell infiltration, hypermutation signature, and gene expression linked to chemokine expression [17–19], but are yet to be validated in prospective clinical trials.

In this study, we explore the prevalence of PD-L1 expression in PDAC using IHC and compare this to clinical characteristics, including MMR status and tumor infiltrating lymphocytes and examine if an association with clinical outcome exists.

Methods

Ethical approval and a waiver of consent for research on this retrospective cohort was obtained from the University of British Columbia Clinical Research Ethics Board (H12–03484).

Sample identification and TMA construction

A tissue microarray was constructed using duplicate 0.6 mm cores from the epithelial component of all available, resected, pathologically confirmed pancreatic ductal adenocarcinomas derived from the archives of the Vancouver Coastal Health Region between 1995 and 2014. All patients received primary surgery with a subset receiving adjuvant chemotherapy with a pyrimidine nucleoside analog. Cores for the tissue microarray were obtained from areas of tumor as determined by routine microscopy on hematoxylin and eosin-stained sections. Cases were excluded if they lacked clinical follow-up data or if clinicopathologic variables were lacking.

Immunohistochemical staining of PD-L1 and mismatch repair markers

Immunohistochemistry was performed on 4-μm-thick formalin-fixed paraffin-embedded sections of tissue microarrays. PD-L1 immunohistochemistry was performed at the Deely Research Centre at the British Columbia Cancer Agency using the Intellipath FLX autostainer (Biocare) platform. Mismatch repair, CD3 and CD8 immunohistochemistry was performed in the clinical laboratory of Vancouver General Hospital using the Ventana Discovery XT and the Ventana Benchmark XT automated system (Ventana Medical Systems, Tucson, AZ).

For PD-L1, slides were incubated with the clone SP142 (Spring Bioscience, Pleasanton, USA) at 1/100 dilution in Da Vinci Green diluent at room temperature for 30 min. Slides were then washed and incubated with Mach2 Rabbit-HRP polymer for 30 min at room temperature and detected with IP DAB chromogen for 5 min. Nuclei were counterstained with a 1/10 dilution of CAT hematoxylin then slides were again washed, air dried and coverslipped with Ecomount. The antibody clone was selected based on its strong concordance to three other PD-L1 clones and RNA in situ hybridization (ISH) in NSCLC [19].

For MMR stains, slides were incubated with MLH1 (mouse monoclonal antibody, 1:50 dilution, cat#: NCL-L- MLH1, clone ID:ES05; Leica Microsystems, New- castle, UK), MSH2 (mouse monoclonal antibody, 1:1000 dilution, cat#: 286 M-16, clone ID:G219–1129; Cellmarque, Rocklin, CA), MSH6 (rabbit monoclonal antibody, 1:200 dilution, cat#: CLAC-0047, clone ID: EP49; Cedarlane

Corporation, Burlington, ON, Canada), and PMS2 (rabbit monoclonal antibody, 1:20 dilution, cat#: CLAC-0049, clone ID:EP51; Cedarlane Corporation) for 32 min at room temperature. For the slides to be stained for PMS2 were additionally prepped with the Epitomics DAB prep kit before antibody incubation.

Antibodies were detected using the Ventana DABMap kit, counterstained with hematoxylin and treated with a proprietary bluing agent (Ventana). Positive and negative controls are performed as part of the routine clinical quality assurance; in addition to the external quality control program (Canadian Immunohistochemistry Quality Control (cIQc), a provider of proficiency testing for Canadian clinical laboratories).

Interpretation of Immunohistochemical stains

PD-L1 status was assessed independently by two anatomical pathologists (BSS and DG) and consensus achieved on all cases. Positivity was evaluated by H-Score, a combination of staining intensity and percentage of tumor cell staining. Staining intensity was scored as 0 (negative), 1 (weak), 2 (moderate), or 3 (strong) based on membranous localization and each score multiplied by the percentage of cells (0% - 100%) staining. Therefore, H-scores ranged from 0 to 300. To account for potential intra-tumoral heterogeneity, the mean of both cores was used to generate the score for each case.

Mismatch repair (MMR) was quantified as per Riazy et al. [20]. Briefly, protein expression for MLH1, MSH2, MSH6, and PMS2 was considered intact (normal) if any percentage of definite positive nuclear staining of the malignant cells was detected on either TMA core. In cases where one or more mismatch repair proteins were interpreted as negative staining, examination utilizing immunohistochemistry on whole sections was performed. Each protein was considered lost (abnormal) if there was complete loss of nuclear staining in the tumor cells and if there was a positive internal control (intact nuclear staining of stromal elements such as inflammatory cells and/or endothelial cells) on whole section. Cases showing a complete absence of nuclear staining pattern of both tumor cells and stromal elements were deemed uninterpretable and thus excluded from the study. Cases that demonstrated loss of any MMR marker on the TMA were subjected to confirmatory whole slide section staining and were scored independently by two pathologists (BSS and DFS), who were blinded to clinical characteristics and patient outcomes. Divergent assessments were reconciled by consensus conference. A case was labeled as mismatch repair deficient (MMRd) if any of the four mismatch repair proteins was completely absent on immunohistochemistry. Cases were classified as mismatch repair proficient (MMRp) if all four proteins stained positive to some degree.

Individual tumor infiltrating lymphocytes were counted and typed in the epithelial and stromal compartments using clinically validated IHC stains for CD3 and CD8. Scoring was performed independently by two anatomical pathologists (BSS and MA-K) and consensus achieved on all cases. To account for potential intra-tumoral heterogeneity, the average of both cores were used to generate the final score for CD8+ and CD3+ tumor infiltrating lymphocytes.

Clinico-pathologic variables and outcome

Standard treatment, clinical and pathologic parameters were collected from the British Columbia Cancer Agency which included: age at surgery, sex, adjuvant chemotherapy agents used, lymphovascular invasion, perineural invasion, pathologic primary tumor (pT) stage, and pathologic regional lymph-node status (pN). The primary outcome measure was defined to be disease-specific survival, where survival time was calculated as the difference between the date of last follow-up and the date of surgery, expressed in years. Patients were censored if they were alive at last follow-up or had died from a cause other than their pancreatic malignancy. Deaths attributable to treatment related toxicities or inter-current diseases were considered censored observations for this analysis.

Statistical analysis

To determine if H-Score or the percent of positive cells for PD-L1 expression yield differential prognostic ability, each scoring method was subjected to an omnibus assessment utilizing the Cox-Proportional Hazards Model to determine if the expression of PD-L1 was a significant prognostic marker in the context of the clinico-pathologic variables outlined previously with the exception of pT-Stage due the fact that the vast majority of the cases in this cohort are pT3. The proportionality assumption for each variable was assessed through examination of Cox-Snell residuals and continuous variables were assessed for linearity. The PD-L1 scoring methodology with the smallest P-value was determined to have the strongest prognostic effect. Parametric survival analysis was used in order to further elucidate the gradient dependent effect of PD-L1 expression on disease specific survival (DSS) for the scoring methodology with the greatest prognostic effect. This procedure modelled the disease specific survival data with 5 different distributions which included: weibull, log-normal, exponential, frechet, and log-logistic. The best distribution to be used for parametric survival analysis was determined by selecting the one with the lowest Bayesian Information Criterion from the model fits. This analysis produces a quantile plot with logSurvival Time plotted against PD-L1 expression which illustrates the gradient dependent relationship between disease specific survival and PD-L1 expression. Based on these findings, a series of three cut-points were created starting with an H-Score or percentage positive cells of 1- as these identify the equivalent cases. Subsequent cut-points were set at increments of 5 which correspond to the increments used for the assessment of percent positive cells. The resultant groups were subjected to univariable survival analysis to quantify differences in disease specific survival using the Kaplan-Meier method. A multivariable approach to disease specific survival, using the Cox Proportional Hazards Model, was used to determine if survival differences between PD-L1 expression categories were independent of adjuvant chemotherapy. Assessment for heterogeneity of clinico-pathologic variables was performed with the following statistical approaches: continuous variables were examined using the Wilcoxon Rank-Sum Test, categorical comparisons were computed using Fisher's exact test. A P-value of <0.05 was considered as statistically significant for all analyses. All analyses were computed with JMP v13.1 (SAS Institute, Cary, NC).

Results

After exclusion criteria were applied, two-hundred fifty-two cases remained (Fig. 1). The demographic information for the cohort were tabulated and are shown in Table 1. The Cox-Proportional Hazards Analysis for PD-L1 H-score and percent positive indicated that the latter was a stronger prognostic indicator with $P = 0.0466$ compared to H-Score with a $P = 0.10$ (Table 2).

Subjecting the survival data to the 5 distribution models outlined in the methods and ranking those fits by the Bayesian Information Criterion revealed that the log-logistic distribution fit best and was used as the basis for parametric disease specific survival

analysis. Parametric disease specific survival of PD-L1 percent positive and H-Score demonstrated an inverse relationship between increased PD-L1 expression and survival time (Fig. 2). As indicated in the multivariable survival analysis, PD-L1 percent positive had a slightly stronger prognostic association compared to H-Score.

Based on the prognostic non-inferiority of PD-L1 percent positive, we elected to pursue this scoring method for the remainder of the study. Cut-points were determined according to our criteria outlined in the methods and resulted in: $> = 1\%$ ($N = 31$; 12.3% of the cohort), $>5\%$ ($N = 17$; 6.7% of the cohort), and $>10\%$ ($N = 12$; 4.8% of the cohort). Univariable survival analysis using these three cut-points showed no disease specific survival differences at the $> = 1$ cut-point ($p = 0.51$) or the >5 cut-point (0.52), but the >10 cut-point yielded statistically significant disease specific survival differences of $p = 0.027$ (Fig. 3). Multivariable DSS analysis of the $>10\%$ positive PD-L1 expression cut-point along with the other clinico-pathologic covariates outlined in Table 2, indicates that this subset of twelve cases has a trend toward inferior prognosis with a Risk Ratio and 95%CI 1.90 [0.96–3.42] ($P = 0.06$). When we sequentially removed statistically insignificant variables from the model (age, histopathologic grade, sex, and lyphovascular Invasion, PD-L1 > 10% became statistically significant Risk Ratio and 95%CI 2.05 [1.03–3.66] ($P = 0.0410$). The remaining statistically significant variables included pN-Stage ($P < 0.0001$), adjuvant chemotherapy ($P = 0.0002$), and perineurial invasion ($P = 0.009$) and resection status ($P = 0.0263$).

Analysis for heterogeneity across clinico-pathologic parameters which included: age, sex, adjuvant chemotherapy use, histopathological grade, lymphovascular invasion, perineural inavasion, pN-Stage, and resection

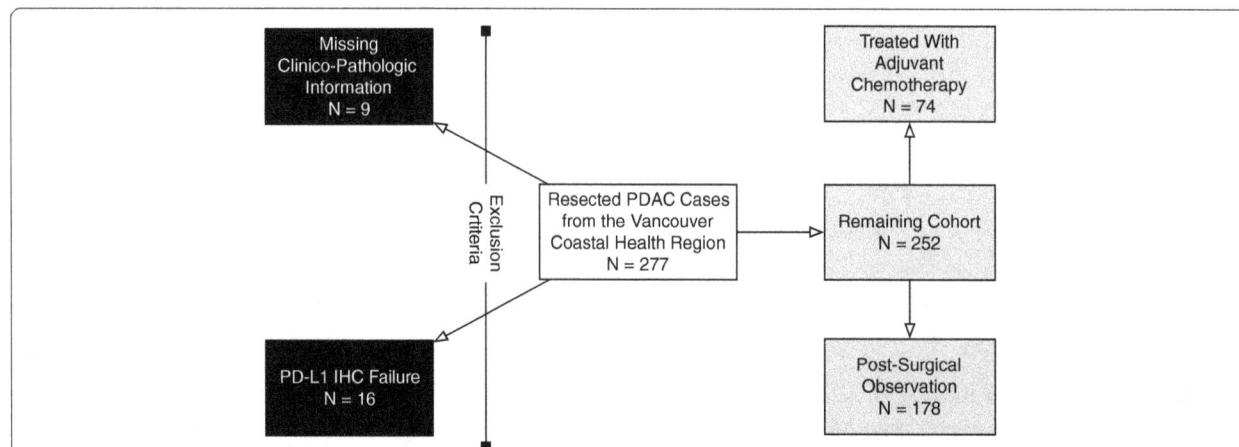

Fig. 1 Patient selection diagram illustrating inclusion and exclusion criteria for this study with final numbers for the cohorts who received adjuvant pyrimidine nucleoside analogs or subjected to post-surgical observation only

Table 1 Demographics of the entire cohort

Variable	Levels	Values
Age	Median [IQR]	66.4 [13.3]
Sex	Male	139 (55.2%)
	Female	113 (44.8%)
Adjuvant Chemotherapy	Given	74 (29.4%)
	Observation	178 (70.6%)
Histologic Grade	1	2 (0.8%)
	2	186 (73.8%)
	3	64 (25.4%)
Lymphovascular Invasion	Present	144 (57.1%)
	Absent	108 (42.9%)
Perineurial Invasion	Present	232 (92.1%)
	Absent	20 (7.9%)
pT Stage	1	2 (0.8%)
	2	11 (4.4%)
	3	238 (94.4%)
	4	1 (0.4%)
pN Stage	0	64 (25.4%)
	1	168 (74.6%)
Resection Status	R0	190 (75.4%)
	R1	62 (24.6%)
CD3 Epithelial	Median [IQR]	0 [0]
CD3 Stromal	Median [IQR]	50 [52]
CD8 Epithelial	Median [IQR]	0 [0]
CD8 Stromal	Median [IQR]	11 [36]
MMR Status	Proficient	211 (84.1%%)
	Deficient	40 (15.9%)
Follow-up Time (Years)	Median [IQR]	1.33 [1.59]
Events	Disease Specific Deaths	200 (79.4%)
	Censorings	52 (20.6%)

status demonstrated a significant relationship between increased PD-L1 expression and higher grade cases (Table 3). The remaining clinico-pathologic variables, mismatch repair, and the stromal or epithelial compartment specific prevalence of CD3+ or CD8+ tumor infiltrating lymphocytes were not associated with the PD-L1 > 10% positive cells cut-point.

Discussion

In this study, we have found a gradient dependent association between PD-L1 expression and inferior disease specific survival in resected pancreatic ductal adenocarcinoma. This finding was independent of the improved prognosis associated with the application of adjuvant chemotherapy with a pyrimidine nucleoside analog.

We assessed multiple scoring methods, H-Score or percent of positive cells, for the quantification of PD-L1 expression and determined that the estimation of percent positive cells yields a stronger association with inferior survival than H-Score. This suggests that the addition of a subjective intensity assessment to generate an H-score may represent an unnecessary step for the quantification of PD-L1 in this disease. Examination of other clinico-pathologic parameters revealed no statistically significant associations with PD-L1 expression at any cut-point, which indicates that PD-L1 expression does not select for any known prognostic variable other than histo-pathologic grade. Due to the limited power associated with our cohort combined with the small fraction of cases that express PD-L1 at a high level, we were limited in our ability to perform multivariable disease specific survival analyses with numerous variables. Exploratory multivariable disease specific survival modeling suggested that our categorized PD-L1 expression utilizing the cut-point of >10% of positive cells is independently associated with inferior disease specific survival and was only surpassed by the presence of regional lymph node metastasis and perineural invasion in terms of negative prognostic variables.

Recent studies have demonstrated that PD-L1 expression is associated with tumor types known to have higher somatic mutation load, as is the case for melanomas, NSCLC and RCC [21, 22]. Considering that PDAC has a lower mutation burden, it is not surprising that we found only 4 to 12% PD-L1 positive tumors compared to the reported 83% in melanoma, 50% in NSCLC and 80% in RCC [10]. Nonetheless, PDAC is associated with tobacco use and *BRCA* loss-of-function, and is predicted to, at least occasionally, show an increased mutation burden as a result of these [23]. Consequently, the lower than average rate of PD-L1 expression in PDAC compared to other malignancies may explain poor response to checkpoint inhibitors in clinical trials since PD-L1 was either not accounted for or the positivity thresholds were only set between 1% and 5% [10, 11]. Although our patient cohort was mostly treatment naive, we were able to identify differential outcomes based on higher PD-L1 expression.

The observed increased trend of lymphocyte tumor infiltration (CD3+) in PD-L1 positive patients has been reported in previous studies [24]. Sanmamed et al. showed that tumor infiltrating lymphocytes release IFN-Gamma as part of the host response to the tumor, which induces upregulation, and expression of, PD-L1 by tumor cells [25]. Our results indicate that a cut-point > = 1% yields the strongest association with CD3+ infiltrating T-cells but due to reduced power associated with increasing the PD-L1 cut-point, statistical significance is lost at higher thresholds.

Table 2 Multivariable disease specific survival analysis for PD-L1 expression quantified by percent positive & H-score

Variable	Comparison	Risk ratio	95%CI	p-value
		PD-L1 H-Score		
PD-L1 H-Score	Per unit change	1.01	0.997–1.02	0.10
Age at Surgery	Per unit change	1.01	0.991–1.02	0.44
Sex	Male v Female	1.14	0.85–1.53	0.37
Adjuvant Chemotherapy	Given v Observation	0.59	0.42–0.81	0.0011
Histopathologic Grade	1 v 2	0.63	0.10–2.10	0.50
	1 v 3	0.49	0.08–1.67	0.28
	2 v 3	0.77	0.55–1.09	0.13
Lymphovascular Invasion	Present v Absent	1.27	0.93–1.74	0.13
Perineural Invasion	Present v Absent	1.66	0.96–3.09	0.07
pN-Stage	1 v 0	1.83	1.27–2.68	0.0010
Resection Status	R0 v R1	0.67	0.49–0.94	0.0202
		PD-L1 Percent Positive		
PD-L1 Percent Positive	Per unit change	1.03	1.0005–1.05	0.0466
Age at Surgery	Per unit change	1.0006	0.99–1.02	0.42
Sex	Male v Female	1.16	0.86–1.55	0.33
Adjuvant Chemotherapy	Given v Observation	0.58	0.42–0.80	0.0008
Histopathologic Grade	1 v 2	0.64	0.10–2.13	0.51
	1 v 3	0.50	0.08–1.71	0.30
	2 v 3	0.78	0.56–1.10	0.15
Lymphovascular Invasion	Present v Absent	1.28	0.94–1.76	0.12
Perineural Invasion	Present v Absent	1.68	0.98–3.13	0.06
pN-Stage	1 v 0	1.85	1.28–2.71	0.0009
Rescetion Status	R0 v R1	0.68	0.49–0.95	0.0189

We found no significant association between MMR and PD-L1 status. Our results are somewhat different from what was observed by Le et al. (2016) who reported that, in a series of 30 cases, PD-L1 was only expressed in MMR deficient (MMRd) tumors, most of which being colorectal carcinomas [11]. This inconsistency might be explained by the lower mutational burden seen in PDAC compared to MMRd colon carcinoma, melanoma, NSCLC and RCC [22]. Tumors with low mutational burden tend to be less immunogenic, making them less likely to develop immune silencing mechanism during their evolution.

There are several limitations to our study, one being the lack of consensus for PD-L1 IHC expression cut-off and gold standard, which our study has attempted to explore. Our IHC protocol for PD-L1 previously showed fairly strong concordance when compared to three other PD-L1 clones and RNA in situ hybridization (ISH), Sheffield et al., in NSCLC [26]. Our sample size is limited given the small percentage of PD-L1 expression and may have been underpowered to detect some more subtle associations, especially in the higher PD-L1 cut-points. Finally, since the IHC was performed on a TMA rather than full section, we might have underrepresented the amount of PD-L1 positive PDAC due to sampling error, although this method approximates the biopsy sampling error in encountered in clinical practice.

The prevalence of PD-L1 positivity in PDAC has been examined in numerous other studies with the percentage of tumor cells staining positive ranging from 4% - 49%. Each of these previous studies utilized different cut-points that varied between 1% - 10% making their results nearly impossible to compare [27–29]. Of particular interest, our results are somewhat different from what has been reported by Nomi et al. who demonstrated a found a 39% PD-L1 positivity in pancreatic cancer using a 10% positivity threshold [28]. Their cohort included 51 cases from Japan, which were stained using Anti-Human CD274, clone MIH1. The difference in PD-L1 expression is notable and although the CD274 is not commonly used in the clinical research setting this result may indicate variability associated with ethnicity.

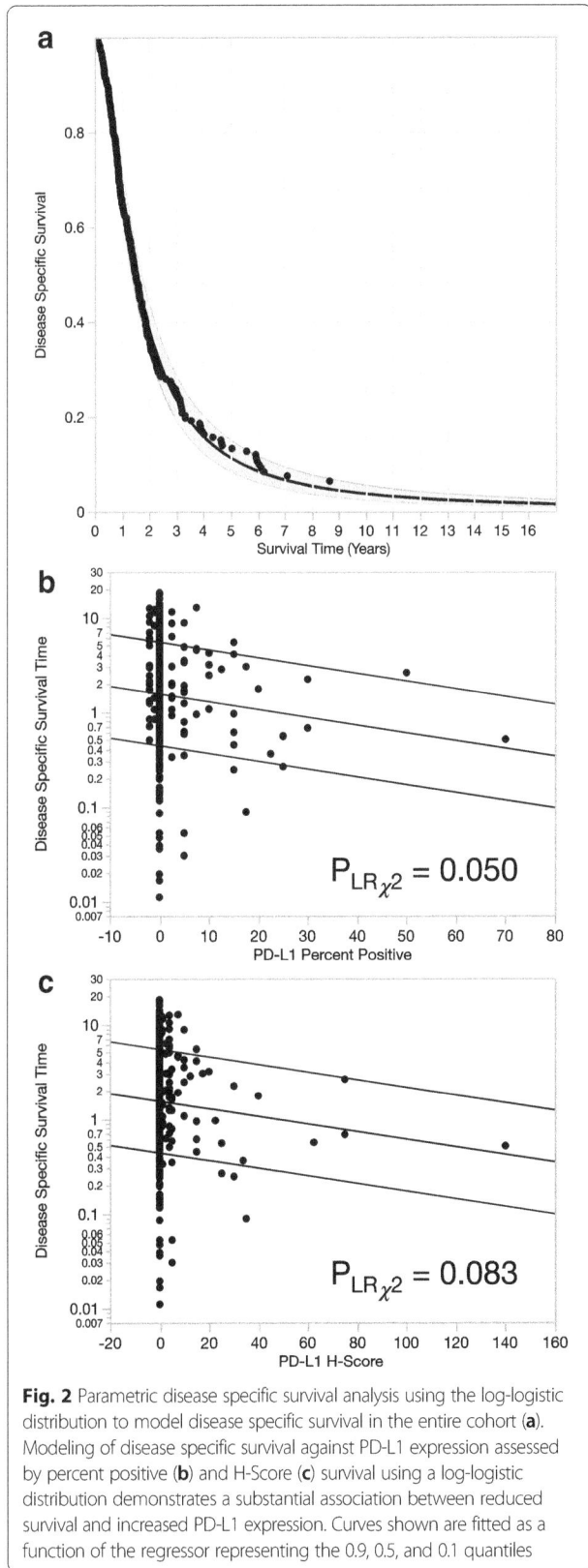

Fig. 2 Parametric disease specific survival analysis using the log-logistic distribution to model disease specific survival in the entire cohort (**a**). Modeling of disease specific survival against PD-L1 expression assessed by percent positive (**b**) and H-Score (**c**) survival using a log-logistic distribution demonstrates a substantial association between reduced survival and increased PD-L1 expression. Curves shown are fitted as a function of the regressor representing the 0.9, 0.5, and 0.1 quantiles

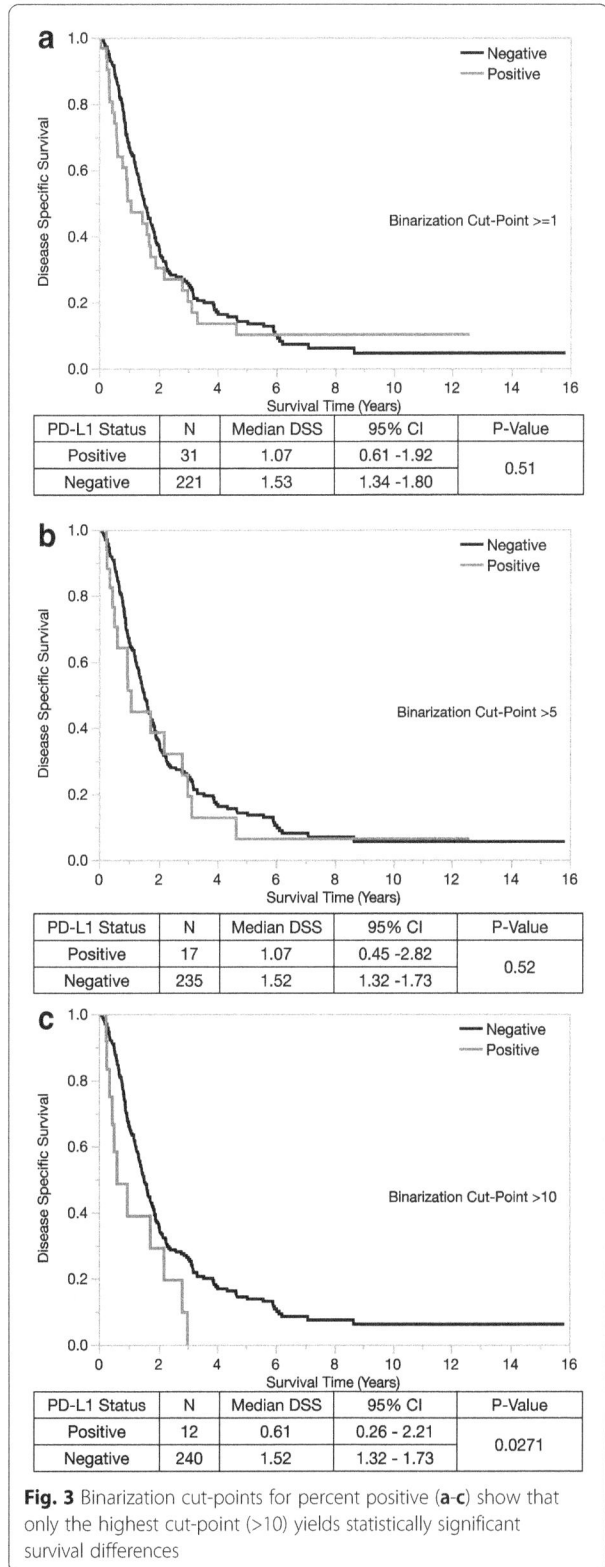

PD-L1 Status	N	Median DSS	95% CI	P-Value
Positive	31	1.07	0.61 -1.92	0.51
Negative	221	1.53	1.34 -1.80	

PD-L1 Status	N	Median DSS	95% CI	P-Value
Positive	17	1.07	0.45 -2.82	0.52
Negative	235	1.52	1.32 -1.73	

PD-L1 Status	N	Median DSS	95% CI	P-Value
Positive	12	0.61	0.26 - 2.21	0.0271
Negative	240	1.52	1.32 - 1.73	

Fig. 3 Binarization cut-points for percent positive (**a-c**) show that only the highest cut-point (>10) yields statistically significant survival differences

Conclusions

In summary, this is the first study to systematically investigate the association between clinical outcome and

Table 3 Assessment for heterogeneity using a percent positive binarization cut-point of >10

Variable	Levels	PD-L1%Positive < 10	PD-L1%Positive > 10	P-Value
Age	Median [IQR]	66.5 [13.1]	65.6 [20.5]	0.96
Sex	Male	132 (55.0%)	7 (58.3%)	1.0
	Female	108 (45.0%)	4 (41.8%)	
Adjuvant Chemotherapy	Given	71 (29.6%)	3 (25.0%)	1.0
	Observation	169 (70.4%)	9 (75.0%)	
Histologic Grade	1	2 (0.8%)	0 (0.0%)	0.029
	2	181 (75.4%)	5 (41.7%)	
	3	57 (23.8%)	7 (58.3%)	
Lymphovascular Invasion	Present	136 (56.7%)	8 (66.7%)	0.56
	Absent	104 (43.3%)	4 (33.3%)	
Perineurial Invasion	Present	221 (92.1%)	11 (91.7%)	1.0
	Absent	19 (7.9%)	1 (9.3%)	
pT Stage	1	2 (0.8%)	0 (0.0%)	0.88
	2	10 (4.2%)	1 (8.3%)	
	3	227 (94.6%)	11 (91.7%)	
	4	1 (0.4%)	0 (0.0%)	
pN Stage	0	62 (25.8%)	2 (16.7%)	0.74
	1	178 (74.2%)	10 (83.3%)	
Resection Status	R0	184 (76.7%)	6 (50%)	0.08
	R1	56 (23.3%)	6 (50%)	
CD3 Epithelial	Median [IQR]	0 [0]	0 [4]	0.16
CD3 Stromal	Median [IQR]	50 [52]	63 [76]	0.52
CD8 Epithelial	Median [IQR]	0 [0]	0 [0]	0.51
CD8 Stromal	Median [IQR]	11 [36]	14 [39]	0.72
MMR Status	Proficient	200 (83.7%)	11 (91.7%)	0.70
	Deficient	39 (16.3%)	1 (8.3%)	

biomarker expression across differing scoring methodologies and cut-points for PD-L1 immunohistochemistry in this disease. We have demonstrated a gradient dependent association between PD-L1 expression and inferior survival that is independent of the prognostic advantage conferred by adjuvant chemotherapy. We postulate that the association presented here may indicate that higher PD-L1 protein expression levels represent a phenotype where PD-1 inhibition may be more effective. However, this hypothesis would have to be tested in the context of a randomized clinical trial. With studies in other diseases also indicating that deficient MMR (MMRd) status has been shown to be a predictive biomarker for immunotherapy, it is entirely plausible that PD-L1 immunohistochemistry is an imperfect biomarker for sensitivity to anti-PD-1 therapy. Interestingly, we found no association between MMRd status and PD-L1 expression in this cohort. More data on the role of PD-1-axis inhibition in PDAC is needed, specifically examining the use of predictive biomarkers in the context of patients treated with immunotherapy. Future studies should endeavor to build predictive models based on multi-marker expression that will serve as tools to triage the PDAC patient population to immunotherapy or other treatment regimens.

Abbreviations

MMRd: Mismatch Repair Deficient; MMRp: Mismatch Repair Proficient; PD1: Programmed Cell Death 1; PDAC: Pancreatic Ductal Adenocarcinoma; PD-L1: Programmed Cell Death Ligand 1

Acknowledgements

We, the authors, would like to recognize the patients and their families for their direct and indirect contributions toward fighting this disease.

Funding

This work was supported through unrestricted research funds provided by the VGH and UBC Hospital Foundation and the BC Cancer Foundation which were administered through the Pancreas Centre BC. The above funders of this research had no influence upon the design of the study, collection, analysis nor interpretation of the data or writing of the manuscript.

Authors' contributions

BTC: Conceived the study, wrote the first draft of the manuscript and had input on revisions after internal review by co-authors. SEK: Conceived the study, performed all statistical analyses and participated in the writing of the manuscript. MA: Developed the method and provided all scoring for immune infiltrates for epithelial and stromal components of each PDAC case. KM: Developed and optimized the immunohistochemical staining procedure for the PD-L1 antibody and was responsible for applying this procedure to the TMA. Contributed to the methods section of the manuscript. DG: Developed the scoring system used for this study and performed the scoring for the PD-L1 antibody. Contributed to the methods section of the manuscript. BHN: Advised on the design of the study and served as an internal reviewer for the manuscript. DJR: Acquired the clinical follow-up for patients included in this TMA case series. Served as an internal reviewer for the manuscript and served in a co-supervisory capacity for the project. BSS: Performed consensus IHC scoring for PD-L1, CD3, CD8, and MMR immunohistochemistry. Advised on study design and helped to improve the manuscript though critical review. DFS: Advised on the study design and aided with the interpretation of the results. Served as an internal reviewer for the manuscript and served in a co-supervisory capacity for the project. Performed original scoring assessment for MMR status. All authors have given final approval of the manuscript in its current form and agree to take responsibility for the accuracy and integrity of it's content. Any errors and omissions are our own.

Competing interests

The authors declare that they have no competing interests.

Author details

[1]Division of Anatomical Pathology, Vancouver General Hospital, Vancouver, British Columbia, Canada. [2]Department of Pathology & Laboratory Medicine, University of British Columbia, Vancouver, British Columbia, Canada. [3]Division of Medical Oncology, University of British Columbia , Vancouver, British Columbia, Canada. [4]Genetic Pathology Evaluation Centre, University of British Columbia, Vancouver, British Columbia, Canada. [5]Pancreas Centre BC, Vancouver, British Columbia, Canada. [6]Deeley Research Centre, British Columbia Cancer Agency, Victoria, British Columbia, Canada. [7]Division of Medical Oncology, British Columbia Cancer Agency, Vancouver, British Columbia, Canada. [8]Department of Biochemistry and Microbiology, University of Victoria, Victoria, British Columbia, Canada. [9]Department of Anatomical Pathology, Abbotosford Regional Hospital and Cancer Centre, Abbotsford, British Columbia, Canada.

References

1. Siegel RL, Miller KD, Jemal A. Cancer statistics, 2016. CA Cancer J Clin. 2016;66:7–30.   –30.
2. Topalian SL, Sznol M, McDermott DF, Kluger HM, Carvajal RD, Sharfman WH, et al. Survival, durable tumor remission, and long-term safety in patients with advanced melanoma receiving nivolumab. J Clin Oncol. 2014;32:1020
3. Brahmer JR, Tykodi SS, Chow LQ, Hwu W-JJ, Topalian SL, Hwu P, et al. safety and activity of anti-PD-L1 antibody in patients with advanced cancer. N Engl J Med. 2012;366:2455–65.
4. De Guillebon E, Roussille P, Frouin E, Tougeron D. Anti program death-1/ anti program death-ligand 1 in digestive cancers. World J Gastrointest Oncol. 2015;7:95–101.
5. Dong H, Strome SE, Salomao DR, Tamura H, Hirano F, Flies DB, et al. Tumor-associated B7-H1 promotes T-cell apoptosis: a potential mechanism of immune evasion. Nat Med. 2002;8:793–800.
6. Dong H, Zhu G, Tamada K, Chen L. B7-H1, a third member of the B7 family, co-stimulates T-cell proliferation and interleukin-10 secretion. Nat Med. 1999;5:1365–9.
7. Freeman GJ, Long AJ, Iwai Y, Bourque K, Chernova T, Nishimura H, et al. Engagement of the PD-1 immunoinhibitory receptor by a novel B7 family member leads to negative regulation of lymphocyte activation. J Exp Med. 2000;192:1027–34.

8. Topalian SL, Drake CG, Pardoll DM. Targeting the PD-1/B7-H1(PD-L1) pathway to activate anti-tumor immunity. Curr Opin Immunol. 2012;24:207–12.
9. Iwai Y, Ishida M, Tanaka Y, Okazaki T, Honjo T, Minato N. Involvement of PD-L1 on tumor cells in the escape from host immune system and tumor immunotherapy by PD-L1 blockade. Proc Natl Acad Sci U S A. 2002;99:12293–7.
10. Topalian SL, Hodi SF, Brahmer JR, Gettinger SN, Smith DC, McDermott DF, et al. Safety, activity, and immune correlates of anti-PD-1 antibody in cancer. N Engl J Med. 2012;366:2443–54.
11. Le DT, Uram JN, Wang H, Bartlett BR, Kemberling H, Eyring AD, et al. PD-1 blockade in tumors with mismatch-repair deficiency. N Engl J Med. 2015; 372:2509–20.
12. Herbst RS, Soria J-CC, Kowanetz M, Fine GD, Hamid O, Gordon MS, et al. predictive correlates of response to the anti-PD-L1 antibody MPDL3280A in cancer patients. Nature. 2014;515:563–7.
13. Powles T, Eder J, Fine GD, Braiteh FS, Loriot Y, Cruz C, et al. MPDL3280A (anti-PD-L1) treatment leads to clinical activity in metastatic bladder cancer. Nature. 2014;515:558–62.
14. Herbst RS, Baas P, Kim D-WW, Felip E, Pérez-Gracia JL, Han J-YY, et al. Pembrolizumab versus docetaxel for previously treated, PD-L1-positive, advanced non-small-cell lung cancer (KEYNOTE-010): a randomised controlled trial. Lancet. 2016;387:1540–50.
15. Meng X, Huang Z, Teng F, Xing L, Yu J. Predictive biomarkers in PD-1/PD-L1 checkpoint blockade immunotherapy. Cancer Treat Rev. 2015;41:868–76.
16. Taube JM, Klein A, Brahmer JR, Xu H, Pan X, Kim JH, et al. Association of PD-1, PD-1 ligands, and other features of the tumor immune microenvironment with response to anti-PD-1 therapy. Clin Cancer Res. 2014;20:5064–74.
17. Ascierto PA, Capone M, Urba WJ, Bifulco CB, Botti G, Lugli A, et al. The additional facet of immunoscore: immunoprofiling as a possible predictive tool for cancer treatment. J Transl Med. 2013;11:54.
18. Messina JL, Fenstermacher DA, Eschrich S, Qu X, Berglund AE, Lloyd MC, et al. 12-chemokine gene signature identifies lymph node-like structures in melanoma: potential for patient selection for immunotherapy? Sci Rep. 2012;2:765.
19. Rizvi NA, Hellmann MD, Snyder A, Kvistborg P, Makarov V, Havel JJ, et al. Cancer immunology. Mutational landscape determines sensitivity to PD-1 blockade in non-small cell lung cancer. Science. 2015;348:124–8.
20. Riaz M, Kalloger SE, Sheffield BS, Peixoto RD, Li-Chang HH, Scudamore CH, et al. Mismatch repair status may predict response to adjuvant chemotherapy in resectable pancreatic ductal adenocarcinoma. Mod Pathol. 2015;28:1383–9.
21. Grosso J, Inzunza D, Wu Q, Simon J, Singh P, Zhang X, et al. Programmed death-ligand 1 (PD-L1) expression in various tumor types. Journal for immunotherapy of cancer. 2013;1:P53.
22. Lawrence MS, Stojanov P, Polak P, Kryukov GV, Cibulskis K, Sivachenko A, et al. Mutational heterogeneity in cancer and the search for new cancer-associated genes. Nature. 2013;499:214–8.
23. Alexandrov LB, Nik-Zainal S, Wedge DC, Aparicio SA, Behjati S, Biankin AV, et al. Signatures of mutational processes in human cancer. Nature. 2013;500:415–21.
24. Furuta J, Inozume T, Harada K, Shimada S. CD271 on melanoma cell is an IFN-γ-inducible immunosuppressive factor that mediates downregulation of melanoma antigens. J Invest Dermatol. 2014;134:1369–77.
25. Sanmamed MF, Chen L. Inducible expression of B7-H1 (PD-L1) and its selective role in tumor site immune modulation. Cancer J. 2014;20:256–61.
26. Sheffield BS, Fulton R, Kalloger SE, Milne K, Geller G, Jones M, et al. Investigation of PD-L1 biomarker testing methods for PD-1 Axis inhibition in non-squamous non-small cell lung cancer. J Histochem Cytochem. 2016;64:587–600.
27. Diana A, Wang L, D'Costa Z, Allen P, Azad A, Silva MA, et al. Prognostic value, localization and correlation of PD-1/PD-L1, CD8 and FOXP3 with the desmoplastic stroma in pancreatic ductal adenocarcinoma. Oncotarget. 2016;7:40992–1004.
28. Nomi T, Sho M, Akahori T, Hamada K, Kubo A, Kanehiro H, et al. Clinical significance and therapeutic potential of the programmed death-1 ligand/ programmed death-1 pathway in human pancreatic cancer. Clin Cancer Res. 2007;13:2151–7.
29. Wang L, Ma Q, Chen X, Guo K, Li J, Zhang M. Clinical significance of B7-H1 and B7-1 expressions in pancreatic carcinoma. World J Surg. 2010;34:1059–65.

A phase-I trial of pre-operative, margin intensive, stereotactic body radiation therapy for pancreatic cancer: the 'SPARC' trial protocol

Daniel L. P. Holyoake[1], Elizabeth Ward[2], Derek Grose[3], David McIntosh[3], David Sebag-Montefiore[4,5], Ganesh Radhakrishna[5], Neel Patel[6], Michael Silva[6], Somnath Mukherjee[1,6], Victoria Y. Strauss[7], Lang'o Odondi[7], Emmanouil Fokas[1], Alan Melcher[8] and Maria A. Hawkins[1*]

Abstract

Background: Standard therapy for borderline-resectable pancreatic cancer in the UK is surgery with adjuvant chemotherapy, but rates of resection with clear margins are unsatisfactory and overall survival remains poor. Meta-analysis of single-arm studies shows the potential of neo-adjuvant chemo-radiotherapy but the relative radio-resistance of pancreatic cancer means the efficacy of conventional dose schedules is limited. Stereotactic radiotherapy achieves sufficient accuracy and precision to enable pre-operative margin-intensive dose escalation with the goal of increasing rates of clear resection margins and local disease control.

Methods/Design: SPARC is a "rolling-six" design single-arm study to establish the maximum tolerated dose for margin-intensive stereotactic radiotherapy before resection of pancreatic cancer at high risk of positive resection margins. Eligible patients will have histologically or cytologically proven pancreatic cancer defined as borderline-resectable per National Comprehensive Cancer Network criteria or operable tumour in contact with vessels increasing the risk of positive margin. Up to 24 patients will be recruited from up to 5 treating centres and a 'rolling-six' design is utilised to minimise delays and facilitate ongoing recruitment during dose-escalation. Radiotherapy will be delivered in 5 daily fractions and surgery, if appropriate, will take place 5–6 weeks after radiotherapy. The margin-intense radiotherapy concept includes a systematic method to define the target volume for a simultaneous integrated boost in the region of tumour-vessel infiltration, and up to 4 radiotherapy dose levels will be investigated. Maximum tolerated dose is defined as the highest dose at which no more than 1 of 6 patients or 0 of 3 patients experience a dose limiting toxicity. Secondary endpoints include resection rate, resection margin status, response rate, overall survival and progression free survival at 12 and 24 months. Translational work will involve exploratory analyses of the cytological and humoral immunological responses to stereotactic radiotherapy in pancreatic cancer. Radiotherapy quality assurance of target definition and radiotherapy planning is enforced with pre-trial test cases and on-trial review. Recruitment began in April 2015.

(Continued on next page)

* Correspondence: maria.hawkins@oncology.ox.ac.uk
[1]CRUK/MRC Oxford Institute for Radiation Oncology, Department of Oncology, University of Oxford, Old Road Campus Research Building, Roosevelt Drive, Oxford OX3 7DQ, UK
Full list of author information is available at the end of the article

(Continued from previous page)

Discussion: This prospective multi-centre study aims to establish the maximum tolerated dose of pre-operative margin-intensified stereotactic radiotherapy in pancreatic cancer at high risk of positive resection margins with a view to subsequent definitive comparison with other neoadjuvant treatment options.

Keywords: Pancreatic cancer, Borderline-resectable, Stereotactic body radiation therapy (SBRT)

Background

Pancreatic cancer is responsible for only 3 % of cancer diagnoses but 5 % of cancer deaths, making it the fifth leading cause of cancer death in the UK (9408 cases in 2013 and 8817 deaths in 2014) [1]. Radical surgical resection represents the only chance of long-term disease control, but was possible for just 8 % of UK patients diagnosed in 2006–2010 [2]. In Europe standard practice for resectable disease is surgery followed by chemotherapy, but for these patients median survival is only 24 months and 50 % of patients will suffer local recurrence [3] suggesting that further improvement in multimodal therapy is required.

The failure to consistently achieve microscopic surgical clearance contributes to the high rates of disease relapse: alongside tumour size, grade and lymph node metastases, resection margin involvement has been repeatedly shown to predict long-term survival [4–6]. Accurate margin assessment requires comprehensive examination of the surgical specimen and rates of margin involvement are higher when a standardised protocol is used [7]. Despite centralization of services and improvement in diagnostic radiology, positive margins were reported in >35 % of patients in the largest multi-national adjuvant trial in pancreatic cancer involving over 1000 patients (ESPAC 3), which again reinforced that patients with positive margins have poor outcome (hazard ratio 1.35, 95 % confidence interval 1.17-1.56, $p < 0.001$) [8].

A small proportion of patients present with pancreatic tumours that can be classified as "borderline-resectable", defined by a limited extent of vascular invasion. For these patients resection is possible but is likely to require vascular reconstruction and there is an especially high risk of positive resection margins, reported to be 62.9 % in the UK [9]. The concept of Borderline Resectable Pancreatic Cancer (BRPC) was initially described in 2001 by Mehta et al., describing 15 cases initially assessed as "marginally resectable" but where resectability was improved with preoperative chemoradiotherapy [10]. The definition of BRPC was refined by an AHPBA/SSO/SSAT consensus statement [11, 12], now adopted by the NCCN [13]:-

- Venous involvement of the SMV or PV with distortion or narrowing of the vein or occlusion of the vein with suitable vessel proximal and distal, allowing safe resection and reconstruction
- Gastro-duodenal artery encasement up to hepatic artery with either short segment encasement or direct abutment of the hepatic artery, without extension to the celiac axis
- Tumour abutment of the SMA not to exceed greater than 180° of the circumference of the vessel wall.

An alternative definition of BRPC by the MDACC has not been as widely recognised [14]. A multidisciplinary team approach is needed to assess the likelihood of attaining negative margins and this should remain the key consideration in determining if a patient is a potential candidate for resection [14, 15].

The management of BPRC is controversial, and there is increased interest in pre-operative treatment strategies that may improve outcomes [16]. Theoretical advantages include a greater chance of delivering full dose treatment, while drawbacks include possible overtreatment of resectable disease, the need for a biopsy and stent to relieve obstruction while awaiting surgery. Many patients presenting with localised disease develop frank metastases shortly after diagnosis and if this occurs during induction therapy these patients can be spared inappropriate and futile surgery [14].

Pre-operative (chemo) radiotherapy aims to treat the tumour in situ to achieve tumour regression and facilitate curative resection. This approach has become standard of care for some tumour sites, having been shown to reduce local recurrence in rectal cancer [17], and increase overall survival in oesophageal cancer [18], but is not established in pancreatic cancer due to limited effectiveness of standard dose schedules, despite potential advantages over postoperative treatment [19]. A complete tumour response is only seen in around 5 % of patients [20], though a larger proportion of patients (35 %) benefit from tumour down-staging to achieve resectability [21] and patients who successfully complete neoadjuvant chemoradiotherapy and go on to have resection tend to have high rates of clear resection margins [22, 23] and reduced rates of local recurrence [24, 25].

Stereotactic body radiation therapy (SBRT) combines rigorous immobilisation and image-guidance with hypofractionation, to reduce radiotherapy planning margins and treat small targeted volumes with greater accuracy and precision, supporting safe delivery of much higher biologically effective doses. It has been shown to be a highly-effective local treatment option in unresectable pancreatic cancer with high rates of local control achieved using treatment delivered in a single exposure [26–29], and when treatment was delivered in 3–5 fractions lower rates of toxicity were seen without compromising disease control [30–35].

The specific goal in treating BRPC with pre-operative radiotherapy will be improve the chances of achieving clear resection margins, reduce risk of local recurrence and achieve chances of long-term survival similar to those for patients with initially resectable tumours. Neoadjuvant treatment has been shown to be deliverable and effective in BRPC, such as in a series of 160 patients described by Katz et al., among whom 78 % completed preoperative therapy and restaging, and 41 % underwent pancreatectomy, with a 94 % rate of clear margins [36].

The premise of the SPARC trial is a Margin-Intense radiotherapy concept where the whole tumour is treated to a minimum dose while a simultaneous integrated boost (SIB) is used to deliver additional dose to the margin of tumour around structures such as the superior mesenteric artery (SMA), SMV or portal vein and retroperitoneal margin. This approach complements surgery as these are the most difficult margins to resect and are at highest risk of positive surgical margins. Prospective dose-escalation aims to establish the maximum tolerated dose for this treatment paradigm for subsequent definitive investigation of efficacy. Once the maximum tolerated dose (MTD) is established this will provide a platform to integrate with optimal systemic treatment.

Methods/Design

Study design

The SPARC trial is a phase I dose-escalation study using the rolling six design [37] to establish MTD of SBRT delivered in the pre-operative setting for borderline resectable pancreatic cancers. This method minimises delays in the dose escalation phase [37]. Patients will complete SBRT in approximately one week and surgery will take place 5–6 weeks after radiotherapy. Patients will be on the study for 36 weeks from registration to end of treatment visit followed by standard care for two years post SBRT day one for the last patient, or when all participants have died.

The trial opened in April 2015 and will recruit up to 24 patients from five UK centres (Oxford, Glasgow, Leeds, Newcastle and Nottingham). The SPARC trial is conducted in accordance with the Helsinki Declaration (1996) and the regulatory requirements for clinical trials of an investigational medicinal product under the European Union Clinical Trials Directive. The trial is approved by the National Research Ethics Service Committee South Central – Oxford B (REC reference: 15/SC/0059) and is sponsored by the University of Oxford, with funding from Cancer Research UK. Data submission for the SPARC trial is via electronic submission into the online database system OpenClinica by site staff. The Oncology Clinical Trial Office (OCTO) coordinates and manages the trial while the Centre for Statistics in Medicine (University of Oxford) will perform all statistical analysis.

Participants

The inclusion and exclusion criteria for the SPARC trial are summarised in Table 1.

Interventions

At registration patients are assigned to the appropriate SBRT dose level (Table 2) and will receive 5 fractions of SBRT over 5–8 days. The dose schedules selected have been designed to achieve approximately equivalent dose to the tumour to that used in conventionally fractionated radical radiotherapy (50-66Gy in 2Gy fractions) while the dose selected for the 'at risk volume' (area at risk of positive margin) is higher, to achieve increased likelihood of ablation of tumour cells. A maximum of 4 dose levels (including one de-escalated dose level) are expected to be needed to establish the MTD.

Dose level assignment will be based on the number of dose limiting toxicities (DLTs) observed, and the number of patients have no DLTs yet, but are still in the DLT assessment period as defined in the outcome measure below (i.e., toxicity data pending/evaluable not yet). In this trial design, the first two patients are treated at level 1. The third patient will be treated at level –1 if two DLTs have been observed. If at least one patients enrolled is not evaluable yet and less than 2 DLTs have been observed, this third patient will be entered at the same dose level, Level 1. For the fourth patient, if toxicity data is pending for at least one of the patients enrolled, the fourth patient will be allocated to the same dose level. But, if there are two or more DLTs when the fourth patient enters the study, the dose level will be de-escalated. The dose level will be escalated if there is no DLT after the first three patients finish the DLT assessment period. This process will be repeated for patients five and six. After the sixth patient is enrolled to a dose cohort, accrual will be only temporarily suspended until toxicity data is fully available for these six patients and/or a decision from the Trial Management Group (TMG) is made. Recruitment will stop once the MTD is identified.

Table 1 SPARC Inclusion/Exclusion criteria

Inclusion criteria	Exclusion criteria
1. Borderline resectable localised tumour of the pancreatic head/uncinate process/body as per NCCN Guidelines (tumours of the tail of pancreas are not eligible for inclusion) or operable tumour in contact with vessels increasing the risk of positive margin as defined by CT +/− MRI +/− PET criteria within 28 +/− 7 days prior to trial entry, de novo or following systemic treatment.	1. Definitive metastatic disease or local disease that cannot be encompassed in the SBRT field.
2. Histologically proven pancreatic ductal adenocarcinoma or cytological proven pancreatic malignancy	2. History of previous or concurrent malignancy diagnoses for which the expected prognosis is likely to be worse than that of the current diagnosis of pancreatic cancer (excludes for example: e.g., localised prostate cancer, early colorectal cancer, early breast cancer, curatively-treated basal cell carcinoma of skin, carcinoma in situ of cervix; curatively treated cancer of other sites who are recurrence free for >3 years).
3. Able to undergo biliary drainage using a stent	
4. Deemed fit and suitable for surgical resection.	
5. No overt metastases or uncertain status with investigations suspicious of possible metastatic disease (e.g., small equivocal pulmonary nodule(s)).	3. Serious medical or psychological condition precluding trial intervention.
6. Male or female, Age ≥16 years	4. Previous upper abdominal or right chest wall radiotherapy where 30 % of the liver has received >15Gy.
7. Life expectancy of at least 6 months	
8. ECOG performance status 0–1	5. Pregnancy: Pregnant or breast-feeding women are ineligible. Women of childbearing potential must use effective methods of contraception.
9. The patient is willing and able to comply with the protocol for the duration of the study, and scheduled follow-up visits and examinations	
10. Written (signed and dated) informed consent and be capable of co-operating with protocol	6. Any other psychological, social or medical condition, physical examination finding or laboratory abnormality that the Investigator considers makes the patient a poor trial candidate or could interfere with protocol compliance or the interpretation of the trial results.
11. Haematological and biochemical indices within specified ranges.	

Outcome measures and definitions

The primary endpoint of the SPARC study is MTD, defined as the highest level of SBRT at which no more than 1 of 6 patients or 0 of 3 patients experiences a DLT in the period from starting SBRT to one month post-surgery or one month after the evaluation in week 3 post-SBRT if no surgery takes place. DLT is defined as these possible adverse events (AEs) (according to CTCAE v4.03), seen in the DLT assessment period:

1. ≥ Grade 3 upper gastro-intestinal (GI) bleeding
2. ≥ Grade 4 nausea/vomiting uncontrolled after 48 h of standard treatment
3. ≥ Grade 4 pancreatitis not stent related
4. Interruption of SBRT >1 week due to SBRT-related AEs
5. ≥ Grade 4 vascular events: SMV thrombosis, bowel ischaemia due to SMA arteritis/stenosis, friable vessels at surgery
6. Other AEs that the TMG agrees to be dose limiting and possibly related to SBRT such as ≥ grade 3 gastrointestinal fistula >30 days after surgery

Secondary outcomes include resection rate, resection margin status rates, rate of pathological complete response, late SBRT toxicity, efficacy and long term safety. Resection rate is defined as the proportion of patients with radical oncological resection of pancreatic cancer over the total enrolled patients. Resection margin status (R0/R1/R2) is defined according to the standards of the Royal College of Pathologists, and response rate is defined as the rate of patients with pathological complete response over the total enrolled patients. Late toxicity is defined as any GI AE/other AE > grade 2 occurring between 1 month and 6 month post-surgery. Additional secondary outcomes include efficacy and long term safety as indicated by progression free survival (PFS) and overall survival (OS). PFS is defined as the time from date of first SBRT dose to the first date of progression or death for any cause, or is censored at the date of last known follow-up date if they are not observed to die during the course of the trial. OS is defined as the time from date of first SBRT dose to the date of death for any cause or is censored at the last known follow-up date. Exploratory outcomes include relationships between imaging and pathology (treatment response and resection margin status) and changes in markers of the innate and adaptive immune response before and during SBRT (cytological assessments and levels of interferon-related RNA).

Table 2 Radiotherapy dose escalation levels

Radiotherapy dose level	Tumour (PTV)				Area at risk of R1 (PTV_R)			
	Dose/# [Gy]	Total dose [Gy]	*BED [Gy$_{10}$]	EQD$_2$ [Gy]	Dose/# [Gy]	Total dose [Gy]	*BED [Gy$_{10}$]	EQD$_2$ [Gy]
Level −1	6	30	50	40	8	40	72	60
Level 1	6	30	50	40	9	45	88	71.5
Level 2	6.5	32.5	56	45	9.5	47.5	92	77.2
Level 3	7	35	62	50	10	50	100	83.3

*BED [Gy$_{10}$] biologically effective dose for acute reacting tissues (α/β = 10), EQD$_2$ equivalent dose in 2-Gy fractions

Sample size considerations

Patient numbers will be determined by the primary end-point of establishing the MTD, which will require a maximum of 24 evaluable patients. An evaluable patient for primary endpoint analysis is defined as one who has received at least one fraction of SBRT and experiences a DLT, or a patient who has received at least four fractions of SBRT and is assessed one month post-surgery (or assessed at similar time for DLT if no surgery). Patients not evaluable for primary endpoint will be replaced, but a patient who does not become evaluable for the primary endpoint may continue to be followed up for surgical outcome, PFS and OS as appropriate, unless consent is withdrawn.

Statistical analysis

All analyses will follow a statistical analysis plan written in accordance with current standard operating procedures. Baseline characteristics will be summarised (number/frequency) for all enrolled patients. Patients who died or withdrew before treatment started or fail to complete the required safety observations will be described separately. Primary MTD analysis will concern the frequency of patients with no DLT according to dose-escalation of SBRT. Descriptive statistics will summarise the DLT's and safety variables with patients grouped according to dose level received. Secondary outcomes (resection rate, resection margin status and response rate) associated with SBRT will be summarised by descriptive statistics along with numbers and percentages. Late toxicity will be summarised by descriptive statistics for all patients who received at least one dose of SBRT treatment. Physical exam, haematology and biochemistry data will be summarised across time. Both PFS and OS estimates at one and two years and 90 % CI will be provided together with median estimates. A Kaplan-Meier curve will be plotted with 90 % CI. A trial summary will record patient recruitment and trial decision-making.

Monitoring committees

The Radiotherapy and Imaging Trials Oversight Committee (RIOC) is the independent committee for SPARC covering both data management committee and oversight responsibilities as delegated by the Sponsor and will meet at least once annually to review and ratify substantial decisions.

Discussion

This study builds on the current evidence base in SBRT for pancreatic cancer, which has so far been largely used in the locally advanced setting with promising results and aims to take it a step further by prospectively evaluating the safety and benefit of pre-operative margin-intense SBRT.

A five-fraction schedule aims to optimise the balance of short duration and tumouricidal biologically-effective dose to the tumour with acceptable risk of late normal tissue injury. Potential clinical benefits of a significantly hypofractionated radiotherapy regimen compared with a protracted conventional 6-week course of chemoradiotherapy include a shorter enforced delay to definitive surgery or alternatively more straightforward integration with systemic therapy regimens.

The concept of margin-intensive therapy aims to further improve local control without increasing toxicity, as the region of integrated boost tends not to overlap with the major dose-limiting organ at risk (duodenum) helping to make safe dose-escalation to this sub-volume possible. Normal-tissue dose-volume constraints retain priority but where there is overlap, only the dose to the overlapping region is constrained as necessary, enabling the non-overlapping portion of the target volume to receive the prescribed dose (see Fig. 1).

The optimal pre-operative therapy in pancreatic cancer has not been identified, and could involve chemotherapy, radiotherapy or both. The national multicentre study ESPAC-5 F is currently open to recruitment in the UK with the primary aim to establish the feasibility of recruiting patients with BRPC to be randomised between two pre-operative chemotherapy regimens (GEMCAP and FOLFIRINOX), pre-operative CRT and standard of care (surgery followed by adjuvant chemotherapy) (38), therapy options which would then require definitive comparative evaluation in a subsequent larger study.

Two single-institution retrospective reviews report outcomes for the use of SBRT in patients with BRPC, both of which show high rates of subsequent successful surgical resection with clear margins [38, 39]. Rajagopalan et al. [38] report on 12 resected patients, of which 7 were deemed BRPC using.

MDACC criteria. Most patients received Gemcitabine-based systemic chemotherapy. The SBRT consisted of 24–36 Gy in 3 fractions, surgery took place at a median 3.3 months (range 1.5 – 6.6 months) and 11/12 patients had an R0 resection. Chuong et al. [39] treated 73 patients (of which 57 were deemed BRPC using NCCN criteria) with systemic Gemcitabine-based chemotherapy and 5-fraction SBRT. Median dose prescribed was 35 Gy to the tumour margin and no less than 25 Gy to the entire pancreatic tumour. 44/57 BRPC cases underwent exploratory resection and 31/32 resected cases had an R0 resection. No acute toxicity > grade 3 occurred and 5.3 % (4 patients with locally advanced inoperable disease) experienced late grade 3 toxicity (3 GI bleeding and 1 anorexia). With a median FU of 10.5 months (2.2-25.9 months) the median OS was 16.4 months in all BRPC patients, with median OS of 19.3 months in resected patients. Disappointing overall survival rates in

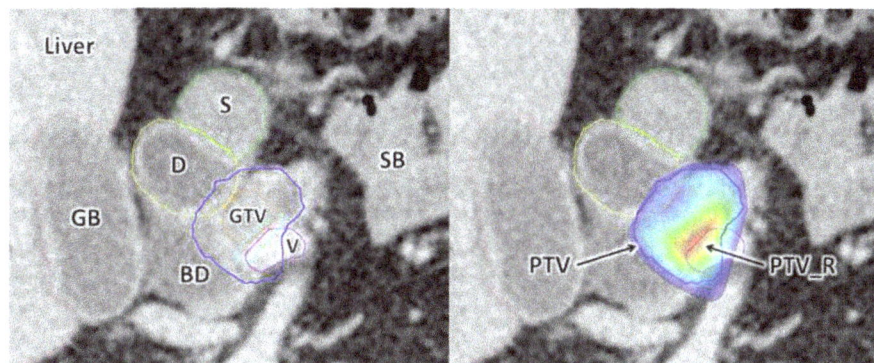

Fig. 1 Axial contrast-enhanced CT of patient with borderline-resectable pancreatic cancer demonstrating SPARC radiotherapy planning. Left-hand image - delineated structures: (*clockwise from left*) GB = gall-bladder, D = duodenum, S = stomach, SB = small-bowel, V = vessel in contact with tumour, GTV = Gross Tumour Volume, BD = bile duct. Right-hand image - radiotherapy plan dose colourwash demonstrating dose levels delivered to PTV_R (*light blue contour*), PTV (*dark blue*) and PTV overlapping with duodenum

published series (median overall survival 5–20 months) are attributed to variable provision of optimal systemic treatment.

Evidence is growing for the importance of Radiation Therapy Quality Assurance (RTQA) for clinical trial interpretation as well as patient outcomes [40]. The SPARC trial incorporates a comprehensive prospective RTQA programme with a detailed radiotherapy protocol and atlas that was supported by a pre-trial workshop for collaborating clinicians, both of which have been shown to reduce variation in target volume definition [41–43]. A pre-trial test case of contouring and planning must be completed satisfactorily by recruiting centres and RTQA will continue with on-trial peer review prior to treatment supported by web-conferencing facilities.

The trial originally opened with eligibility criteria that excluded patients with suspicion of metastatic disease, those who may not be fit for surgical resection, and those who had received induction chemotherapy, which has become more common practice since the study was initially designed. Many patients presenting to our centre with BRPC were rendered ineligible for these reasons, and during the first year that the trial was open only one patient was successfully recruited. The primary endpoint of the study is the assessment of the safety and tolerability of the intervention, and therefore the patient eligibility inclusion and exclusion criteria for the study were revised to the current version published here, with the aim of improving patient recruitment.

Exploratory immunological investigations

Preclinical evidence suggests radiotherapy generates an immunological response, which can contribute to the efficacy of treatment. Direct damage and local inflammation increases antigen presentation to stimulate adaptive immune responses, and radiotherapy delivered in larger fractions has been shown to particularly enhance this

effect [28]. In the SPARC study a panel of immunological tests to examine innate and adaptive immune responses to pancreatic SBRT. These preliminary data will be explored for their utility as predictive bio-markers in future studies.

Conclusion

The non-interventional phase of follow-up after the last patient last visit at the end of study will permit an estimate of the efficacy of pre-operative SBRT on overall survival and progression free survival to be observed. Once the MTD has been defined in this phase I trial, a phase II study will definitively evaluate efficacy endpoints. If positive, subsequent randomised phase III investigations will be required to assess superiority of this treatment strategy alone or integrated with pre-operative systemic treatment over surgery alone for this patient group.

Abbreviations

AHPBA: American Hepato-Pancreato-Biliary Association; ALP: Alkaline phosphatase; AST: Aspartate transaminase; BED: Biologically effective dose; BRPC: Borderline resectable pancreatic cancer; CI: Confidence interval; CRT: Chemo-radiotherapy; CRUK: Cancer Research United Kingdom; CSM: University of Oxford Centre for Statistics in Medicine; CT: Computed tomography; CTAAC: Cancer Research UK Clinical Trials Award and Advisory Committee; DLT: Dose-limiting toxicity; ESPAC: European study group for pancreatic cancer; EQD$_2$: Equivalent dose in 2-Gy fractions; FOLFIRINOX: Folinic acid-5-fluourouracil-irinotecan-oxaliplatin; FU: Follow-up; GEMCAP: Gemcitabine-capecitabine; HR: Hazard ratio; MDACC: MD Anderson Cancer Centre; MDT: Multi-disciplinary team; MRI: Magnetic resonance imaging; MTD: Maximum tolerated dose; NCCN: National comprehensive cancer network; OCTO: Oncology clinical trials office; OCTRU: Oxford clinical trials research unit; OIRO: CRUK/MRC Oxford Institute for Radiation Oncology; OS: Overall survival; PFS: Progression-free survival; PV: Portal vein; REC: Research ethics committee; RIOC: Radiotherapy and imaging trials oversight committee; RTQA: Radiation therapy quality assurance; SBRT: Stereotactic body radiation therapy; SMA: Superior mesenteric artery; SMV: Superior mesenteric vein; SSAT: Society for surgery of the alimentary tract; SSO: Society of surgical oncology

Acknowledgements

The SPARC clinical trial is sponsored by the University of Oxford.

Trial Management Group:
Prof David Sebag-Montefiore, Dr Ganesh Radhakrishna, Mr Andrew Smith (Leeds Teaching Hospital NHS Trust).
Dr Derek Grose, Dr David McIntosh (Beatson Cancer Centre, Glasgow).
Dr Somnath Mukherjee, Dr Neel Patel, Mr Michael Silva, Mr Maxwell Robinson (Oxford University Hospitals NHS Trust, Oxford).
Dr Victoria Strauss, Dr Lang'o Odondi (Centre for Statistical Medicine, Oxford).
Translational research team: Dr Emmanouil Fokas (Oxford Institute for Radiation Oncology, Oxford), Professor Alan Melcher (The Institute of Cancer Research, London).

Funding
The trial is funded by Cancer Research UK (grant number C43735/A18787). DLPH is funded by a CRUK Nuffield Clinical Research Fellowship, grant code C5255. MAH is funded by the MRC (Medical Research Council), grant code MC_PC_12001/2.

Authors' contributions
DLPH drafted the manuscript and participated in trial design and coordination. VS & LO developed the trial design and helped to draft the manuscript. MAH conceived the study, participated in its design and coordination and helped to draft the manuscript. All authors were involved in the trial design and have read and approved the final manuscript.

Competing interests
The authors declare that they have no competing interests.

Author details
[1]CRUK/MRC Oxford Institute for Radiation Oncology, Department of Oncology, University of Oxford, Old Road Campus Research Building, Roosevelt Drive, Oxford OX3 7DQ, UK. [2]Oncology Clinical Trials Office, Department of Oncology, University of Oxford, Old Road Campus Research Building, Roosevelt Drive, Oxford OX3 7DQ, UK. [3]The Beatson West of Scotland Cancer Centre, 1053 Great Western Rd, Glasgow G12 0YN, UK. [4]The University of Leeds, Cancer Research UK Leeds Centre,14 Leeds Institute of Cancer and Pathology, Cancer Genetics Building, St James's University Hospital, 15 Beckett Street, Leeds, West Yorkshire LS9 7TF, UK. [5]Leeds Cancer Centre, Leeds Teaching Hospitals NHS Trust, Bexley Wing, Beckett Street, Leeds LS9 7TF, UK. [6]Oxford University Hospitals NHS Foundation Trust, Old Road, Headington, Oxford OX3 7LE, UK. [7]Centre for Statistics in Medicine, Nuffield Department of Orthopaedics, Rheumatology and Musculoskeletal Sciences, University of Oxford, Botnar Research Centre, Windmill Road, Oxford OX3 7LD, UK. [8]The Institute of Cancer Research, Chester Beatty Laboratories, 237, Fulham Rd, London SW3 6JB, UK.

References
1. Pancreatic cancer statistics. [http://www.cancerresearchuk.org/health-professional/cancer-statistics/statistics-by-cancer-type/pancreatic-cancer]. Accessed 9 Sept 2016.
2. National Cancer Intelligence Network and Cancer Research UK. Major resections by cancer site, in England; 2006–2010. London: Public Health England; 2015. http://www.ncin.org.uk/view?rid=2972. Accessed 9 Sept 2016.
3. Oettle H, Neuhaus P, Hochhaus A, Hartmann JT, Gellert K, Ridwelski K, et al. Adjuvant chemotherapy with gemcitabine and long-term outcomes among patients with resected pancreatic cancer: the CONKO-001 randomized trial. JAMA. 2013;310(14):1473–81.
4. Sohn TA, Yeo CJ, Cameron JL, Koniaris L, Kaushal S, Abrams RA, et al. Resected adenocarcinoma of the pancreas-616 patients: results, outcomes, and prognostic indicators. J Gastrointest Surg. 2000;4(6):567–79.
5. Howard TJ, Krug JE, Yu J, Zyromski NJ, Schmidt CM, Jacobson LE, et al. A margin-negative R0 resection accomplished with minimal postoperative complications is the surgeon's contribution to long-term survival in pancreatic cancer. J Gastrointest Surg. 2006;10(10):1338–45. discussion 1345-1336.

6. Ghaneh P, Costello E, Neoptolemos JP. Biology and management of pancreatic cancer. Gut. 2007;56(8):1134–52.
7. Verbeke CS, Menon KV. Redefining resection margin status in pancreatic cancer. HPB (Oxford). 2009;11(4):282–9.
8. Neoptolemos JP, Stocken DD, Bassi C, Ghaneh P, Cunningham D, Goldstein D, et al. Adjuvant chemotherapy with fluorouracil plus folinic acid vs gemcitabine following pancreatic cancer resection: A randomized controlled trial. JAMA. 2010;304(10):1073–81.
9. Ravikumar R, Sabin C, Abu Hilal M, Bramhall S, White S, Wigmore S, et al. Portal vein resection in borderline resectable pancreatic cancer: a United Kingdom multicenter study. J Am Coll Surg. 2014;218(3):401–11.
10. Mehta VK, Fisher G, Ford JA, Poen JC, Vierra MA, Oberhelman H, et al. Preoperative chemoradiation for marginally resectable adenocarcinoma of the pancreas. J Gastrointest Surg. 2001;5(1):27–35.
11. Callery MP, Chang KJ, Fishman EK, Talamonti MS, William Traverso L, Linehan DC. Pretreatment assessment of resectable and borderline resectable pancreatic cancer: expert consensus statement. Ann Surg Oncol. 2009;16(7):1727–33.
12. Vauthey JN, Dixon E. AHPBA/SSO/SSAT Consensus Conference on Resectable and Borderline Resectable Pancreatic Cancer: rationale and overview of the conference. Ann Surg Oncol. 2009;16(7):1725–6.
13. National Comprehensive Cancer Network. Pancreatic Adenocarcinoma Version 2.2015. 2015. Accessed 31st Dec 2015.
14. Varadhachary GR, Tamm EP, Abbruzzese JL, Xiong HQ, Crane CH, Wang H, et al. Borderline resectable pancreatic cancer: definitions, management, and role of preoperative therapy. Ann Surg Oncol. 2006;13(8):1035–46.
15. Talamonti M. Borderline resectable pancreatic cancer: a new classification for an old challenge. Ann Surg Oncol. 2006;13(8):1019–20.
16. Heestand GM, Murphy JD, Lowy AM. Approach to patients with pancreatic cancer without detectable metastases. J Clin Oncol. 2015;33(16):1770–8.
17. Sauer R, Liersch T, Merkel S, Fietkau R, Hohenberger W, Hess C, et al. Preoperative versus postoperative chemoradiotherapy for locally advanced rectal cancer: results of the German CAO/ARO/AIO-94 randomized phase III trial after a median follow-up of 11 years. J Clin Oncol. 2012;30(16):1926–33.
18. van Hagen P, Hulshof MC, van Lanschot JJ, Steyerberg EW, van Berge Henegouwen MI, Wijnhoven BP, et al. Preoperative chemoradiotherapy for esophageal or junctional cancer. N Engl J Med. 2012;366(22):2074–84.
19. Stessin AM, Meyer JE, Sherr DL. Neoadjuvant Radiation Is Associated With Improved Survival in Patients With Resectable Pancreatic Cancer: An Analysis of Data From the Surveillance, Epidemiology, and End Results (SEER) Registry. Int J Radiat Oncol Biol Phys. 2008;72(4):1128–33.
20. Moutardier V, Magnin V, Turrini O, Viret F, Hennekinne-Mucci S, Goncalves A, et al. Assessment of pathologic response after preoperative chemoradiotherapy and surgery in pancreatic adenocarcinoma. Int J Radiat Oncol Biol Phys. 2004;60(2):437–43.
21. Gillen S, Schuster T, Meyer Zum Buschenfelde C, Friess H, Kleeff J. Preoperative/neoadjuvant therapy in pancreatic cancer: a systematic review and meta-analysis of response and resection percentages. PLoS Med. 2010;7(4):e1000267.
22. Sasson AR, Wetherington RW, Hoffman JP, Ross EA, Cooper H, Meropol NJ, et al. Neoadjuvant chemoradiotherapy for adenocarcinoma of the pancreas: Analysis of histopathology and outcome. Int J Gastrointest Cancer. 2004;34(2–3):121–7.
23. White RR, Xie HB, Gottfried MR, Czito BG, Hurwitz HI, Morse MA, et al. Significance of histological response to preoperative chemoradiotherapy for pancreatic cancer. Ann Surg Oncol. 2005;12(3):214–21.
24. Breslin TM, Hess KR, Harbison DB, Jean ME, Cleary KR, Dackiw AP, et al. Neoadjuvant chemoradiotherapy for adenocarcinoma of the pancreas: treatment variables and survival duration. Ann Surg Oncol. 2001;8(2):123–32.
25. Greer SE, Pipas JM, Sutton JE, Zaki BI, Tsapakos M, Colacchio TA, et al. Effect of neoadjuvant therapy on local recurrence after resection of pancreatic adenocarcinoma. J Am Coll Surg. 2008;206(3):451–7.
26. Koong AC, Le QT, Ho A, Fong B, Fisher G, Cho C, et al. Phase I study of stereotactic radiosurgery in patients with locally advanced pancreatic cancer. Int J Radiat Oncol Biol Phys. 2004;58(4):1017–21.
27. Koong AC, Christofferson E, Le QT, Goodman KA, Ho A, Kuo T, et al. Phase II study to assess the efficacy of conventionally fractionated radiotherapy followed by a stereotactic radiosurgery boost in patients with locally advanced pancreatic cancer. Int J Radiat Oncol Biol Phys. 2005;63(2):320–3.

A phase-I trial of pre-operative, margin intensive, stereotactic body radiation therapy for pancreatic...

117

28. Schellenberg D, Goodman KA, Lee F, Chang S, Kuo T, Ford JM, et al. Gemcitabine chemotherapy and single-fraction stereotactic body radiotherapy for locally advanced pancreatic cancer. Int J Radiat Oncol Biol Phys. 2008;72(3):678–86.

29. Schellenberg D, Kim J, Christman-Skieller C, Chun CL, Columbo LA, Ford JM, et al. Single-fraction stereotactic body radiation therapy and sequential gemcitabine for the treatment of locally advanced pancreatic cancer. Int J Radiat Oncol Biol Phys. 2011;81(1):181–8.

30. Polistina F, Costantin G, Casamassima F, Francescon P, Guglielmi R, Panizzoni G, et al. Unresectable locally advanced pancreatic cancer: a multimodal treatment using neoadjuvant chemoradiotherapy (gemcitabine plus stereotactic radiosurgery) and subsequent surgical exploration. Ann Surg Oncol. 2010;17(8):2092–101.

31. Mahadevan A, Miksad R, Goldstein M, Sullivan R, Bullock A, Buchbinder E, et al. Induction gemcitabine and stereotactic body radiotherapy for locally advanced nonmetastatic pancreas cancer. Int J Radiat Oncol Biol Phys. 2011; 81(4):e615–22.

32. Lominska CE, Unger K, Nasr NM, Haddad N, Gagnon G. Stereotactic body radiation therapy for reirradiation of localized adenocarcinoma of the pancreas. Radiat Oncol. 2012;7(1):74.

33. Tozzi A, Comito T, Alongi F, Navarria P, Iftode C, Mancosu P, et al. SBRT in unresectable advanced pancreatic cancer: preliminary results of a mono-institutional experience. Radiat Oncol. 2013;8(1):148.

34. Gurka MK, Kim C, He AR, Charabaty A, Haddad N, Turocy J, et al. Stereotactic Body Radiation Therapy (SBRT) Combined With Chemotherapy for Unresected Pancreatic Adenocarcinoma. Am J Clin Oncol. 2014.

35. Herman JM, Chang DT, Goodman KA, Dholakia AS, Raman SP, Hacker-Prietz A, et al. Phase 2 multi-institutional trial evaluating gemcitabine and stereotactic body radiotherapy for patients with locally advanced unresectable pancreatic adenocarcinoma. Cancer. 2015;121(7):1128–37.

36. Katz MH, Pisters PW, Evans DB, Sun CC, Lee JE, Fleming JB, et al. Borderline resectable pancreatic cancer: the importance of this emerging stage of disease. J Am Coll Surg. 2008;206(5):833–46. discussion 846–838.

37. Skolnik JM, Barrett JS, Jayaraman B, Patel D, Adamson PC. Shortening the timeline of pediatric phase I trials: the rolling six design. J Clin Oncol. 2008; 26(2):190–5.

38. Rajagopalan MS, Heron DE, Wegner RE, Zeh HJ, Bahary N, Krasinskas AM, et al. Pathologic response with neoadjuvant chemotherapy and stereotactic body radiotherapy for borderline resectable and locally-advanced pancreatic cancer. Radiat Oncol. 2013;8(1):254.

39. Chuong MD, Springett GM, Freilich JM, Park CK, Weber JM, Mellon EA, et al. Stereotactic body radiation therapy for locally advanced and borderline resectable pancreatic cancer is effective and well tolerated. Int J Radiat Oncol Biol Phys. 2013;86(3):516–22.

40. Willett CG, Moughan J, O'Meara E, Galvin JM, Crane CH, Winter K, et al. Compliance with therapeutic guidelines in Radiation Therapy Oncology Group prospective gastrointestinal clinical trials. Radiother Oncol. 2012;105(1):9–13.

41. Dewas S, Bibault JE, Blanchard P, Vautravers-Dewas C, Pointreau Y, Denis F, et al. Delineation in thoracic oncology: a prospective study of the effect of training on contour variability and dosimetric consequences. Radiat Oncol. 2011;6(1):118.

42. Khoo EL, Schick K, Plank AW, Poulsen M, Wong WW, Middleton M, et al. Prostate contouring variation: can it be fixed? Int J Radiat Oncol Biol Phys. 2012;82(5):1923–9.

43. Nijkamp J, de Haas-Kock DF, Beukema JC, Neelis KJ, Woutersen D, Ceha H, et al. Target volume delineation variation in radiotherapy for early stage rectal cancer in the Netherlands. Radiother Oncol. 2012;102(1):14–21.

Cytoplasmic TRAIL-R1 is a positive prognostic marker in PDAC

Jan-Paul Gundlach[1†], Charlotte Hauser[1†], Franka Maria Schlegel[2], Christine Böger[3], Christian Röder[2], Christoph Röcken[3], Thomas Becker[1], Jan-Hendrik Egberts[1], Holger Kalthoff[2] and Anna Trauzold[1,2*] (iD)

Abstract

Background: The death receptors TRAIL-R1 and TRAIL-R2 are frequently overexpressed in cancer and there is an emerging evidence for their important role in malignant progression, also in the case of pancreatic ductal adenocarcinoma (PDAC). In their canonical localization at the plasma membrane, TRAIL-R1/–R2 may induce cell death and/or pro-inflammatory signaling leading to cell migration, invasion and metastasis. Although, they have repeatedly been found intracellular, in the cytoplasm and in the nucleus, their functions in intracellular locations are still not well understood. Likewise, studies dealing with the prognostic relevance of TRAIL-Rs located in particular cellular compartments are very rare. For PDAC, the correlation of nuclear TRAIL-R2 with worse patients' prognosis has been shown recently. Corresponding data on TRAIL-R1 are not available so far.

Methods: In the present study we analyzed the expression of TRAIL-R1 in 106 PDACs and 28 adjacent, peritumoral non-malignant pancreatic ducts with special emphasis on its cytoplasmic and nuclear localization and correlated the immunohistochemical findings with clinico-pathological patient characteristics.

Results: TRAIL-R1 was found in 93.4% of all PDAC samples. Cytoplasmic staining was present with very similar intensity in tumor and normal tissue. In contrast, nuclear TRAIL-R1 staining was significantly stronger in tumor compared to normal tissue ($p = 0.006$). Interestingly, we found that the number of cells with cytoplasmic TRAIL-R1 staining negatively correlates with tumor grading ($p = 0.043$). No such correlation could be detected for nuclear TRAIL-R1. Neither, cytoplasmic nor nuclear TRAIL-R1 staining showed a correlation with other clinico-pathological parameter such as pTNM categories. However, Kaplan-Meier analyses revealed significantly prolonged median survival of patients with positive cytoplasmic TRAIL-R1 expression in more than 80% of tumor cells compared to patients with tumors containing a smaller quantity of cells positively stained for cytoplasmic TRAIL-R1 (20 vs. 8 months; $p = 0.004$).

Conclusion: Cytoplasmic TRAIL-R1 is a positive prognostic marker for patients with PDAC. Our findings indicate that loss of cytoplasmic TRAIL-R1 results in recurrent disease with more malignant phenotype thus suggesting anti-tumor activities of cytoplasmic TRAIL-R1 in PDAC.

Keywords: TRAIL-R1, Death receptor, Immunhistology, Pancreatic cancer

* Correspondence: atrauzold@email.uni-kiel.de
†Jan-Paul Gundlach and Charlotte Hauser contributed equally to this work.
[1]Department of General Surgery, Visceral, Thoracic, Transplantation and Pediatric Surgery, University Hospital Schleswig-Holstein (UKSH), Campus Kiel, Arnold-Heller Str. 3, Haus 18, 24105 Kiel, Germany
[2]Institute for Experimental Cancer Research, University of Kiel, Arnold-Heller Str. 3 (Haus 17), D-24105 Kiel, Germany
Full list of author information is available at the end of the article

Background

Despite tremendous efforts in molecular and clinical oncology, pancreatic ductal adenocarcinoma (PDAC) still remains one of the deadliest cancers with a mortality rate almost equal to its incidence rate [1]. Its dismal prognosis results from the lack of early diagnostic options, its highly aggressive growth and a resistance to current radio- and chemotherapeutic treatments [2]. Thus, identification of new prognostic markers provides a strategy to uncover still unknown players driving PDAC malignancy and potentially to identify novel therapeutic targets.

TNF-related apoptosis inducing ligand (TRAIL) and its death inducing receptors TRAIL-R1 and TRAIL-R2 are promising candidates for the development of such novel targeted strategies. The rationale behind this assumption is the original observations that i) TRAIL induces apoptosis preferentially in tumor cells leaving normal healthy cells alive; ii) tumor cells usually express high levels of either TRAIL-R1 or TRAIL-R2 or both. These facts led to the development of different TRAIL formulations as well as agonistic TRAIL-R1- or TRAIL-R2-specific antibodies for treatment of human malignancies. However, relatively soon it has been recognized that many tumor cells are resistant to TRAIL induced apoptosis, the fact explaining the disappointing results from clinical trials [3]. In addition, it became evident that TRAIL-R1 and TRAIL-R2 may respond to TRAIL - apart from apoptosis induction - with activation of different non-apoptotic signal transduction pathways like NF-kB, ERK1/ERK2, JNK, Src and AKT [4], which can lead to the inhibition of apoptosis as well as to cell proliferation, migration and invasion. Most importantly, TRAIL receptor signaling may enhance cancer cell invasion and metastasis in vivo [5–7]. Thus, therapeutic concepts are needed which combine TRAIL receptor targeting agents with agents sensitizing tumor cells and reducing the unwanted, non-death-inducing signaling of the receptors. The important concern regarding TRAIL-receptor based anti-tumor therapy is also the observed preference for the usage of the particular TRAIL death receptor for the transmission of the TRAIL-mediated signaling in tumor cells. Generalized predictions on main death receptor responsibility for apoptosis induction in given cancer types are difficult. It is widely accepted that the preference for either TRAIL-R1 or TRAIL-R2 is a cell type specific feature. A comprehensive compilation of tumor cell lines together with their preferences for usage of the particular TRAIL death receptor is provided by Roosmalen et al. [8]. In PDAC cells, others and we have shown that regardless of the simultaneous presence of TRAIL-R1 and TRAIL-R2 at the cell surface, these cells use predominantly TRAIL-R1 when treated with recombinant TRAIL [9, 10].

Consequently, TRAIL-R1-targeting variants of TRAIL and agonistic TRAIL-R1 specific antibodies were expected to have higher therapeutic effects in the treatment of PDAC than they in fact do [3]. Interestingly, a recent report revealed that some PDAC cell lines show preference for TRAIL-R2 in inducing cell death [11] pointing to an unexpected high diversity of TRAIL receptor preference even in the same tumor entity.

Of note, under physiological conditions TRAIL has been shown to be an important effector molecule in the tumor immunosurveillance [12, 13]. On the other hand, malignant cells themselves can produce TRAIL and this may lead to an increase of their invasive and migratory properties [7]. Thus, the expression levels of TRAIL receptors as well as the preference for the usage of TRAIL-R1 or TRAIL-R2 in TRAIL-induced apoptotic/non-apoptotic signaling may be an essential factor determining both, the tumor initiation and progression.

The biological responses to TRAIL are attributed to the function of TRAIL receptors at the plasma membrane. Interestingly, although the intracellular presence of TRAIL-R1 and/or TRAIL-R2 has repeatedly been noticed, only recently the question of biological relevance and eventually specific functions of intracellular receptors began to be addressed. Obviously, sequestration of the receptors in the cytoplasm or in the nucleus, frequently observed in cancer, could represent one of the strategies used by these cells to escape TRAIL-induced apoptosis. Indeed, such mechanisms have been proposed for both cytoplasmic [14–16] and nuclear TRAIL receptors [16–18]. More recently, specific function of nuclear TRAIL-R2 has also been uncovered [19]. In the nucleus, TRAIL-R2 interacts with the microprocessor complex and impairs the maturation of the miRNA let-7. This leads to the increased levels of the malignancy promoting factors HMGA2 and Lin28B and enhances tumor cell proliferation in vitro and in vivo [19]. Likewise, specific functions of cytoplasmic TRAIL death receptors have also been proposed lately. Concrete, in response to endoplasmic reticulum (ER) stress, as a part of unfolded protein response (UPR), cytoplasmic TRAIL-R1 and TRAIL-R2 both are able to aggregate and induce cell death [20, 21].

Interestingly, although numbers of immunohistological studies addressed the issue of the impact of differentially expressed TRAIL death receptors in tumor and corresponding normal healthy tissue, the clinical relevance of TRAIL receptors present in particular intracellular compartment, cytoplasm or nucleus was analyzed only sporadically. For PDAC we reported recently that high levels of nuclear TRAIL-R2 correlates with worse prognosis for PDAC patients suffering from early stage PDACs [19]. The level of TRAIL-R2 in the cytoplasm of PDAC cells, although significantly higher than in healthy tissue, did not correlate with any clinico-pathological parameter. To the best of our knowledge, no corresponding data for TRAIL-R1 are available so far. To fill this gap, we evaluated the clinical relevance of high levels of TRAIL-R1 in tumor tissues of PDAC patients with special emphasis to the possible differential impact of its cytoplasmic and nuclear localization.

Methods

We retrieved formalin fixed and paraffin embedded PDAC and adjacent, peritumoral non-malignant tissue samples from the archives of the Institute of Pathology of the University Hospital Schleswig-Holstein and Christian-Albrechts-University Kiel, resected between 1999 and 2010. Follow-up data were retrieved from the Epidemiological Cancer Registry Schleswig–Holstein, Germany, hospital records and general practitioners. Patients were included if histology confirmed an adenocarcinoma of the pancreas. pTNM stage was determined according to the 8th edition of the Union for International Cancer Control (UICC) guidelines [22]. This study was approved by the local institutional review board of the Medical Faculty of the Christian-Albrechts-University of Kiel (A-110/99).

Immunohistochemical staining

For immunohistochemistry 3 μm paraffin sections were deparaffinized in xylol and re-hydrated in a descending alcohol series. Antigen retrieval was achieved by heating for 15 min at 89 °C in citrate-buffer (pH 6.0). Intrinsic biotin and avidin binding sites were blocked with Avidin-Biotin Blocking Kit (Vector Laboratories, Burlingham, CA), endogenous peroxidase-activity with Hydrogen-Peroxide Block (15 min, RT; Thermo Scientific, Fremont, CA) and unspecific background was reduced with Ultra-Vision Block (5 min, RT; Thermo Scientific, Fremont, CA, USA). Slides were incubated with primary antibodies as previously described (clone TR1.02; Ganten et al., 2009 [23]). Bound antibodies were detected by a Super Sensitive IHC Detection System (BioGenex, San Ramon, USA). For color development, a Fast Red system (Sigma, Deisenhofen, Germany) was used. Washing steps were done with Tris-buffered saline supplemented with Tween (TBST). All slides were counterstained with hemalum and cover slipped.

Microscopic evaluations and histopathological scoring

Evaluation of the staining was performed on a Leica DM 1000-Microscope (Leica, Wetzlar, Germany) and a two-dimensional scoring system was applied to semi-quantitatively assess the TRAIL-R1 expression data. The intensity of the staining was judged on an arbitrary scale of 0 to 3 with 0: no staining; 1: weak staining; 2: moderate staining and 3: strong staining. In samples with varying staining intensities, strongest values were stated. In

addition, the percentage of stained cells was quantified and scaled from 0 to 4 with 0: no positive cells; 1: 1–10%; 2: 10–50%; 3: 51–80%; and 4: 81–100% positively stained cells. Both values were summarized in a sum score (Table 1) and separately assessed for cytoplasm and nuclei by two independent pathologists.

Statistical analyses

Statistical analyses were done using SPSS 23.0 (SPSS, IBM Corporation, Armonk, NY, USA). For the correlation of the clinico-pathological patient characteristics and TRAIL-R1 expression, data were dichotomized and Kendall's Tau (τ) was used. Only patients with existing follow-up data were included. Patients who died within 14 days after surgery and patients who received neoadjuvant treatment were excluded. Consequently, for these analyses 97 out of 106 patients were included. Out of these, 19 patients were censored because they were either alive or lost in follow up. The overall postoperative survival was analyzed. Staining intensities of tumor and normal tissues were compared using the Wilcoxon test as a nonparametric test for paired samples. Survival analyses were performed by Kaplan-Meier estimates and statistical evaluations were done by log-rank tests. P values ≤0.05 were considered significant.

Results

Patient collective

To investigate the significance of TRAIL-R1 for pancreatic cancer biology, we analyzed the staining intensity, the percentage of stained cells and the intracellular distribution of this receptor in sections of 106 tumors and 28 morphologically normal corresponding peritumoral ducts from 106 patients suffering from PDAC. Out of 106 patients, 51 (48.1%) were female and median age was 65 years (range 47–85 years). Cancer of the pancreatic head, corpus and tale were found in 75/106 (70.8%), 7/106 (6.6%) and 8/106 (7.5%) cases, respectively. In 16/106 cases (15.1%), the localization was not specified. The detailed clinico-pathological patient characteristics are summarized in Table 2. Most of the patients have undergone surgery at stage T3 (94/106; 88.7%) and had already developed lymph node metastases (84/106, 79.2%), whereas no patient was operated at stage T1. Resected tumors were well or moderately

Table 1 Histomorphological evaluation score

Staining intensity	Points	Number of positive cells	Points
Negative	0	0%	0
Weak positive	1	< 10%	1
Moderate positive	2	10–50%	2
Strong positive	3	51–80%	3
–	–	81–100%	4

Table 2 Clinico-pathological patient characteristics on the basis of the TNM status (according to the UICC Classification of Malignant Tumors). Given are the total number of patients and the percentage (%)

Feature	n	%
T – category		
T1	0	0.0
T2	3	2.8
T3	94	88.7
T4	9	8.5
N - category		
N0	22	20.8
N1	84	79.2
NX	0	0.0
M - category		
M0	69	65.1
M1	11	10.4
MX	26	24.5
Venous invasion		
V0	79	74.5
V1	19	17.9
V2	3	2.8
VX	5	4.7
Perineural invasion		
Pn0	39	36.8
Pn1	59	55.7
PnX	8	7.5
Lymphatic invasion		
L0	30	28.3
L1	71	67.0
LX	5	4.7
R - status		
R0	74	69.8
R1	28	26.4
R2	2	1.9
RX	2	1.9
Histopathological grading		
G1	11	10.4
G2	59	55.7
G3	35	33.0
G4	1	0.9

T1: Tumor < 2 cm within pancreas; T2: > 2 cm, T3 over pancreas without infiltration of A. mes. Sup. or Truncus coeliacus, T4: vessel infiltration

differentiated in 66.1% of the cases. In 89.6% (95/106), patients were free of distant metastases at the time of resection. Resection without residual tumor load was achieved in 74/106 patients (69.8%).

Expression of TRAIL-R1 in PDAC and non-malignant adjacent tissue

TRAIL-R1 was expressed in 93.4% (99/106) of all PDAC samples (Table 3a). Analysis of its intracellular distribution revealed a cytoplasmic and nuclear localization, whereas plasma membrane staining was not distinct and therefore not evaluable. Representative images showing expression pattern of TRAIL-R1 in tumor tissue and non-malignant, adjacent tissue are shown in Fig. 1.

In the cytoplasm, we found weak, moderate and strong TRAIL-R1 expression in 51.9, 22.6 and 18.9% (55/106; 24/106 and 20/106) of the cases, respectively (Table 3b). In 78.3% of the tumors, over 50% of the carcinoma cells showed positive cytoplasmic expression (Fig. 1). Cytoplasmic staining of TRAIL-R1 was present with very similar intensity in tumor and normal tissue.

In contrast, apparent differences in the nuclear TRAIL-R1 staining frequency and intensity were observed in tumor versus normal tissue (Table 3b, $p = 0.006$). Whereas overall 34% of tumors showed nuclear presence of TRAIL-R1 with either weak (26.4%; 28/106) or moderate (7.6%; 8/106) staining intensity, only 7.1% (2/28) of normal ducts expressed TRAIL-R1 in the nucleus and this with only weak intensity.

Correlation of TRAIL-R1 expression with clinico-pathological parameters and patient survival

Next, we correlated the expression level of TRAIL-R1 and its intracellular distribution (cytoplasm and nucleus) with diverse clinico-pathological parameters like tumor stage (T), nodal spread (N), distant metastasis (M), grading (G), lymphatic invasion (L), venous invasion (V) and perineural invasion. As shown in Table 4, we found a significant negative correlation of the amount of cells positively stained for TRAIL-R1 in the cytoplasm with a tumor grading ($\tau = -0.228$; $p = 0.043$). Apart from that, no other correlation was found for cytoplasmic or nuclear staining with any of the parameters.

Further we explored whether the TRAIL-R1 expression pattern could be of prognostic value. To address this issue, we dichotomized the results for intensity and amount of positive cells as well as the sum score in a group with strong and in a group with weak expression of TRAIL-R1 (see Table 5) and analyzed these data by Kaplan-Meier analysis. Cumulative survival was compared by log rank test and p values ≤ 0.05 were considered significant.

Neither the intensity of cytoplasmic staining nor the sum score showed a significant correlation with the patient survival. Likewise, nuclear staining showed no prognostic relevance.

Since the immunostaining revealed differences in number of stained cells per tumor, we wondered whether this parameter could be of prognostic relevance for the patients. Importantly, we found that patients with

Table 3 Cytoplasmic and nuclear TRAIL-R1 expression in malignant and non-malignant ducts

a)	cytoplasm		nuclei	
	n	%	n	%
Positive tumor cells				
0%	7	6.6	70	66.0
< 10%	5	4.8	9	8.5
11–50%	11	10.4	16	15.1
51–80%	22	20.8	10	9.4
> 80%	61	57.5	1	0.9
Staining intensity				
Negative	7	6.6	70	66.0
Weak positive	55	51.9	28	26.4
Moderate positive	24	22.6	8	7.5
Strong positive > 80%	20	18.9	0	0.0
Sum score				
0	7	6.6	70	66.0
2	4	3.8	9	8.5
3–4	25	23.6	21	19.8
5–6	57	53.8	6	5.7
7	13	13.0	0	0.0

b)	tumor		non-malignant		tumor		non-malignant	
	n	%	n	%	n	%	n	%
Staining intensity								
Negative	7	6.6	3	10.7	70	66.0	26	92.9
Weak positive	55	51.9	14	50.0	28	26.4	2	7.1
Moderate positive	24	22.6	6	21.5	8	7.5	0	0.0
Strong positive	20	18.9	5	17.9	0	0.0	0	0.0
Staining pattern: tumor vs. non-malignant	no difference ns, $p = 0.698$				$p = 0.006$			

a) number of positive cells, staining intensity and corresponding sum score are shown for cytoplasm and nucleus separately. Additionally, particular staining intensity in relation to histologic specification (tumor vs. peritumoral non-malignant) and for cytoplasmic vs. nuclear staining are provided (b)

Discussion

tumors in which > 80% of the cells express TRAIL-R1 in the cytoplasm have significantly prolonged median survival compared to the patients whose tumors show TRAIL-R1 positivity in less than 80% cells (20 vs. 8 months; $p = 0.004$; Fig. 2).

Discussion

Identification of the prognostic factors related to survival of cancer patients represents a strategy to understand the molecular mechanisms driving tumor progression and therapy resistance, and may consequently support the development of novel therapeutic strategies. The expression levels of TRAIL-R1 and TRAIL-R2 were shown to be of prognostic relevance for different tumor entities. In addition to their localization at the plasma membrane, TRAIL-R1 and TRAIL-R2 are also found in the cytoplasm and in the nucleus of several cell types. Especially in tumor cells, diminished plasma membrane but enhanced intracellular presence of these receptors was frequently observed. Importantly, despite these observations and emerging evidences for distinct compartment-specific functions of TRAIL-Rs, their cumulative expression levels - regardless of their intracellular distribution - are mainly taken into account when immunohistochemical studies are evaluated. However, recent studies on the TRAIL-R2-expression in PDAC tissues suggest the necessity of considering the intracellular distribution of TRAIL-Rs. Thus, the expression levels of TRAIL-R2 may emerge as either a positive or a negative prognostic marker, depending on the subcellular distribution (plasma membrane vs. nucleus) [19, 24].

Immunohistochemical studies described high cytoplasmic levels of TRAIL receptors in different cancer types, e.g. colorectal cancer [25–27], breast cancer cell lines [23, 28], renal cell carcinoma [29], NSCLC [30, 31], melanoma [32, 33], PDAC [19, 24], hepatocellular

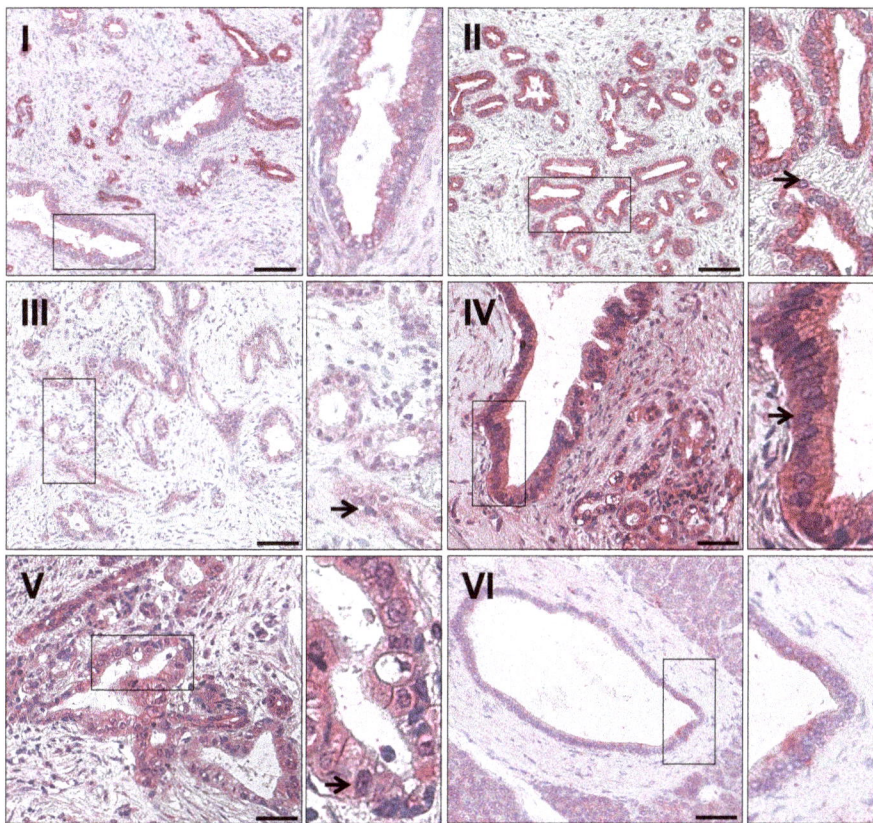

Fig. 1 Representative images of TRAIL-R1 staining in PDAC tissue (I-V) and non-neoplastic pancreatic duct (VI). I: Tumors with strong cytoplasmic TRAIL-R1 staining in 51–80% cells and no nuclear TRAIL-R1 staining. II: Tumors with strong positive cytoplasm in > 80% cells with negative nuclear staining. III: Tumors with weak positive cytoplasmic staining intensity in > 80% of the cells. Weak positive staining in 10–50% of the nuclei. IV: Tumors with moderate positive cytoplasmic staining in > 80% cells. Weak positive nuclei in 51–80% cells. V: Tumors with moderate positive nuclei in 51–80% of the nuclei. Weak positive cytoplasmic staining in > 80% of the cells. VI: Non-neoplastic duct with weak to moderate positive cytoplasm staining and without positive nuclei. Magnifications corresponding to the rectangles in the large pictures are shown in the small windows. Arrows indicate exemplary nuclear staining. Scale bar marks 100 μm (I – III + VI) or 50 μm (IV – V)

Table 4 Correlation of TRAIL-R1 expression with clinico-pathological parameters

Staining parameter	Tumor stage	Lymph nodes	Metastasis	Grading	Lymph vessels	Venous invasion	Perineural invasion
Intensity cytoplasm	$\tau = -0.018$ $p = 0.880$	$\tau = 0.045$ $p = 0.703$	$\tau = -0.096$ $p = 0.413$	$\tau = -0.099$ $p = 0.382$	$\tau = 0.127$ $p = 0.277$	$\tau = 0.096$ $p = 0.404$	$\tau = -0.033$ $p = 0.779$
Number pos. cytoplasm	$\tau = -0.115$ $p = 0.327$	$\tau = -0.080$ $p = 0.496$	$\tau = 0.070$ $p = 0.548$	$\tau = -0.228$ $p = 0.043$	$\tau = -0.018$ $p = 0.877$	$\tau = 0.044$ $p = 0.705$	$\tau = 0.104$ $p = 0.375$
Sum score cytoplasm	$\tau = 0.012$ $p = 0.918$	$\tau = -0.006$ $p = 0.960$	$\tau = -0.062$ $p = 0.598$	$\tau = -0.105$ $p = 0.351$	$\tau = 0.071$ $p = 0.542$	$\tau = 0.096$ $p = 0.407$	$\tau = -0.015$ $p = 0.896$
Intensity nuclei	$\tau = -0.210$ $p = 0.073$	$\tau = -0.006$ $p = 0.960$	$\tau = 0.129$ $p = 0.272$	$\tau = -0.079$ $p = 0.482$	$\tau = -0.064$ $p = 0.584$	$\tau = 0.096$ $p = 0.407$	$\tau = 0.154$ $p = 0.188$
Number pos. nuclei	$\tau = -0.100$ $p = 0.392$	$\tau = 0.172$ $p = 0.142$	$\tau = 0.021$ $p = 0.858$	$\tau = -0.057$ $p = 0.611$	$\tau = -0.005$ $p = 0.963$	$\tau = 0.100$ $p = 0.385$	$\tau = 0.148$ $p = 0.205$
Sum score nuclei	$\tau = -0.028$ $p = 0.831$	$\tau = -0.010$ $p = 0.929$	$\tau = 0.142$ $p = 0.224$	$\tau = 0.079$ $p = 0.483$	$\tau = 0.125$ $p = 0.285$	$\tau = 0.134$ $p = 0.245$	$\tau = 0.147$ $p = 0.210$

Abbreviations: τ Kendall's τ, *p* p value
Shown are correlation coefficients Kendall's τ as well as the significance of the correlation

Table 5 Impact of TRAIL-R1 expression pattern on survival of PDAC patient

Staining parameter	Total number of patients	Number of deceased patients	Median survival ± SD (95% CI) in months	p - value
Intensitiy cytoplasm				
Negative to weak positive	60	48	15 ± 3.611 (7.922–22.078)	
Moderate to strong positive	37	30	17 ± 3.513 (10.115–23.885)	0.735
Number of cells with positively stained cytoplasm				
≤ 80%	40	37	8 ± 3.041(2.041–13.959)	
> 80%	57	41	20 ± 3.855 (12.444–27.556)	0.004
Sum score cytoplasm				
≤ 5	65	52	15 ± 3.733 (7.682–22.318)	
> 5	32	26	17 ± 3.992 (9.177–24.823)	0.552
Staining intensity nuclei				
Negative to weak positive	89	70	15 ± 1.573 (11.918–18.082)	
Moderate to strong positive	8	8	13 ± 4.950 (3.298–22.702)	0.431
Number of cells with positively stained nucleus				
≤ 50%	88	69	15 ± 1.430 (12.198–17.802)	
> 50%	9	9	12 ± 4.472 (3.235–20.765)	0.687
Sum score nuclei				
≤ 3	19	17	8 ± 1.023 (5.995–10.005)	
> 3	78	61	16 ± 1.622 (12.821–19.179)	0.109

Abbreviations: *SD* standard deviation, *CI* confidence interval
P-values were estimated by log-rank-test with p ≤ 0.05 considered as significant

carcinoma [14], and glioblastoma multiforme [34]. Notably, the levels of just these intracellular receptors turned out to be of prognostic relevance in different tumor types [16]. Intriguingly, whereas high intracellular levels of TRAIL-R1 mainly correlated with positive patient's prognosis, increased levels of TRAIL-R2 often correlated with shorter patient's survival (for review [16]). These observations point to the existence of different, receptor-specific activities of cytoplasmic TRAIL death receptors and, in addition, suggest anti-tumor activities of intracellular TRAIL-R1, at least in some tumor entities.

In our present study, we identified cytoplasmic TRAIL-R1 as a positive prognostic marker for patients with PDAC. Interestingly, whereas overall staining intensity showed no prognostic relevance, the number of TRAIL-R1 positive cells per tumor turned out to be important for patient's outcome. Noteworthy, we used an antibody for immunochemistry which is able to detect membrane expressed TRAIL-R1 as it has been shown before [23]. Specifically, patients with tumors in which more than 80% of cells showed cytoplasmic TRAIL-R1 staining had significantly prolonged survival compared to patients whose tumors presented with less than 80% cells positively stained for TRAIL-R1. In line with these findings, a significant negative correlation between number of cells with positive stained TRAIL-R1

in the cytoplasm and tumor grading was found. These results indicate that loss of cytoplasmic TRAIL-R1 may support recurrent disease with more malignant phenotype.

Little is known about the origin and sub-cytoplasmic localization of intracellular TRAIL death receptors. Cytoplasmic TRAIL death receptors have been detected in Golgi vesicles [32], endosomes [32] and autophagosomes [35]. In addition, their presence in soluble cytoplasmic fractions was also reported [19].

Likewise, the function(s) of cytoplasmic TRAIL receptors is still not fully understood. Sequestration of these receptors in autophagosomes could act as a strategy by which tumor cells escape TRAIL-induced apoptosis [17, 18]. On the other hand, internalization of TRAIL death receptors in response to TRAIL-treatment has been demonstrated, and may represent a part of TRAIL-induced signal transduction pathway [36]. Recently, the importance of cytoplasmic TRAIL-R1 in inducing cell death as a consequence of unresolved unfolded protein response (UPR) has been demonstrated [20, 21]. Noteworthy, in this case TRAIL-R1 mediated cell death is independent of TRAIL. Efficient UPR activation represents a characteristic feature of many human cancers. It allows the tumor cells to survive and adapt to adverse environmental conditions, promotes dormancy and also tumor growth, progression

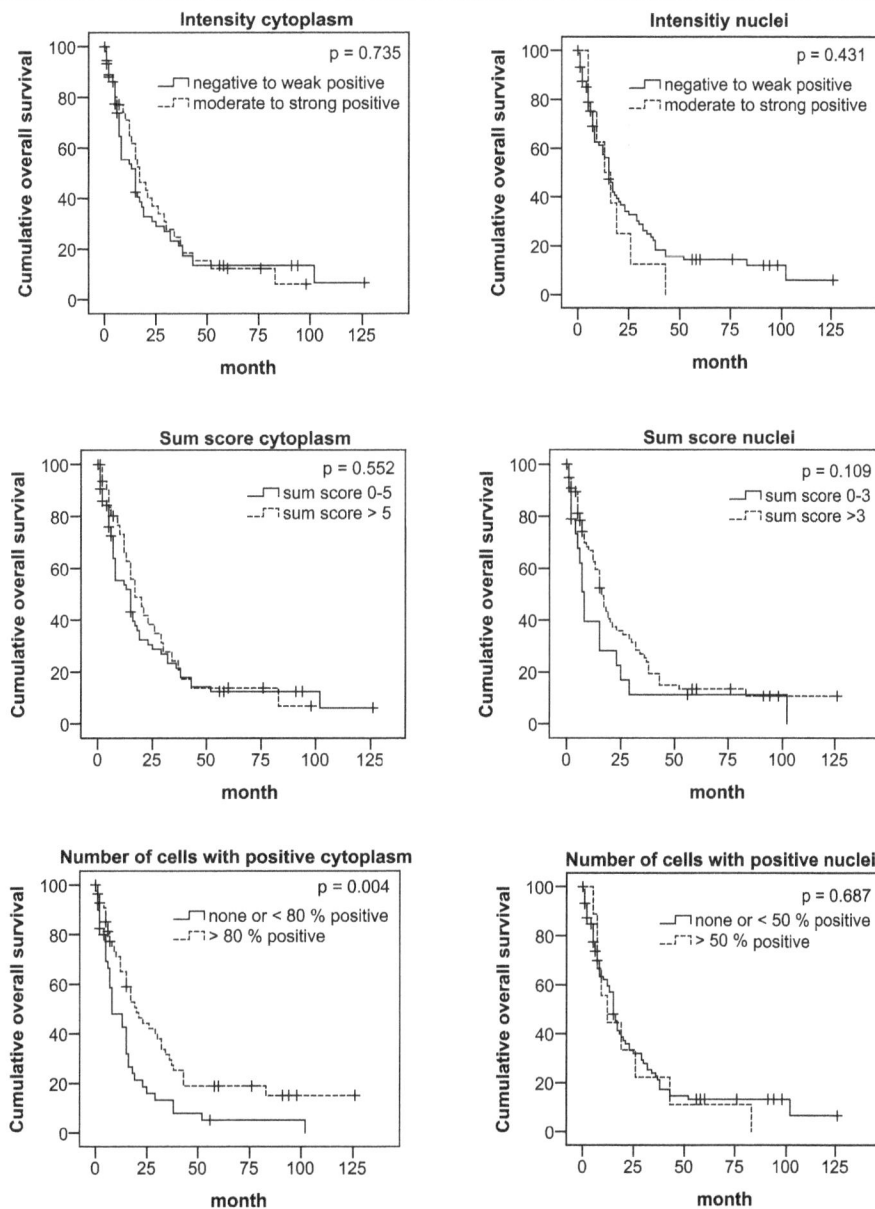

Fig. 2 Kaplan-Meier analyses of the cumulative survival of patients with differential expression of TRAIL-R1. *P*-values were calculated by the log rank test and *p* ≤ 0.05 was considered significant

and therapy resistance. In this context, loss of cytoplasmic TRAIL-R1 would select cancer cells which are resistant to UPR-induced apoptosis and thus cells with more aggressive phenotype.

The TRAIL-TRAIL-R system has been shown to be of crucial importance in the tumor immune surveillance [12, 13]. Cytoplasmic TRAIL death receptors may represent a reservoir of receptors, which upon stimulation localize to the plasma membrane and boost the primary response of cells to TRAIL. Since PDAC cells preferentially utilize TRAIL-R1 to induce apoptosis in response to TRAIL, loss of TRAIL-R1 could lead to an escape of

immune surveillance and accelerate the recurrent tumor growth.

Alternatively, it is also possible that cytoplasmic TRAIL-R1, via direct protein-protein interaction, sequesters TRAIL-R2 in the cytoplasm thus inhibiting its malignancy-promoting nuclear functions. According to this scenario, cells, which have lost cytoplasmic TRAIL-R1, would also present with a more aggressive phenotype.

Which, if any of these potential cytoplasmic TRAIL-R1 functions, accounts for the obviously anti-tumoral functions of cytoplasmic TRAIL-R1 remains to be elucidated.

The existence of further, still unknown functions of intracellular TRAIL receptors is very likely.

Likewise, the cellular pathways leading to the observed loss of TRAIL-R1 in a subset of PDAC cells are not known yet. Recently, several mechanisms negatively regulating the cellular levels of TRAIL-R1, but not TRAIL-R2, have been registered in cancer cells. Thus, hypermethylation of TRAIL-R1 promotor leading to an epigenetic silencing of TRAIL-R1 gene was detected in ovarian cancer cells [37]. Furthermore, at the transcriptional level, negative regulation of TRAIL-R1 promotor by GLI3 as well as miR-25-dependent decrease of TRAIL-R1 levels were reported for cholangiocarcinoma cells [38, 39]. At the post-translational level, specific degradation of TRAIL-R1 protein was described in breast cancer and melanoma cells. Here, membrane-associated RING-CH (MARCH)-8 ubiquitin ligase targeted TRAIL-R1, but not TRAIL-R2, for lysosomal degradation. Interestingly, plasma levels of miR-25 are significantly elevated in PDAC and evaluation of the levels of miR-25 together with MIC-1 and CA19–9 was shown to be able to distinguish between PDAC, benign pancreatic disorders and other GI cancers [40].

Conclusion

We show that cytoplasmic TRAIL-R1 may serve as a novel prognostic marker for PDAC patients. In addition, our data point to the necessity to investigate the evidently underestimated biological functions of intracellular TRAIL receptors.

Abbreviations
CI: Confidence interval; GI: Gastrointestinal; IHC: Immunohistochemistry; PDAC: Pancreatic ductal adenocarcinoma; SD: Standard deviation; TRAIL: TNF-related apoptosis inducing ligand; UPR: Unfolded protein response

Acknowledgements
We thank Gökhan Alp and Sandra Krüger for excellent technical assistance.

Funding
The study was financially supported by Erich und Gertrud Roggenbuck-Stiftung and intramural funding given to CH.

Authors' contributions
JPG and CH wrote the manuscript, prepared the figures and evaluated the data. FS and CB performed the histological examination and where together with JPG and C Röder major contributor to the data analyses. CR, TB, JHE and HK supported infrastructure and organizational issues. AT designed the study, analyzed the data, designed and wrote the manuscript. All authors read and approved the final manuscript. Some of the data are part of the doctoral thesis of FS.

Competing interests
The authors declare that they have no competing interests.

Author details
[1]Department of General Surgery, Visceral, Thoracic, Transplantation and Pediatric Surgery, University Hospital Schleswig-Holstein (UKSH), Campus Kiel, Arnold-Heller Str. 3, Haus 18, 24105 Kiel, Germany. [2]Institute for Experimental Cancer Research, University of Kiel, Arnold-Heller Str. 3 (Haus 17), D-24105 Kiel, Germany. [3]Department of Pathology, University Hospital Schleswig-Holstein (UKSH), Campus Kiel, Arnold-Heller Str. 3, Haus 14, 24105 Kiel, Germany.

References
1. Siegel RL, Miller KD, Jemal A. Cancer statistics, 2017. CA Cancer J Clin. 2017; 67(1):7–30.
2. Ansari D, Gustafsson A, Andersson R. Update on the management of pancreatic cancer: surgery is not enough. World J Gastroenterol. 2015; 21(11):3157–65.
3. Lemke J, von Karstedt S, Zinngrebe J, Walczak H. Getting TRAIL back on track for cancer therapy. Cell Death Differ. 2014;21(9):1350–64.
4. Azijli K, Weyhenmeyer B, Peters GJ, de Jong S, Kruyt FAE. Non-canonical kinase signaling by the death ligand TRAIL in cancer cells: discord in the death receptor family. Cell Death Differ. 2013;20(7):858–68.
5. Trauzold A, Siegmund D, Schniewind B. TRAIL promotes metastasis of human pancreatic ductal adenocarcinoma. Oncogene. 2006;25(56):7434–9.
6. Hoogwater FJH, Nijkamp MW, Smakman N, EJa S, Emmink BL, Westendorp BF, DaE R, Sprick MR, Schaefer U, Van Houdt WJ, et al. Oncogenic K-Ras turns death receptors into metastasis-promoting receptors in human and mouse colorectal cancer cells. Gastroenterology. 2010;138(7):2357–67.
7. Karstedt SV, Conti A, Nobis M, Montinaro A, Hartwig T, Lemke J, Legler K, Annewanter F, Campbell A, Taraborrelli L, et al. Cancer-cell-autonomous TRAIL-R signaling promotes KRAS-driven cancer progression, invasion and metastasis. Cancer Cell. 2015;27(4):561–73.
8. van Roosmalen IA, Quax WJ, Kruyt FA. Two death-inducing human TRAIL receptors to target in cancer: similar or distinct regulation and function? Biochem Pharmacol. 2014;91(4):447–56.
9. Stadel D, Mohr A, Ref C, MacFarlane M, Zhou S, Humphreys R, Bachem M, Cohen G, Moller P, Zwacka RM, et al. TRAIL-induced apoptosis is preferentially mediated via TRAIL receptor 1 in pancreatic carcinoma cells and profoundly enhanced by XIAP inhibitors. Clin Cancer Res. 2010;16(23):5734–49.
10. Lemke J, Noack A, Adam D, Tchikov V, Bertsch U, Roder C, Schutze S, Wajant H, Kalthoff H, Trauzold A. TRAIL signaling is mediated by DR4 in pancreatic tumor cells despite the expression of functional DR5. J Mol Med (Berl). 2010;88(7):729–40.
11. Mohr A, Yu R, Zwacka RM. TRAIL-receptor preferences in pancreatic cancer cells revisited: both TRAIL-R1 and TRAIL-R2 have a licence to kill. BMC Cancer. 2015;15:494.
12. Takeda K, Smyth MJ, Cretney E, Hayakawa Y, Kayagaki N, Yagita H, Okumura K. Critical role for tumor necrosis factor-related apoptosis-inducing ligand in immune surveillance against tumor development. J Exp Med. 2002;195(2):161–9.
13. Cretney E, Takeda K, Yagita H, Glaccum M, Peschon JJ, Smyth MJ. Increased susceptibility to tumor initiation and metastasis in TNF-related apoptosis-inducing ligand-deficient mice. J Immunol. 2002;168(3):1356–61.
14. Kriegl L, Jung A, Engel J, Jackstadt R, Gerbes AL, Gallmeier E, Reiche JA, Hermeking H, Rizzani A, Bruns CJ, et al. Expression, cellular distribution, and prognostic relevance of TRAIL receptors in hepatocellular carcinoma. Clin Cancer Res. 2010;16(22):5529–38.
15. Chen JJ, Shen HC, Rivera Rosado LA, Zhang Y, Di X, Zhang B. Mislocalization of death receptors correlates with cellular resistance to their cognate ligands in human breast cancer cells. Oncotarget. 2012;3(8):833–42.
16. Bertsch U, Röder C, Kalthoff H, Trauzold A. Compartmentalization of TNF-related apoptosis-inducing ligand (TRAIL) death receptor functions: emerging role of nuclear TRAIL-R2. Cell Death Dis. 2014;5:–e1390.
17. Kojima Y, Nakayama M, Nishina T, Nakano H, Koyanagi M, Takeda K, Okumura K, Yagita H. Importin beta1 protein-mediated nuclear localization of death receptor 5 (DR5) limits DR5/tumor necrosis factor (TNF)-related apoptosis-inducing ligand (TRAIL)-induced cell death of human tumor cells. J Biol Chem. 2011;286(50):43383–93.

18. Bai X, Williams JL, Greenwood SL, Baker PN, Aplin JD, Crocker IP. A placental protective role for trophoblast-derived TNF-related apoptosis-inducing ligand (TRAIL). Placenta. 2009;30(10):855–60.

19. Haselmann V, Kurz A, Bertsch U, Hübner S, Olempska-Müller M, Fritsch J, Häsler R, Pickl A, Fritsche H, Annewanter F, et al. Nuclear death receptor TRAIL-R2 inhibits maturation of let-7 and promotes proliferation of pancreatic and other tumor cells. Gastroenterology. 2014;146(1):278–90.

20. Lu M, Lawrence DA, Marsters S, Acosta-Alvear D, Kimmig P, Mendez AS, Paton AW, Paton JC, Walter P, Ashkenazi A. Opposing unfolded-protein-response signals converge on death receptor 5 to control apoptosis. Science. 2014;345(6192):98–101.

21. Dufour F, Rattier T, Constantinescu AA, Zischler L, Morle A, Ben Mabrouk H, Humblin E, Jacquemin G, Szegezdi E, Delacote F, et al. TRAIL receptor gene editing unveils TRAIL-R1 as a master player of apoptosis induced by TRAIL and ER stress. Oncotarget. 2017;8(6):9974–85.

22. Brierley JD GM, Wittekind C. (ed.): TNM Classification of Malignant Tumours, 8th Edition; 2016.

23. Ganten TM, Sykora J, Koschny R, Batke E, Aulmann S, Mansmann U, Stremmel W, Sinn H-P, Walczak H. Prognostic significance of tumour necrosis factor-related apoptosis-inducing ligand (TRAIL) receptor expression in patients with breast cancer. J Mol Med (Berl). 2009;87(10):995–1007.

24. Gallmeier E, Bader DC, Kriegl L, Berezowska S, Seeliger H, Goke B, Kirchner T, Bruns C, De Toni EN. Loss of TRAIL-receptors is a recurrent feature in pancreatic cancer and determines the prognosis of patients with no nodal metastasis after surgery. PLoS One. 2013;8(2):e56760.

25. Strater J, Hinz U, Walczak H, Mechtersheimer G, Koretz K, Herfarth C, Moller P, Lehnert T. Expression of TRAIL and TRAIL receptors in colon carcinoma: TRAIL-R1 is an independent prognostic parameter. Clin Cancer Res. 2002; 8(12):3734–40.

26. Granci V, Bibeau F, Kramar A, Boissiere-Michot F, Thezenas S, Thirion A, Gongora C, Martineau P, Del Rio M, Ychou M. Prognostic significance of TRAIL-R1 and TRAIL-R3 expression in metastatic colorectal carcinomas. Eur J Cancer. 2008;44(15):2312–8.

27. Bavi P, Prabhakaran SE, Abubaker J, Qadri Z, George T, Al-Sanea N, Abduljabbar A, Ashari LH, Alhomoud S, Al-Dayel F, et al. Prognostic significance of TRAIL death receptors in middle eastern colorectal carcinomas and their correlation to oncogenic KRAS alterations. Mol Cancer. 2010;9:203.

28. McCarthy MM, Sznol M, DiVito KA, Camp RL, Rimm DL, Kluger HM. Evaluating the expression and prognostic value of TRAIL-R1 and TRAIL-R2 in breast cancer. Clin Cancer Res. 2005;11(14):5188–94.

29. Macher-Goeppinger S, Aulmann S, Tagscherer KE, Wagener N, Haferkamp A, Penzel R, Brauckhoff A, Hohenfellner M, Sykora J, Walczak H, et al. Prognostic value of tumor necrosis factor-related apoptosis-inducing ligand (TRAIL) and TRAIL receptors in renal cell cancer. Clin Cancer Res. 2009;15(2):650–9.

30. Spierings DC, de Vries EG, Timens W, Groen HJ, Boezen HM, de Jong S. Expression of TRAIL and TRAIL death receptors in stage III non-small cell lung cancer tumors. Clin Cancer Res. 2003;9(9):3397–405.

31. Cooper WA, Kohonen-Corish MR, Zhuang L, McCaughan B, Kennedy C, Screaton G, Sutherland RL, Lee CS. Role and prognostic significance of tumor necrosis factor-related apoptosis-inducing ligand death receptor DR5 in nonsmall-cell lung cancer and precursor lesions. Cancer. 2008;113(1):135–42.

32. Zhang XD, Franco AV, Nguyen T, Gray CP, Hersey P. Differential localization and regulation of death and decoy receptors for TNF-related apoptosis-inducing ligand (TRAIL) in human melanoma cells. J Immunol. 2000;164(8):3961–70.

33. Zhuang L, Lee CS, Scolyer RA, McCarthy SW, Zhang XD, Thompson JF, Screaton G, Hersey P. Progression in melanoma is associated with decreased expression of death receptors for tumor necrosis factor-related apoptosis-inducing ligand. Hum Pathol. 2006;37(10):1286–94.

34. Kuijlen JM, Mooij JJ, Platteel I, Hoving EW, van der Graaf WT, Span MM, Hollema H, den Dunnen WF. TRAIL-receptor expression is an independent prognostic factor for survival in patients with a primary glioblastoma multiforme. J Neuro-Oncol. 2006;78(2):161–71.

35. Di X, Zhang G, Zhang Y, Takeda K, Rivera Rosado LA, Zhang B. Accumulation of autophagosomes in breast cancer cells induces TRAIL resistance through downregulation of surface expression of death receptors 4 and 5. Oncotarget. 2013;4(9):1349–64.

36. Akazawa Y, Mott JL, Bronk SF, Werneburg NW, Kahraman A, Guicciardi ME, Meng XW, Kohno S, Shah VH, Kaufmann SH et al. Death receptor 5 internalization is required for lysosomal permeabilization by TRAIL in malignant liver cell lines. *Gastroenterology* 2009, **136**(7):2365–2376 e2361–2367.

37. Horak P, Pils D, Haller G, Pribill I, Roessler M, Tomek S, Horvat R, Zeillinger R, Zielinski C, Krainer M. Contribution of epigenetic silencing of tumor necrosis factor-related apoptosis inducing ligand receptor 1 (DR4) to TRAIL resistance and ovarian cancer. Mol Cancer Res. 2005;3(6):335–43.

38. Kurita S, Mott JL, Almada LL, Bronk SF, Werneburg NW, Sun SY, Roberts LR, Fernandez-Zapico ME, Gores GJ. GLI3-dependent repression of DR4 mediates hedgehog antagonism of TRAIL-induced apoptosis. Oncogene. 2010;29(34):4848–58.

39. Razumilava N, Bronk SF, Smoot RL, Fingas CD, Werneburg NW, Roberts LR, Mott JL. miR-25 targets TNF-related apoptosis inducing ligand (TRAIL) death receptor-4 and promotes apoptosis resistance in cholangiocarcinoma. Hepatology. 2012;55(2):465–75.

40. Yuan W, Tang W, Xie Y, Wang S, Chen Y, Qi J, Qiao Y, Ma J. New combined microRNA and protein plasmatic biomarker panel for pancreatic cancer. Oncotarget. 2016;7(48):80033–45.

Treatment recommendations within the leeway of clinical guidelines: A qualitative interview study on oncologists' clinical deliberation

I. Otte[1*†], S. Salloch[2†], A. Reinacher-Schick[3] and J. Vollmann[1]

Abstract

Background: Recommending the optimal treatment for an individual patient requires a well-balanced consideration of various medical, social and ethical factors. The interplay of these factors, interpretation of the patient's situation and understanding of the existing clinical guidelines can lead to divergent therapy recommendations, depending on the attending physician. Gaining a better understanding of the individual process of medical decision-making and the differences occurring will support the delivery of optimal individualized care within the clinical setting.

Methods: A case vignette of a 64-year-old patient with locally advanced pancreatic adenocarcinoma was discussed with oncologists in 14 qualitative, semi-structured interviews at two academic institutions. Relevant factors that emerged were ranked by the participants using the Q card sorting method. Qualitative data analysis and descriptive statistics were performed.

Results: Oncologists recommend different therapeutic approaches within the leeway of the relevant clinical guidelines. One group of participants endorses a rather aggressive and potentially curative approach with a combination chemotherapy following the FOLFIRINOX protocol to provide the patient with the best chances of resectability. The second group suggests a milder chemotherapy approach with gemcitabine, highlighting the palliative approach and the patient's quality of life. Clinical guidelines are generally seen as an important point of reference, but are complicated to apply in highly individual cases.

Conclusion: The physician's individual assessment of factors, such as biological age, general condition or prognosis, plays a decisive role in treatment recommendations, particularly in those cases which are not fully covered by guidelines. Judgment and discretion remain crucial in clinical decision-making and cannot and should not be fully ruled out by evidence-based guidelines. Therefore, a more comprehensive reflection on the interaction between evidence-based medicine and the physician's estimation of each individual case is desirable. Knowledge of existing barriers can enhance the implementation of guidelines, for example, through medical education.

Keywords: Pancreatic carcinoma, Treatment recommendation, Clinical deliberation, Clinical guidelines, Clinical decision-making, Qualitative research

* Correspondence: ina.otte@rub.de
†Equal contributors
[1]Institute for Medical Ethics and History of Medicine, Ruhr University
Bochum, Markstr. 258a, D-44795 Bochum, Germany
Full list of author information is available at the end of the article

Background

Choosing and recommending a suitable treatment option for an oncological patient is a complex task which requires a well-balanced consideration of various factors. A physician's professional knowledge and experience, the newest scientific findings and clinical guidelines, are among these factors. However, institutional, social, legal and ethical factors also influence the final treatment recommendation.

Empirical evidence suggests that a physician's personal beliefs play a key role in the development of an initial hypothesis, the ways in which they search for evidence and the mechanisms involved in deriving a final treatment plan [1]. The use of clinical guidelines by physicians was also shown to be linked to several factors, such as the evidence incorporated in these guidelines, the physician's expertise, their relationship to the patient, and the patient's medical and social situation [2–4]. Research has further shown that the decision-making process and treatment selection can also be influenced by patient-sided factors, such as a patient's demographics or socioeconomic status [5–8].

While research has identified the influence of these factors, the way in which physicians weigh and prioritize them concretely during decision-making processes has not yet been well documented. The reasons for preferring one treatment over the other remain especially unclear [9]. Differences in treatment recommendations are, however, of great practical importance, as patients may receive divergent treatment offers depending on their choice of attending physician. This situation is aggravating in situations with multiple treatment options which are highly preference-sensitive [10], or in situations in which not only the treatment offer, but also the intended therapy goal may vary. Analyzing the individual process of weighing one factor against another is, therefore, key to a better understanding of differences in medical decision-making. Gaining more knowledge and insight into this process could support the delivery of optimal individualized care within the clinical setting.

Decisions about the intensity of oncologic care are highly influenced by national contexts and health care systems. Health care coverage in Germany is universal and mandatory for all citizens. Approximately 85% of the population is covered by the statutory health insurance (SHI), which covers all medical services and procedures that are adequate, practicable and cost-effective. Private health insurance covers a benefit package similar to SHI, but can also include additional options. Therefore, the German population, with rare exemptions, receives funding for all cancer treatments which are judged as beneficial from a medical and efficiency perspective.

Methods

We conducted a qualitative interview study on oncologists' treatment recommendations in individual cases to gain a better understanding of the process of clinical deliberation. Following approval from the ethics committee of the Medical Faculty of the Ruhr-University Bochum (Reg. No. 5025–14), 14 semi-structured qualitative interviews were conducted, each of which included the same case vignette (see Table 1).

The case vignette was discussed by using the card sorting method (Q methodology), which is suitable for semi-quantitative factor analysis [11]. While rating the different factor cards (on a scale with 5 being the highest influence on medical decision-making and 0 being no influence at all) regarding the case vignette, the participants were asked to explain the rationale underlying their ratings verbally. Consequently, the card sorting was also used as a discussion prompter to start an in-depth narration which enabled us to elaborate further on the underlying attitudes and values behind the participants' treatment choices.

The focus of the interviews was on thematic aspects, such as intuition, evidence-based medicine (EBM), work experience, clinical guidelines and their perceived importance for medical decision-making (Table 2). Based on the literature review, factor cards were developed to represent four categories of possible influences on medical decision-making: colleagues, patient and family, EBM-related factors (guidelines, scientific literature) and personal values. The factor cards were pretested during the first interviews, giving the interviewees the opportunity to add relevant factors to the card set. Together with the qualitative semi-structured interview part (see Additional file 1 for the interview guide), we reached a level of detail which is usually not obtainable by using only a purely traditional statistical technique.

A purposive sample was drawn from three departments of two German university hospitals, both of which are comprehensive cancer centers for pancreatic malignancies. The main criterion for participants being included in the study was their current employment in the unit of medical oncology. Variation was sought regarding gender and professional experience in the treatment of oncological patients.

Analysis

Interviews were transcribed verbatim. All transcripts were read and reread to ensure familiarity with the data. The coding process followed Mayring's nine steps of content analysis: a) The relevant data was defined; b) the context of the appearance of the data registered; c) a formal characterization of the data material described; d) the course of analysis specified; e) a theory-lead differentiation checked; f) the technique of analysis defined (summarization, explication, structuring); g) the unit of analysis defined; h) the data material analyzed; and, finally, i) the data material interpreted [12]. The data

Table 1 Case vignette

Patient demographics	M, 64 yrs.; married
Status praesens	Nausea and pain in the upper abdomen, back pain, unintended weight loss of 6 kg, condition stable, but generally restricted.
Past medical history (PMH)	Three-vessel CAD; s/p CABG occasionally AP on exertion-controlled arterial hypertension, COPD GOLD II, under medication.
Family history (FH)	Unknown
Social History (SH)	Smoker (60 pack-years), lives at home with his wife who supports him with domestic activities; he formerly worked as a butcher, now unfit for work.
Allergies (ALL)	None
Physical examination (PE) and test results	- Slightly diminished general condition, BMI 27, 3, 140/95, heart and lungs: NAD, neurology: NAD - Endoscopic ultrasound: mass located in the pancreatic head, inhomogeneous - MRI scan abdomen: 3.5 cm mass in processus uncinatus, multiple peripancreatic lymph nodes - MR angiography: primary cancer not resectable: full vessel involvement and infiltration of SMA - Histology (endosonography): high-grade pancreatic ductal adenocarcinoma, no metastases detected - LAB: Hemoglobin 13.2 g/dl; Leukocyte 5200/µl; Thrombozyten 150,000/µl Creatinin: 1.2 mg/dl Bilirubin: 1.1 mg/dl Amylase: 100 U/l Lipase: 55 U/l CA19–9 (carbohydrate antigen 19.9): 1350 U/ml
Diagnosis	Locally advanced, pancreatic ductal adenocarcinoma cT4N1M0 (UICC stage III)

was repeatedly coded, moving from concrete passages to abstract levels of coding, deriving themes from the data and searching for repeated concepts. All findings were critically tested and discussed in team meetings. Any disagreements were resolved by discussion. Since the coding system remained the same for the last interviews and the findings did not add something significantly new to the interviews conducted previously, we concluded that we had reached saturation.

Table 2 Factors rated regarding their influence on physicians' decision-making

Factor cards	Rated importance (5 > 0) mean:
Patient's wishes and preferences	4.86
Clinical guidelines	4.29
Patient's general condition	4.2
Medical literature	4.14
Supervisors	4.07
Medical co-workers	3.93
Nurses	3.77
Patient's age	3.46
Professional experience	3.43
Support from relatives/ social environment	3.36
Intuition	3.21
Physician's own values	3.20
Institutional guidelines	3.07
Psycho-oncologist	2.85
Wishes and interests of patient's relatives	2.57

5 being the greatest influence and 0 no influence at all

Results

The sample consisted of eight male and six female oncologists aged between 30 and 53 years (median age: 38 years), with a median clinical experience of 9 years. Six participants were still in their residency. The participants rated different factors which influenced their decision-making:

The participating oncologists recommended different therapeutic approaches in the second part of the interviews, while also providing insights into their clinical deliberation and decision-making routine. Whereas a minority of the participants assumed that there was still a chance to reach operability in the case vignette, most thought that reaching operability was unlikely and a palliative approach was the better option for the patient. The analysis revealed that the participants' recommendations could be divided into two major groups in which the physicians recommended either an aggressive type of chemotherapy with the FOLFIRINOX regimen or the more moderate form of a monotherapy with gemcitabine. Two participants recommended approaches diverging from these schemes: One physician recommended a merely supportive therapy and the other physician suggested initial laparoscopic surgery for diagnostic purposes.

Treatment recommendation A: Combination chemotherapy with Oxaliplatin, Leucovorin, Irinotecan and 5-FU (FOLFIRINOX protocol)

Physicians in this group recommended an aggressive type of cytostatic therapy with FOLFIRINOX, because they believe it offers a better probability of shrinking the primary cancer to achieve resectability.

IP 3: "I would recommend chemotherapy with FOLFIRINOX, because I can see that the patient could

reach resectability with this chemotherapy using FOLFIRINOX."

Their hope was that by shrinking the primary cancer, the chances for a surgical removal would increase, resulting in a possibly curative approach.

IP 14: "And he is not bedridden, so when we start with chemotherapy following the FOLFIRINOX regimen, it could be that the pancreatic tumor shrinks in a certain way, which means, that probably in the future, it could become operable, so that surgery could be an option, but, in any case, you would start with an intensive, strong chemotherapy following the FOLFIRINOX regimen."

The participants from this group, furthermore, think that the patient is relatively young and, therefore, in a sufficiently good condition to undergo this rather aggressive regimen.

IP9: "So the patient is of a relatively young age and has a severe carcinoma with a very poor prognosis. That means I would offer him chemotherapy with FOLFIRINOX in view of a possible resectability of the tumor."

Treatment recommendation B: Palliative monochemotherapy with gemcitabine

Physicians who recommended a mild type of chemotherapy with gemcitabine often aim at a palliative approach, with a stronger focus on quality of life rather than on resectability, since they assess the chances of reducing the tumor mass as rather low. They further believe that the general condition of the patient is not good enough to endure an aggressive form of chemotherapy and, therefore, select a regimen that they think would be better tolerated by the patient:

IP 4: "So (..) he is in a moderate condition; there is this FOLFIRINOX which you could give, but many do not tolerate it well. When I look at the case, he has COPD, he has a cardiac disease. (...) it is questionable if he could tolerate it."

While acknowledging that there are potentially curative approaches, participants of this group rather suggest going with a milder form of chemotherapy to prolong the time of survival, while still offering the patient a good quality of life:

IP 5: "I'd say I would decide between a system therapy with gemcitabine mono or, what we could also think about is a combination of gemcitabine, maybe he can tolerate it in reduced doses. It is a bit difficult, because his carcinoma is theoretically shrinkable, but it is cT4, and the chances that this ends in resectability are very low, especially since he is probably limited in his ability to tolerate therapy due to his pre-existing condition."

In contrast to the previous group, the oncologists in the second group thought the patient was "not the youngest" and, therefore, probably not capable of undergoing a more aggressive protocol.

IP 12: "One therapy option would be palliative chemotherapy with gemcitabine, which could, in the case of pancreatic carcinomas, be at least effective regarding the total time of overall survival. (...) He is not the youngest, so that I fear this patient would not be offered FOLFIRINOX."

Dealing with guidelines

While discussing and deciding their therapy recommendations, the physicians mentioned guidelines as an important factor and a framework on which they could orientate their decision-making. Clinical guidelines were the second highest factor influencing the physicians' decision-making in the card-sorting part of the interview. The participants were asked to explain how they use clinical guidelines in their decision-making process and what possible difficulties they could face in guideline implementation, to gain more insight into the role and the importance of guidelines. One of the difficulties named repeatedly was that guidelines often refer to a prototype of patient who might differ from the actual person the physician is treating:

IP12: "Guidelines often refer to a standard patient and we do not deal with a standard patient in the concrete situation. So we have to adapt the guidelines to the concrete patient we are treating."

This can be particularly difficult when the guidelines are based on studies which included significantly younger patients with a better general condition:

IP7: "Guidelines, for example, are based on some studies that were conducted on young and rather healthy patients and these results aren't always transferrable to older patients or patients in a severe state, so we have to adapt the guidelines to match our cases. Typical situations would be the FOLFIRINOX regimen, which causes the patient, Mr. M, from the case vignette, for example, a lot of side effects, but the studies that were conducted on younger and healthier patients, well, these patients could deal with the side effects much better and experienced fewer of them."

Furthermore, the physicians stated that they face situations in which guidelines do not provide clear guidance, for example, in cases of recurring disease or therapy failure:

IP4: "There are cases in which guidelines do not apply, where you have a relapse and there is no third-line therapy or fourth-line therapy available, right, when you have already tried so much (..) Or in cases where the first-line therapy is not well tolerated and in which we have to try something different. Something weaker which might not have as good an outcome, but which does not kill or unnecessarily weaken the patient. It depends on the general condition of the patient, but there are also cases that are so rare that there hasn't been any research yet."

Sometimes the implementation was also found to be difficult because the guidelines are presented in an oversimplified way:

IP3: "Well, in the end, guidelines are very generic, which means they address certain age groups or patients that have benefited from a certain type of chemotherapy in a certain way. And this does not cover all the different factors (...), like patient preferences or social environment, sometimes the guidelines cover the age, but overall it is all very simplified."

The interview analysis generally demonstrates that the concrete treatment recommendation physicians make to an oncologic patient depends highly on their subjective estimation of the patient's biological age and prognosis. Clinical guidelines are seen as an important point of reference, but cease being helpful in highly individual cases.

Discussion

German oncologists generally adhere to the German S3 guidelines, which are consensus guidelines based on an elaborate formal evidence assessment where official evidence tables are published together with the guideline. International guidelines, such as the ASCO or ESMO guideline, are also taken into consideration in the process of the German guideline development, with the goal of an international harmonization of the guidelines. The German guideline for pancreatic cancer [13], which was published in 2013, is presently being revised in an elaborate process. In the meantime, many German oncologists refer to international guidelines, such as the NCCN guidelines, for more recent recommendations [14].

The case vignette in our study referred to a 64-year-old patient with locally advanced pancreatic adenocarcinoma (LAPC) and a supposed Eastern Cooperative Oncology Group (ECOG) performance status between 1 and 2. According to US guidelines, patients who have LAPC and an ECOG of 0 or 1 together with a favorable comorbidity profile and a support system for aggressive medical therapy should receive an initial systemic therapy with combination regimens [4, 5]. However, there is no clear evidence to support one regimen over another, and it is recommended that physicians offer therapy on the basis of extrapolation from data derived from studies in the metastatic setting [5]. Newer regimens such as fluorouracil, leucovorin, irinotecan and oxaliplatin, and gemcitabine plus nanoparticle albumin-bound paclitaxel have not been evaluated in randomized controlled trials (RCTs) involving LAPC, but these combination regimens are being frequently used by clinicians and, thus, may be recommended for patients with LAPC with good performance status (ECOG 0 and 1) [14]. For patients with LAPC, regimens with gemcitabine only, or gemcitabine plus capecitabine (GEMCAP) alone or in combination are potentially better tolerated and might be considered a better

option in patients with a borderline ECOG or based on patient preference. The German S3 guideline on exocrine pancreatic adenocarcinoma more generally suggests that patients with a performance status from 0 to 2 should receive palliative chemotherapy [3].

This spectrum of therapeutic options which could be applied in adhering to guidelines is mirrored in the study participants' answers regarding the case vignette. The qualitative interviews also give some indication about when oncologists tend to suggest a more or less aggressive treatment. The most important factors that influence the choice of an aggressive or less aggressive treatment are the general condition of the patient, often in combination with their age. While participants who suggest the more aggressive option judge the patient to be in an overall good general condition and rather young, oncologists who suggest a milder version believe that the patient is "not the youngest" and that his preexisting medical conditions would limit his tolerance and ability to undergo this regimen. These findings are in accordance with previous research, which demonstrates that younger patients are more likely to receive aggressive care near the end of life [15, 16]. The present interview study, however, sheds light on the fact that the factor of the "patient's age" depends highly on the attending physician's estimation. The study also demonstrates that the diverging clinical judgement of the probability of reaching resectability has an immense impact on the decision-making and the final treatment recommendation. Oncologists who assessed the chance to reach operability in the case vignette presented as rather low, focused on time-prolonging measures, while those who thought that operability was attainable, suggested the aggressive protocol with a higher chance of resectability and a more severe set of side effects. Assessment of resectability is, thus, identified as another factor which influences treatment aggressiveness in addition to other, known, factors, such as comorbidity [17] and socioeconomic variables [18].

Participants also explained their difficulties with the implementation of clinical guidelines. While some of the difficulties named by the oncologists were already known to exist for general practitioners (GPs), such as differences between actual patients and the research population or contradictive patient preferences [4, 19], our study adds insight to the implementation process of guidelines in the oncological setting, as well as new barriers that are related to it. Whereas Carlsen and Norheim showed that GPs find clinical guidelines to be too detailed [3], the oncologists in our study often found them too generic and, therefore, not applicable to their patients. They said it was particularly difficult to use guidelines when they were based on research that focus on younger and healthier patients, making it difficult to predict how patients in a more severe state would respond to such therapy or cope with its side effects. The absence of clinical guidelines in cases of relapse or third- or fourth-line therapy was also said to be problematic.

Conclusions

In our study, the physician's individual assessment of factors, such as biological age, general condition or prognosis, plays a decisive role in treatment recommendations, particularly in those cases which are not fully covered by guidelines. Physician's judgment and discretion remain crucial in clinical decision-making and cannot be fully ruled out by evidence-based guidelines. Therefore, a more comprehensive reflection on the interaction between evidence-based guidelines and the physician's assessment of each individual case are desirable, since knowledge of existing local, regional or international peculiarities or ethical barriers can assist the enhancement of the implementation of guidelines.

Abbreviations

ALL: Allergies; AP: Angina pectoris; BMI: Body mass index; CA19–9: Carbohydrate antigen 19.9; CABG: Coronary artery bypass grafting; CAD: Coronary artery disease; COPD: Chronic obstructive pulmonary disease; EBM: Evidence-based medicine; ECOG: Eastern Cooperative Oncology Group; FH: Family history; FOLFIRINOX: Combination chemotherapy protocol with oxaliplatin, irinotecan and 5-FU; GEMCAP: Combination chemotherapy protocol with gemcitabine plus capecitabine; GOLD: Global Initiative for Chronic Obstructive Lung Disease; GPs: General practitioners; HPI: History of present illness; LAPC: Locally advanced pancreatic adenocarcinoma; MRI: Magnetic resonance imaging; NAD: Nothing abnormal detected; PE: Physical examination; PMH: Past medical history; SH: Social history; SHI: Statutory health insurance; UICC: Union for International Cancer Control

Acknowledgements

We would like to thank all participants for their time and consideration in taking part in this study.

Funding

This work was supported by FoRUM: Forschungsförderung Ruhr-University Bochum Medical Faculty (grant number F818–2014). Furthermore, we acknowledge support by the DFG Open Access Publication Funds of the Ruhr-Universität Bochum. The funding body had no influence on the design of the study, the collection, analysis, and interpretation of data and the manuscript.

Authors' contributions

Study design and interview guideline were developed by IO, SS, ARS and JV. Data was collected and analyzed by IO and SS. The manuscript was drafted by IO and SS. ARS and JV revised it critically for important intellectual content. IO, SS, ARS and JV read and approved the final manuscript and are accountable for all aspects of the work.

Competing interests

The authors declare that they have no competing interests.

Author details

[1]Institute for Medical Ethics and History of Medicine, Ruhr University Bochum, Markstr. 258a, D-44795 Bochum, Germany. [2]Institute for Ethics and History of Medicine, University Medicine Greifswald, Ellernholzstr. 1-2, D-17487 Greifswald, Germany. [3]Department for Hematology, Oncology and Palliative Care, St. Josef-Hospital, Ruhr-University Bochum, Gudrunstr. 56, D-44791 Bochum, Germany.

References

1. Konstantara E, Vandrevala T, Cox A, Creagh-Brown BC, Ogden J. Balancing professional tension and deciding upon the status of death: making end-of-life decisions in intensive care units. Health Psychol Open. 2016;3(1):2191–6.
2. Zwolsman SE, van Dijk N, te Pas E, Wieringa-de WM. Barriers to the use of evidence-based medicine: knowledge and skills, attitude, and external factors. Perspect Med Educ. 2013;2(1):4–13.
3. Carlsen B, Norheim OF. "what lies beneath it all?" an interview study of GPs attitudes to the use of guidelines. BMC Health Serv Res. 2008;8:218.
4. Freeman AC, Sweeney K. Why general practitioners do not implement evidence: qualitative study. BMJ. 2001;323(1):1–5.
5. Yellen SB, Cella DF, Leslie WT. Age and clinical decision making in oncology patients. J Natl Cancer Inst. 1994;86(23):1766–70.
6. McKinlay JB, Potter DA, Feldman HA. Non-medical influences on medical decision-making. Soc Sci Med. 1996;42(5):769–76.
7. Petrisek AC, Laliberte LL, Allen SM, Mor V. The treatment decision-making process: age differences in a sample of women recently diagnosed with nonrecurrent, early-stage breast cancer. Gerontologist. 1997;37(5):598–608.
8. Bridges J, Hughes J, Farrington N, Richardson A. Cancer treatment decision-making processes for older patients with complex needs: a qualitative study. BMJ Open. 2015;5(12):e009674.
9. Jiwa M, Meng X, O'Shea C, Magin P, Dadich A, Pillar V. How do general practitioners manage patients with cancer symptoms? A video-vignette study. BMJ Open. 2015;5(9):e008525.
10. Redelmeier DA, Shafir E. Medical decision making in situations that offer multiple alternatives. JAMA. 1995;273(4):302–5.
11. Cross RM. Exploring attitudes: the case for Q methodology. Health Educ Res. 2005;20(2):206–13.
12. Mayring P. Qualitative Content Analysis. Theoretical Foundation, Basic Procedures and Software Solution. Social Science Open Access Repository. 2014. http://nbn-resolving.de/urn:nbn:de:0168-ssoar-395173. Accessed 17 Nov 2017.
13. Leitlinienprogramm Onkologie der AWMF, Deutschen Krebsgesellschaft e.V. und Deutschen Krebshilfe e.V. S3-Leitlinie zum exokrinen Pankreaskarzinom. Version 1.0 - Oktober 2013. AWMF-Registriernummer: 032/010OL. Leitlinie (Langversion). In: Leitlinienprogramm Onkologie. 2014. http://leitlinienprogramm-onkologie.de/uploads/tx_sbdownloader/LL_Pankreas_OL_Langversion.pdf. Accessed 27 Mar 2017.
14. National Comprehensive Cancer Network (NCCN). NCCN Clinical Practice Guidelines in Oncology (NCCN Guidelines): Pancreatic Adenocarcinoma. Version 2.2016. In: Translational Research Informatics Center Kobe. 2016. https://www.tri-kobe.org/nccn/guideline/pancreas/english/pancreatic.pdf. Accessed 27 Mar 2017.
15. Miesfeldt S, Murray K, Lucas L, Chang CH, Goodman D, Morden NE. Association of age, gender, and race with intensity of end-of-life care for medicare beneficiaries with cancer. J Palliat Med. 2012;15(5):548–54.
16. Sheffield KM, Boyd CA, Benarroch-Gampel J, Kuo YF, Cooksley CD, Riall TS. End-of-life care in medicare beneficiaries dying with pancreatic cancer. Cancer. 2011;117(21):5003–12.
17. Ho TH, Barbera L, Saskin R, Lu H, Neville BA, Earle CC. Trends in the aggressiveness of end-of-life cancer care in the universal health care system of Ontario. J Clin Oncol. 2011;29(12):1587–91.
18. Virnig BA, Morgan RO, Persily NA, DeVito CA. Racial and income differences in use of the hospice benefit between the medicare managed care and medicare fee-for-service. J Palliat Med. 1999;2(1):23–31.
19. Zwolsman S, te Pas E, Hooft L, Wieringa-de Waard M, van Dijk N. Barriers to GPs' use of evidence-based medicine: a systematic review. Br J Gen Pract. 2012;62(600):511–21.

Evaluation of pancreatic cancer cell migration with multiple parameters in vitro by using an optical real-time cell mobility assay device

Akira Yamauchi[1]* [ID], Masahiro Yamamura[2], Naoki Katase[3], Masumi Itadani[1], Naoko Okada[2], Kayoko Kobiki[1], Masafumi Nakamura[4], Yoshiyuki Yamaguchi[2] and Futoshi Kuribayashi[1]

Abstract

Background: Migration of cancer cell correlates with distant metastasis and local invasion, which are good targets for cancer treatment. An optically accessible device "TAXIScan" was developed, which provides considerably more information regarding the cellular dynamics and less quantity of samples than do the existing methods. Here, we report the establishment of a system to analyze the nature of pancreatic cancer cells using TAXIScan and we evaluated lysophosphatidic acid (LPA)-elicited pancreatic cell migration.

Methods: Pancreatic cancer cell lines, BxPC3, PANC-1, AsPC1, and MIAPaCa-2, were analyzed for adhesion as well as migration towards LPA by TAXIScan using parameters such as velocity and directionality or for the number of migrated cells by the Boyden chamber methods. To confirm that the migration was initiated by LPA, the expression of LPA receptors and activation of intracellular signal transductions were examined by quantitative reverse transcriptase polymerase reaction and western blotting.

Results: Scaffold coating was necessary for the adhesion of pancreatic cancer cells, and collagen I and Matrigel were found to be good scaffolds. BxPC3 and PANC-1 cells clearly migrated towards the concentration gradient formed by injecting 1 μL LPA, which was abrogated by pre-treatment with LPA inhibitor, Ki16425 (IC$_{50}$ for the directionality ≈ 1. 86 μM). The LPA dependent migration was further confirmed by mRNA and protein expression of LPA receptors as well as phosphorylation of signaling molecules. LPA$_1$ mRNA was highest among the 6 receptors, and LPA$_1$, LPA$_2$ and LPA$_3$ proteins were detected in BxPC3 and PANC-1 cells. Phosphorylation of Akt (Thr308 and Ser473) and p42/44MAPK in BxPC3 and PANC-1 cells was observed after LPA stimulation, which was clearly inhibited by pre-treatment with a compound Ki16425.

Conclusions: We established a novel pancreatic cancer cell migration assay system using TAXIScan. This assay device provides multiple information on migrating cells simultaneously, such as their morphology, directionality, and velocity, with a small volume of sample and can be a powerful tool for analyzing the nature of cancer cells and for identifying new factors that affect cell functions.

Keywords: Migration, Chemotaxis, Lipid mediator, Inhibitor, TAXIScan, Metastasis

* Correspondence: akiray@med.kawasaki-m.ac.jp
[1]Department of Biochemistry, Kawasaki Medical School, 577 Matsushima, Kurashiki, Okayama 701-0192, Japan
Full list of author information is available at the end of the article

Background

Migration of cancer cells correlates with distant metastasis and local invasion. This phenomenon involves various molecules including chemoattractants, trophic growth factors and their receptors, adhesion molecules, intracellular signaling molecules, motor proteins, and the cytoskeleton [1]. These molecules are orchestrated to help cells migrate to specific parts of the body or even spontaneously without an apparent destination. As cancer metastasis is directly associated with prognosis, controlling cancer cell migration is an effective strategy for treating the disease. Pancreatic cancer is among those with the poorest prognosis [2]. The treatment for this type of cancer is currently restricted as there are few effective drugs and knowledge regarding the nature of this cancer type is insufficient. New insights regarding this cancer and novel approaches for its treatment have long been awaited.

Lysophosphatidic acid (LPA) is a highly bioactive lipid mediator and is known to be involved in cancer cell migration, proliferation, and production of angiogenic factors [3]. In the process of cell migration, LPA works as a potent chemoattractant for various kinds of cells. Six receptors of LPA (LPA_1, LPA_2, LPA_3, LPA_4, LPA_5, and LPA_6) are known and all of them are G-protein coupled [4–9]. Some cells express one of these receptors, while others express multiple receptors for LPA [10]. Several articles have reported that pancreatic cancer cell lines express LPA receptors and the cells migrate towards LPA, using Boyden chamber and/or Transwell culture methods, which involve counting the number of migrated cells [11–13].

TAXIScan is an assay device for studying cell dynamics in vitro and has been used in the analysis of both suspension (mostly hematopoietic) and adherent cells [14–22]. The device functions as an optically accessible system and provides two-dimensional images of cell migration. TAXIScan provides markedly more information including morphology as well as quantitative analysis compared to existing methods such as Boyden chamber method. This device consists of an etched silicon substrate and a flat glass plate, both of which form horizontal channels each with a micrometer-order depth and forms 2 compartments on either side of a channel. Cells are placed and aligned on one side, while a stimulating factor is injected to the other side (typically 1 μL each of the cells and the stimulant). The cells react to the stable concentration gradient of the stimulant inside the horizontal channel [14]. The cell images are observed thereafter and filmed with a charge-coupled device camera located beneath the glass. By analyzing the cell images, many parameters can be determined including velocity, directionality, etc. [23–26].

The objective of this study is to establish TAXIScan as a system for pancreatic cancer research by using pancreatic cancer cell lines and to evaluate cancer cell migration in vitro for understanding the characteristics of this cancer cell type and for identifying new drugs to regulate cancer cell migration. Here, we show the adherence of cells to the scaffolds as well as LPA-elicited migration by TAXIScan, and by an existing method, the modified Boyden chamber method (Transwell). The LPA-elicited migration was confirmed by checking the expression of LPA receptors and the effect of an LPA inhibitor Ki16425.

Methods

Reagents

Fetal bovine serum (FBS) was obtained from Nichirei Biosciences Inc. (Tokyo, Japan); RPMI1640 and D-MEM were from Sigma-Aldrich (St. Louis, MO, USA); Collagen I, Matrigel (growth factor reduced), fibronectin, laminin, and collagen I pre-coated coverslips were obtained from Becton Dickinson (San Jose, CA, USA); fatty-acid-free bovine serum albumin (BSA) from Nacalai Tesque (Kyoto, Japan); LPA from Enzo Life Sciences Inc. (Farmingdale, NY, USA); Opti-MEM from Thermo Fisher Scientific Inc. (Waltham, MA, USA); Anti- LPA_1, LPA_3, LPA_5, and LPA_6 rabbit polyclonal antibodies from GeneTex Inc. (Irvine, CA, USA); anti-LPA $_2$ rabbit polyclonal antibody from Abgent (San Diego, CA, USA); and anti-LPA_4 rabbit polyclonal antibody from Acris Antibodies Inc. (San Diego, CA, USA); Ki16425 was purchased from Cayman Chemical (Ann Arbor, MI, USA).

Maintenance of cells

Human pancreatic cancer cell lines BxPC3 (ATCC CRL-1687), PANC-1 (ATCC CRL-1469), and AsPC1 (ATCC CRL-1682) were obtained from the American Type Culture Collection (ATCC), and MIAPaCa-2 (RCB2094) and KATOIII (RCB2088) from Riken Cell Bank. PC3 and 211H were kindly provided by Dr. Masakiyo Sakaguchi. Cells were cultured and maintained in RPMI1640 with 10% FBS or in D-MEM with 10% FBS on 10-cm diameter dishes as the standard procedure. Passaging of the cells was performed using PBS and Trypsin/EDTA solution when they were 80-90% confluent. All samples were handled according to the Declaration of Helsinki.

Migration assay

The Real-time cell mobility assay was performed by optical real-time cell mobility assay device "EZ-TAXIScan" (ECI, Inc., Kawasaki, Japan) as described previously [20], except for assembling the TAXIScan holder together with a coverslip pre-coated with the extracellular matrix. Briefly, coverslips were coated with collagen I (100 μg/mL), Matrigel (1/30 diluted solution with culture medium), fibronectin (100 μg/mL), laminin (100 μg/mL), or the culture medium, by incubating 100 μL of each solution on a coverslip at room temperature for 1 h before assembling the TAXIScan holder. After collagen I was selected as the scaffold, collagen I pre-coated coverslips were used for the

TAXIScan method. The pre-coated coverslip was washed once with 0.5 mL of PBS and was placed on the glass plate for TAXIScan. The TAXIScan holder was assembled according to the manufacturer's instructions. Cells were harvested by detaching from culture flasks using the same conditions as passaging. One µL of suspension prepared in the culture medium containing 2×10^6 cells/mL was applied to the cell-injection side of TAXIScan holder and the cells (100 or less in most of the cases) were aligned at the edge of the micro-channel. After obtaining the first round of images, 1 µL of the chemoattractant solution prepared in the chemotaxis buffer was added to the ligand-injection side of the device to initiate migration. The assay conditions were as follows: duration, 4 h; interval, 5 min; micro-channel depth, 10 µm; and temperature, 37 °C. Time-lapse images of cell migration were stored as electronic files on a computer hard disk and analyzed when needed. The morphologies of migrating cells were depicted by tracing the edge of cells and then superimposing the resulting outlines onto the initial image. Movies of the images were made and quantification of velocity and directionality was carried out through the "TAXIScan analyzer 2" software. The trajectory of each cell on the image was traced by clicking the center portion of each cell on the computer display. The velocity (V) and the directionality (D) of each cell were calculated using the traced data as described previously [20, 23]. The statistical analysis for the velocity and the directionality was done by the Kruskal-Wallis Test (Non-parametric ANOVA) followed by the Dunn's Multiple Comparisons Test, as the data did not show normal distribution in most cases [20].

The modified Boyden chamber method was performed using collagen I-coated polycarbonate membrane inserts (8 µm pore size) in a 24-well plate (CytoSelect 24-Well Cell Haptotaxis Assay kit, Cell Biolabs, Inc. San Diego, CA, USA) or Transwell Plate with non-coated polycarbonate membrane (Corning Incorporated, Corning, NY, USA), per the manufacturer's protocols. Briefly, the cells grown on a culture dish were detached with Trypsin/EDTA solution, washed with PBS, and re-suspended in RPMI1640/HEPES buffer with 0.1% fatty-acid-free BSA (the chemotaxis buffer) to attain a density of 0.5×10^6 cells/mL. A total of 1.5×10^5 cells per well were placed in the upper chamber; the chemotaxis buffer with or without LPA was injected to the lower chamber, and then the plate was incubated at 37 °C for 2 h. The migrated cells were stained with the staining solution (supplied with the kit), observed under the microscope, and then lysed with the lysis solution (supplied with the kit) to quantify the number of migrated cells by measuring the absorbance at 560 nm. The absorbance was calibrated with the numbers of cells by using the standard curve with a series of different cell numbers (0, 10, 32, 100, 320, 1000, 3200, and 10,000 cells).

Quantitative reverse transcriptase polymerase reaction (qRT-PCR)

Total RNA was extracted from the cells using the RNeasy kit (QIAGEN, Hilden, Germany). Cells were seeded on 10 cm-diameter dishes until 80-90% confluency was attained. On the day of the experiment, the medium was removed, and the cells were washed with 5 mL PBS, followed by addition of lysis solution, per the manufacture's recommended procedure. Template DNA was prepared with extracted total RNA of each sample using Ready-To-Go You-Prime First-Strand Beads kit (GE Healthcare, Little Chalfont, UK) and 0.5 µL each of 1st strand DNA per sample was used for quantitative polymerase reaction (qPCR) with Fast SYBR Green Master Mix reagent (Life Technologies, Carlsbad, CA, USA). Analysis was done after preparing samples in a 96-well plate; signal during PCR was detected by Step One Plus Real-time PCR system (Life Technologies). The primers used are given in Additional file 1: Table S1. β-actin was used as an internal control for normalization of data. Data were analyzed by the software accompanied with the PCR system.

Protein expression and phosphorylation detection

Cells were seeded on 10-cm-diameter dishes until 80-90% confluency was attained. On the day of the experiment, cells were rinsed once with 5 mL of serum free Opti-MEM and then stimulated with 1 µM LPA prepared in the chemotaxis assay buffer (0.1%BSA in RPMI1640) pre-warmed at 37 °C for 30 s, 2 min, or 5 min. Immediately after stimulation, the medium was replaced with ice-cold chemotaxis assay buffer and cells were kept on ice until lysis was done. Cells were lysed with ice-cold lysis buffer from the PathScan RTK Signaling Antibody Array kit (Cell Signaling Technology, Danvers, MA, USA) per the manufacture's procedure. Cell lysate was kept at −70 °C until the PathScan phosphorylation array or SDS-PAGE/western blotting was performed. For western blotting, each cell lysate was subjected to SDS-PAGE, blotting, and antibody reaction. The pre-stained protein marker (Bio-Rad, Hercules, CA, USA) or the CruzMarker protein marker (Santa Cruz Biotechnology, Santa Cruz, CA, USA) was used to estimate the molecular weight of probed bands. Protein bands were visualized with ECL prime (GE Healthcare) and detected by LAS-4000 mini device (GE Healthcare). The list of the phosphorylated proteins for the array is shown in Additional file 2: Table S2.

Results

Establishing the optical real-time migration assay system for pancreatic cancer cells

We established the assay system for pancreatic cells using optically accessible horizontal cell mobility assay device, EZ-TAXIScan. This device has been used for monitoring chemotaxis assays mostly for hematopoietic cells such as neutrophils, monocytes/macrophages, dendritic cells, eosinophils, and lymphocytes [14–25]. In the case of adherent cells, like the cancer cells, additional procedures may be required for retrieving the optimal response from cells, such as scaffold coating [26]. Therefore, we compared different coatings on glass for facilitating pancreatic cell migration. Human collagen I, fibronectin, laminin, and Matrigel (growth factor reduced) were examined as scaffold substances coated on the glass plate inside the TAXIScan chamber. Among these materials, collagen I and Matrigel showed good performances (Fig. 1) (An additional movie file shows this in more detail [see Additional file 3]). Without coating, the cells did not attach well onto the glass plate (Fig. 1a) and did not show good migration (Fig. 1b). On the glass coated with collagen I or Matrigel, most cells attached and spread well even without a stimulant such as the chemoattractant (Fig. 1a). On the glass coated with collagen I or Matrigel, BxPC3 cells migrated towards LPA (Fig. 1b).

LPA is known as a chemoattractant for cancer cells. To observe chemotactic migration of the pancreatic cancer cells towards LPA using the TAXIScan system, we used different concentrations of LPA to seek an optimal concentration for migration and observed that 1 μM of LPA was optimal for BxPC3 and PANC-1 cells (Fig. 2a) (An additional movie file shows this in more detail [see Additional file 4]). In the case of AsPC1 and MIAPaCa-2 cells, very few cells migrated towards LPA at the concentration ranging from 0.1 nM to 10 μM (only the 1 μM data is shown in Fig. 2a, an additional movie file shows this in more detail [see Additional file 5]).

BxPC3 cells were the most responsive to LPA of all the cell lines studied. Therefore, we quantitated the directionality and velocity of migration of BxPC3 cells in response to different concentrations of LPA. The directionality in response to LPA increased in a dose-dependent manner (Fig. 2b left panel). The velocity also increased in a dose-dependent manner in the dose range of 1 to 10 μM LPA (Fig. 2b right panel). These results were in agreement the TAXIScan images (Fig. 2a). We confirmed the same phenomenon by an existing assay method, the Boyden chamber method. In the Boyden chamber method, BxPC3 cells showed good response to LPA in a dose-dependent manner (Fig. 2c, left). The concentrations of LPA that elicited the migration of BxPC3 cells were observed to be similar in both methods.

Expression of receptors for LPA on pancreatic cancer cells

To confirm if the migration of cells was due to the LPA-dependent phenomenon, we evaluated the expression of LPA receptors. Because most published reports showed either only mRNA expression or only protein expression [12, 13, 27], we attempted to show both mRNA and protein expression systematically by using qRT-PCR and western blotting. As LPA_1, LPA_2, LPA_3, LPA_4, LPA_5, and LPA_6 are the known receptors for LPA; we used primers for these receptor isoforms (Additional file 1: Table S1) [27] to compare their mRNA expressions. In BxPC3 cells, based on the results of qRT-PCR, LPA_1 was the most highly expressed receptor among all the 6 receptors (Fig. 3a), whereas LPA_2, LPA_3, and LPA_6 were moderately expressed and LPA_5 showed the lowest expression. In PANC-1 cells, LPA_1 and LPA_3 were the major receptors expressed. In AsPC1 cells, the mRNA expression of LPA_1, LPA_2, and LPA_6 were detected, and in MIAPaCa-2 cells, the mRNA expression of most LPA receptors was extremely low. LPA_3 expression was highest among the receptors for the MIAPaCa-2 cells (Fig. 3a).

We also evaluated the expression of these receptors at the protein level in the 4 pancreatic cell lines by western blotting using anti-LPA antibodies. All cell lines express a certain amount of LPA_1, LPA_2 and LPA_3 receptors, however, very low expression of LPA_4, LPA_5, and LPA_6 receptors was observed in lysates of all cell lines compared to 211H, KATOIII or PC3 which were used as positive controls (Fig. 3b). The data from the migration assay and western blotting indicated that BxPC3 and PANC-1 cells express the LPA receptors and the migration images of the cells reflects the LPA-elicited migration.

Signal transduction during migration of pancreatic cancer cells towards LPA

To further confirm that the migration was LPA-dependent, we determined phosphorylation of various molecules in BxPC3 and PANC-1 cells using the PathScan array, which enabled us to simultaneously evaluate the phosphorylation of 39 different molecules (Additional file 2: Table S2). We carried out phosphorylation assays at the time points 0.5, 2, and 5 min following LPA stimulation, due to uniform stimulation of cells by LPA on culture dishes, which precludes the use of an LPA concentration gradient similar to that of the TAXI Scan device. Using this array system, we observed that Akt (Thr308 and Ser473), p44/42MAPK, IRS-1, InsR, c-kit, EphA2, and Tie2 were phosphorylated after LPA stimulation in both BxPC3 (Fig. 4a, b) and PANC-1 cells (Fig. 4c, d). Of these phosphorylated proteins, Akt and MAPK are known to be key molecules involved in migration and proliferation. The phosphorylation of these signaling molecules after uniform stimulation was further observed by western blotting. The results obtained showed that Akt (Thr308 and Ser473), p44/42MAPK were phosphorylated after LPA stimulation, as expected, in both BxPC3 and PANC-1 cell lines within 5 min (Figs. 4e and 5c). For the record, we also checked longer time points, such as 15, 30, 60, 120, and 240 min which were similar to the time points used in the TAXIScan experiments, but no additional increase in phosphorylation of these molecules

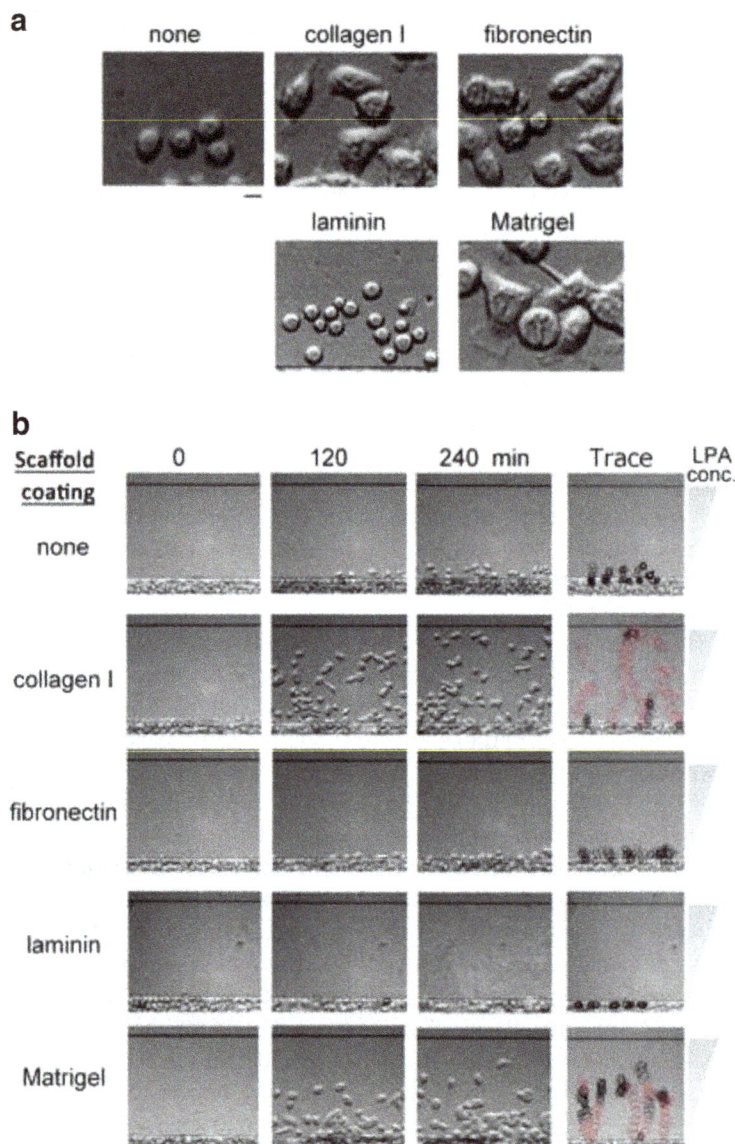

Fig. 1 Adhesion and migration of pancreatic cancer cells monitored by TAXIScan. **a** Morphology of BxPC3 pancreatic cancer cells after adherence to each scaffold material coated on the coverslip without chemoattractant. Images were taken 240 min after starting the assay. Scale bar: 10 μm. **b** Chemotaxis of BxPC3 pancreatic cancer cells towards 100 nM LPA with or without various kinds of scaffold-coating. Images taken at time 0, 120 and 240 min are shown. The morphologies of 4 or 5 representative migrating cells throughout the assays are shown on the "Trace" column. The outlines of the migrating cells were traced every 10 min in this column. Cells migrating at more than 1 μm/min are shown in *red*. All data are representative of 3 independent experiments. Scale bar: 100 μm

was observed (Fig. 4e). These data further support the establishment of the assay system of cancer cell migration towards LPA.

Effect of inhibitor on migration towards LPA

We also tested the effect of an LPA inhibitor, Ki16425 [28], on LPA-elicited migration of BxPC3 cells. When the cells were treated with Ki16425, the migration of the cells towards LPA was abrogated in a dose-dependent manner (Fig. 5a, b, an additional movie file shows this in more detail [see Additional file 6]). The half maximal

inhibitory concentration (IC_{50}) value for directionality was ≈ 1.86 μM (Fig. 5b, left graph). Owing to weak inhibition of velocity by Ki16425, the IC_{50} value for velocity was >100 μM (Fig. 5b, right graph). When the cells were treated 50 μM Ki16425, the phosphorylation of Akt and MAPK was reduced, as observed during western blot analysis (Fig. 5c). The pancreatic cancer cells showed LPA-elicited chemotactic migration with clarity in the TAXIScan chamber, and this phenomenon was vigorously supported by the inhibition of the intracellular signaling with Ki16425.

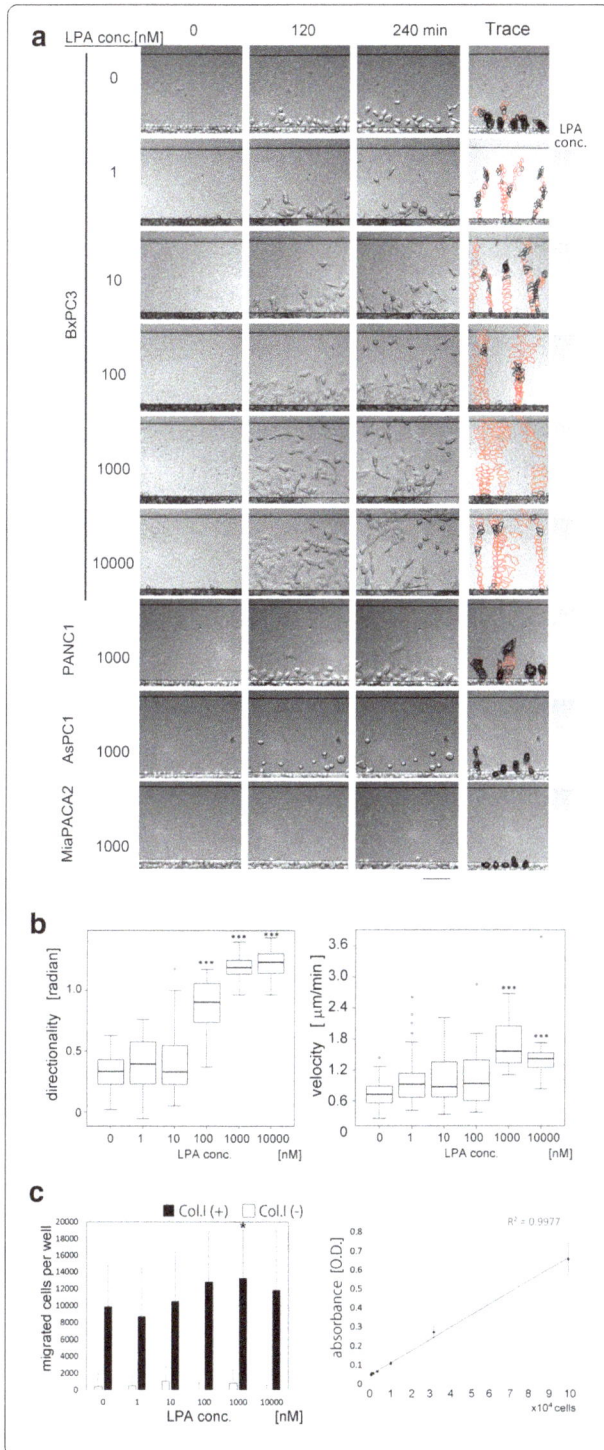

Fig. 2 Chemotaxis of pancreatic cancer cells towards LPA detected by TAXIScan (**a** and **b**) or Boyden chamber (**c**). **a** Four pancreatic cancer cell lines were used for the TAXIScan method. Dose-dependency of BxPC3 chemotaxis towards LPA is observed. The migration images of PANC-1, AsPC1, and MIAPaCa-2 cells in the optimal conditions are also shown. Images taken at time 0, 120 and 240 min are shown. The morphologies of 4 or 5 representative migrating cells throughout the assays are shown on the "Trace" column. The outlines of the migrating cells were recorded every 10 min in this column. Cells migrating at more than 1 μm/min are shown in *red*. Data are representative of 3 independent experiments. Scale bar: 100 μm. **b** Quantitation of the directionality and velocity of migration of BxPC3 cells towards various concentrations of LPA. The graph on the left indicates the directionality and the graph on the right indicates velocity. *White circles* are outliers. Statistical analysis was done by the Kruskal-Wallis Test (Nonparametric ANOVA) followed by the Dunn's Multiple Comparisons Test. Data are representative of 3 independent experiments. **c** Migration of BxPC3 cells towards LPA using Boyden chamber assay kit. The migrated cells were stained with the staining solution and the numbers of the migrated cells were estimated by measuring OD 560 nm based on the standard curve (*the graph on the right*). The assay results with the collagen I coated membrane (*black bar*) or the plain membrane (*white bar*) are shown in the graph on the left. Mean values of data are shown and the error bars represents the standard error ($n = 6$). Statistical analysis was conducted using the Student's t-test. *$p < 0.05$ (vs. data without LPA)

Discussion

In this study, we established a pancreatic cancer cell migration assay system by using the TAXIScan device. We found that coating of scaffolds such as collagen and Matrigel on glass, similar to that in some published studies using other methods, was necessary for successful adhesion and migration. BxPC3 and PANC-1 cells migrated towards LPA in a dose-dependent manner, which was clearly inhibited by an LPA inhibitor, Ki16425. This is the first report of pancreatic cancer cell migration monitored by the TAXIScan system that enables analysis of multiple parameters, including directionality, velocity, and cell morphology. Additionally, this is the first report simultaneously comparing the TAXIScan and Boyden chamber methods. The Boyden chamber method has been used for over 50 years [29], the limitations of this method have been pointed out by several researchers. In this method, a membrane of 10 μm thickness, having holes of 8 μm diameter (in this study) with random density, separates the upper and lower wells (see Additional file 7). It is thought that cells are able to sense differences in the chemoattractant concentration between these two wells. Although this method appears simple, it has certain limitations. (I) The density of holes may not be uniform. (II) The microstructure inside the hole, e.g., a micro-channel of 10 μm length × 8 μm diameter, is unknown, and the chemo-attractant gradient is not measurable. (III) A large number of cells is necessary for this assay (1.5×10^5 cells per well in this study). (IV) A considerable amount of chemo-attractant is necessary (500 μL per well in this study), which is expensive. (V) The process of cell migration is not visible. (VI) The device only displays the numbers of migrated cells. (VII) The obtained data may have high background noise. (VIII) The density of cells migrating to the lower side of the membrane is not uniform. A few advantage of this method are as follows: (I) It has a simple structure; (II) the apparatus itself (without coating

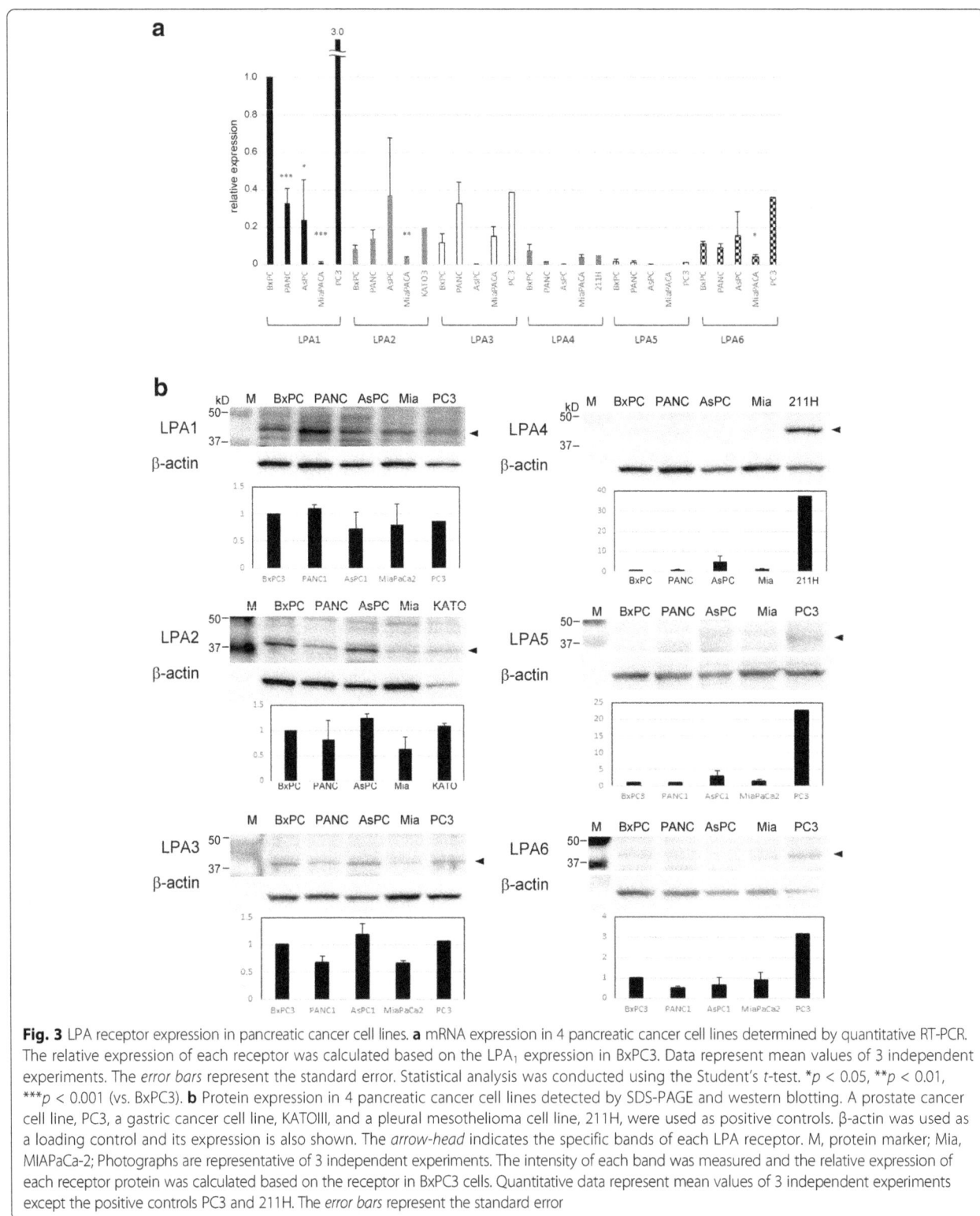

Fig. 3 LPA receptor expression in pancreatic cancer cell lines. **a** mRNA expression in 4 pancreatic cancer cell lines determined by quantitative RT-PCR. The relative expression of each receptor was calculated based on the LPA$_1$ expression in BxPC3. Data represent mean values of 3 independent experiments. The *error bars* represent the standard error. Statistical analysis was conducted using the Student's *t*-test. *$p < 0.05$, **$p < 0.01$, ***$p < 0.001$ (vs. BxPC3). **b** Protein expression in 4 pancreatic cancer cell lines detected by SDS-PAGE and western blotting. A prostate cancer cell line, PC3, a gastric cancer cell line, KATOIII, and a pleural mesothelioma cell line, 211H, were used as positive controls. β-actin was used as a loading control and its expression is also shown. The *arrow-head* indicates the specific bands of each LPA receptor. M, protein marker; Mia, MIAPaCa-2; Photographs are representative of 3 independent experiments. The intensity of each band was measured and the relative expression of each receptor protein was calculated based on the receptor in BxPC3 cells. Quantitative data represent mean values of 3 independent experiments except the positive controls PC3 and 211H. The *error bars* represent the standard error

materials) is inexpensive; and (III) it is well known and widely used. On the other hands, the advantages of TAXI-Scan are as follows [14] (see also Additional file 8): (I) it has an uniform micro-channel (260 μm length × 1000 μm width × 8 μm height); (II) the chemoattractant, which is placed on one end of the micro-channel, defuses uniformly through the channel, resulting in a stable concentration gradient [14]; (III) a small number of cells

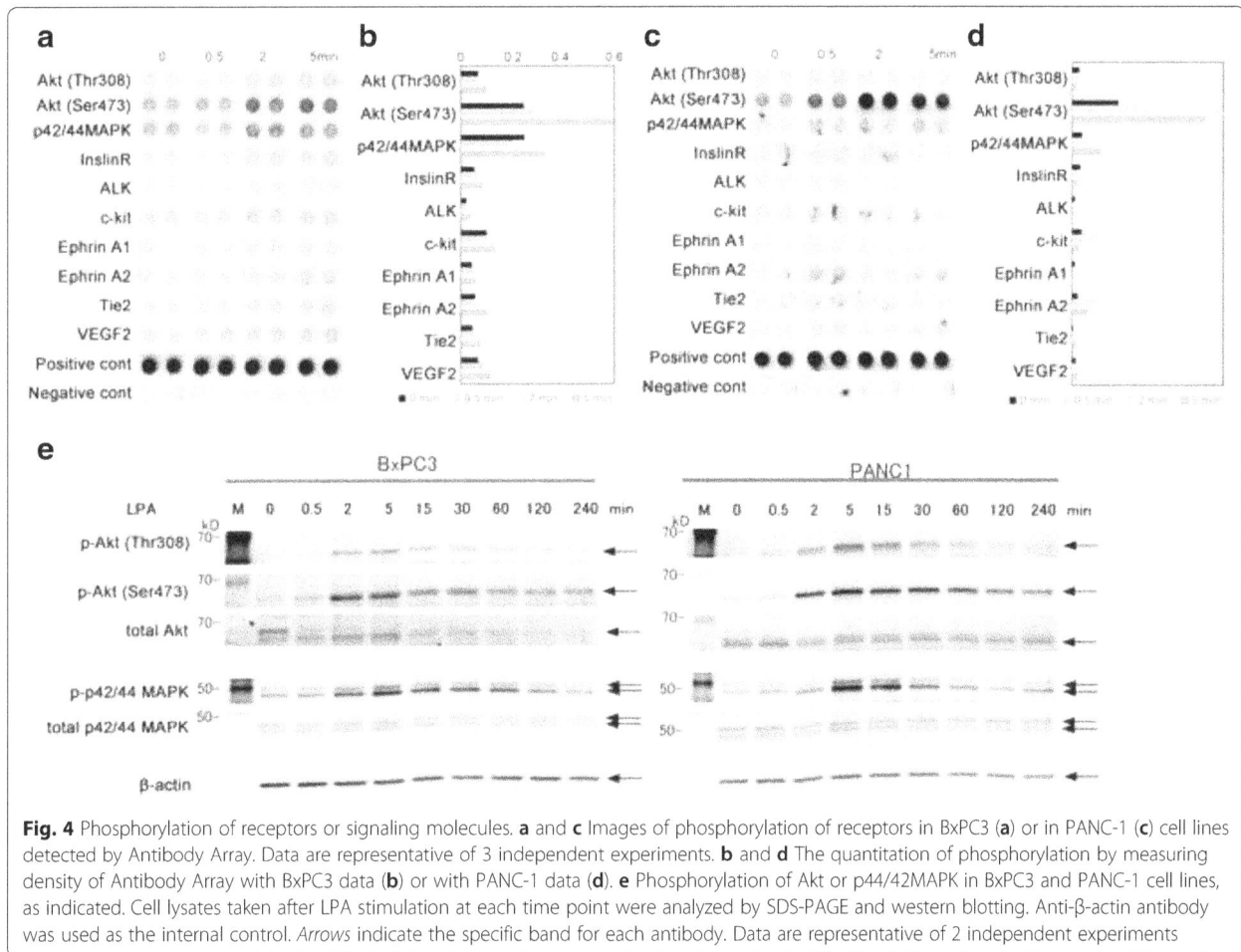

Fig. 4 Phosphorylation of receptors or signaling molecules. **a** and **c** Images of phosphorylation of receptors in BxPC3 (**a**) or in PANC-1 (**c**) cell lines detected by Antibody Array. Data are representative of 3 independent experiments. **b** and **d** The quantitation of phosphorylation by measuring density of Antibody Array with BxPC3 data (**b**) or with PANC-1 data (**d**). **e** Phosphorylation of Akt or p44/42MAPK in BxPC3 and PANC-1 cell lines, as indicated. Cell lysates taken after LPA stimulation at each time point were analyzed by SDS-PAGE and western blotting. Anti-β-actin antibody was used as the internal control. *Arrows* indicate the specific band for each antibody. Data are representative of 2 independent experiments

is required for analysis (100 or less cells per channel); (IV) a small and inexpensive amount of chemoattractant is necessary (1 μL per channel); (V) migrating cells are observable; (VI) images obtained during migration are recorded automatically; (VII) data obtained from this assay including that on morphology, behavior, directionality, and velocity, are more informative. However, some demerits of TAXIScan are as follows: (I) although the running cost is low, the initial cost is high, and (II) it is not well-known yet. In fact, it may not be appropriate to position TAXI-Scan as an alternate to the Boyden method, because both methods utilize completely different equipment and data collection methods, and the quality of data obtained using these methods is entirely different (Additional files 7 and 8). However, because of lower requirement of samples and the collection of more informative data, the approach to cancer cell migration using TAXIScan is more useful than analysis using existing techniques such as the Boyden chamber method. With the TAXIScan system, the characteristics of pancreatic cancer cells can be analyzed in detail. Moreover, our system can be adopted for migration studies in other types of cancer cells.

In the Boyden chamber method, a certain number of cells without LPA was observed to migrate, indicating a high background (Fig. 2c), similar to that reported previously [30–33]. This high background with the Boyden chamber method is considered to be due to the thickness of the membrane (10 μm in this study). In TAXIScan method, cells without LPA were observed to migrate for more than 10 μm (up to 100 μm) (Fig. 2a), explaining this phenomenon. From this point of view, we could argue that TAXIScan has a wider dynamic range to detect cell migration.

Herein, 4 pancreatic cancer cell lines were analyzed and only 2 of these cell-lines, BxPC3 and PANC-1, showed good migration towards LPA with reasonable co-evidence on the expression of LPA receptors. The reason why AsPC1 and MIAPaCa-2 cells do not migrate towards LPA is still unknown. BxPC3 and PANC-1 do express LPA_1, LPA_2, and LPA_3; however, these cell lines do not express LPA_4, LPA_5, and LPA_6 as observed during western blotting (Fig. 3b). The latter 3 receptors are likely not involved in cell migration but might be involved in other cellular functions.

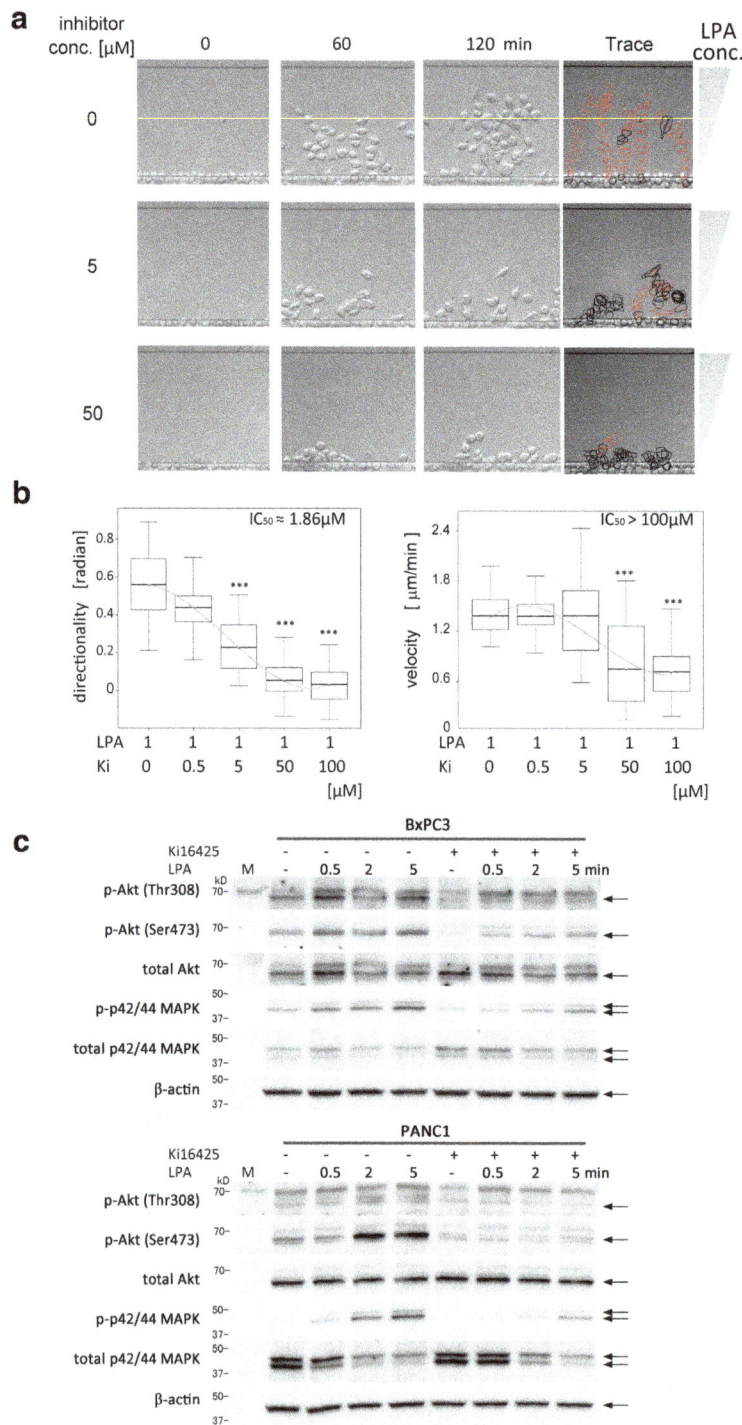

Fig. 5 Inhibition of BxPC3 chemotaxis towards LPA by Ki16425. **a** BxPC3 chemotaxis towards 1 μM LPA with various concentrations of Ki16425. Cells were pre-incubated with Ki16425 for 24 h and the chemotaxis assay was performed using TAXIScan. Data are representative of 3 independent experiments. **b** Box-plots of the directionality and the velocity in BxPC3 migration towards LPA with Ki16425. The graph on the left indicates directionality and that on the right indicates velocity. The half maximal inhibitory concentration (IC$_{50}$) values are also shown. Statistical analysis was done by the Kruskal-Wallis Test (Non-parametric ANOVA) followed by the Dunn's Multiple Comparisons Test. ***$p < 0.0001$ (vs. data with 1 μM LPA and without Ki16425). Data are representative of 3 independent experiments. **c** Inhibition of phosphorylation of Akt or p44/42MAPK by Ki16425 in BxPC3 and PANC-1 cell lines, as indicated. Cell lysates taken after LPA stimulation at each time point were analyzed by SDS-PAGE and western blotting. Anti-β-actin antibody was used as the internal control. *Arrows* indicate the specific band for each antibody. Data are representative of 3 independent experiments

LPA inhibitor, Ki16425, shown in this study is believed to block human LPA_1 and LPA_3 receptors [28]; 10 μM of Ki16425 significantly blocked the migration of cancer cells [13]. In our system, Ki16425 clearly inhibited BxPC3 cell migration towards LPA at 5-50 μM concentrations, indicating that TAXIScan and BxPC3 cells are the best tools for screening inhibitors of pancreatic cell migration. Utilizing such a new method, new molecules for regulating pancreatic cancer metastasis can be identified, and the limited treatment options and the poor prognosis of this disease can be overcome. Studies on neutrophils have tested various kinds of compounds and found that some compounds inhibit neutrophil function, leading to the successful selection of several effective molecules [34]. Collectively, it can be concluded that the system established in our study can be a powerful tool for cancer research and drug discovery in seeking effectors and inhibitors for analyzing cancer cell function. We are currently looking for and screening such molecules that can regulate pancreatic cancer cell migration; some promising molecules will be reported in the near future.

Conclusions

We established a novel pancreatic cancer cell migration assay system that provides optical and quantitative information simultaneously. Using this system, we demonstrated that BxPC3 and PANC-1 cells showed good migration towards LPA. The effect of an LPA inhibitor, Ki16425, was detected clearly in this system, which was confirmed by the reduction in the phosphorylation of signal transduction molecules, Akt and MAPK. As this method provides a large amount of information on migrating cells simultaneously, such as their morphology, directionality, and velocity, with a small volume of sample, it can be a powerful tool for analyzing the characteristics of cancer cells and for evaluating factors affecting cellular functions.

Additional files

Additional file 1: Table S1. Primers used for the quantitative RT-PCR. Total 6 pairs of primers for LPA receptors (LPA1, LPA2, LPA3, LPA4, LPA 5, and LPA6) were used for this study, based on the information reported previously (27).

Additional file 2: Table S2. Targets for PathScan RTK signaling array. The phosphorylation of 39 different molecules in BxPC3 and PANC-1 cells was evaluated using the PathScan array. Details are described in Methods section.

Additional file 3: Chemotaxis of BxPC3 pancreatic cancer cells towards 100 nM LPA with or without various kinds of scaffold-coating. Images were taken every 5 min for 4 h and movies were created by TAXIScan Analyzer2 software. Representative of 3 independent experiments. Scale bar: 100 μm.

Additional file 4: Chemotaxis of BxPC3 pancreatic cancer cells towards various concentrations of LPA on a collagen I coated coverslip. Images

were taken every 5 min for 4 h and movies were created by TAXIScan Analyzer2 software. Representative of 3 independent experiments. Scale bar: 100 μm.

Additional file 5: Chemotaxis of four kinds of pancreatic cancer cells towards 1 μM LPA on a collagen I coated coverslip. Images were taken every 5 min for 4 h and movies were created by TAXIScan Analyzer2 software. Representative of 3 independent experiments. Scale bar: 100 μm.

Additional file 6: Inhibition of BxPC3 chemotaxis towards LPA by Ki16425. Cells were pre-incubated with Ki16425 for 24 h and the chemotaxis assay towards 1 μM LPA was performed using TAXIScan. Images were taken every 5 min for 4 h and movies were created by TAXIScan Analyzer2 software. Representative of 3 independent experiments. Scale bar: 100 μm.

Additional file 7: The modified Boyden chamber assay. A) Schematic diagram (sagittal section) of one well of the modified Boyden chamber assay (Transwell). Cells in the chemotaxis buffer are located in the upper chamber and the chemoattractant the chemotaxis buffer is added to the lower chamber. B) Schematic diagram of the membrane part of the modified Boyden chamber. The membrane separates the upper and the lower chamber. The matrix is coated on the lower side of the membrane. C) Photographs of the lower side of the membrane after the assay. Cells are stained with the staining solution accompanied with the assay kit. Magnification: 400×.

Additional file 8: The TAXIScan assay. A) Schematic diagram (sagittal section) of one channel of the TAXIScan chamber. The chamber is filled with the chemotaxis buffer (light brown color). Cells are located on the one side of the micro-channel and the chemoattractant (red color) is placed on the other side of the micro-channel. B) Schematic diagram (sagittal section) of the micro-channel. The chemoattractant is defused in the micro-channel, which forms the stable concentration gradient. Cells on the matrix-coated coverslip migrates towards the gradient of the chemoattractant in the micro-channel. C) Photograph of cells migrating towards the chemoattractant. The image is taken from underneath of the TAXIScan chamber.

Abbreviations
BSA: Bovine serum albumin; EDTA: Ethylenediamine tetraacetic acid; EGF: Epidermal growth factor; Eph: Ephrin; FBS: Fetal bovine serum; IC50: The half maximal inhibitory concentration; InsR: Insulin receptor; IRS-1: Insulin receptor substrate 1; LPA: Lysophosphatidic acid; MAPK: Mitogen-activated protein kinase; RTK: Receptor tyrosine kinase; SDS-PAGE: Sodium dodecyl sulfate-polyacrylamide gel electrophoresis; Tie2: Tyrosine kinase with Ig-like loops and epidermal growth factor homology domains-2

Acknowledgements
We would like to thank Dr. Masakiyo Sakaguchi for providing materials, Editage (www.editage.jp) for English language editing, and the central research center of Kawasaki Medical School for technical supports.

Funding
This study was supported by JSPS KAKENHI Grant Number JP15K10201 (to AY), JP25861742 / JP16K11470 (to NK), and JP15K09671 (to FK), Wesco Scientific Promotion Foundation (to AY), Kawasaki Medical foundation for Medicine and Medical Welfare (to AY), and Kawasaki Medical School project-research fund (to AY, MY, and NK). There was no role with all funding bodies above in the design of the study or collection, analysis, or interpretation of the data or writing the manuscript.

Availability of data and materials
All data and materials are available upon reasonable request to the corresponding author. The data in this study were not deposited in publicly available repositories since there is no suitable repository service for the data.

Authors' contributions
AY and MY overviewed and designed this study and analyzed data. NK, MI, KK, and NO collected and analyzed data. MN, YY, and FK critically discussed and corrected the manuscript. All authors have read and approved the manuscript.

Competing interests
There is no competing interest regarding the publication of this paper.

Author details
[1]Department of Biochemistry, Kawasaki Medical School, 577 Matsushima, Kurashiki, Okayama 701-0192, Japan. [2]Department of Clinical Oncology, Kawasaki Medical School, Okayama, Japan. [3]Department of Molecular and Developmental Biology, Kawasaki Medical School, Okayama, Japan. [4]Department of Surgery and Oncology, Graduate School of Medical Sciences, Kyushu University, Fukuoka, Japan.

References
1. Roussos ET, Condeelis JS, Patsialou A. Chemotaxis in cancer. Nat Rev Cancer. 2011;11(8):573–87.
2. Dorsam RT, Gutkind JS. G-protein-coupled receptors and cancer. Nat Rev Cancer. 2007;7(2):79–94.
3. Murph M, Tanaka T, Liu S, Mills GB. Of spiders and crabs: the emergence of lysophospholipids and their metabolic pathways as targets for therapy in cancer. Clin Cancer Res. 2006;12(22):6598–602.
4. Hecht JH, Weiner JA, Post SR, Chun J. Ventricular zone gene-1 (vzg-1) encodes a lysophosphatidic acid receptor expressed in neurogenic regions of the developing cerebral cortex. J Cell Biol. 1996;135(4):1071–83.
5. An S, Bleu T, Hallmark OG, Goetzl EJ. Characterization of a novel subtype of human G protein-coupled receptor for lysophosphatidic acid. J Biol Chem. 1998;273(14):7906–10.
6. Bandoh K, Aoki J, Hosono H, Kobayashi S, Kobayashi T, Murakami-Murofushi K, Tsujimoto M, Arai H, Inoue K. Molecular cloning and characterization of a novel human G-protein-coupled receptor, EDG7, for lysophosphatidic acid. J Biol Chem. 1999;274(39):27776–85.
7. Noguchi K, Ishii S, Shimizu T. Identification of p2y9/GPR23 as a novel G protein-coupled receptor for lysophosphatidic acid, structurally distant from the Edg family. J Biol Chem. 2003;278(28):25600–6.
8. Kotarsky K, Boketoft A, Bristulf J, Nilsson NE, Norberg A, Hansson S, Owman C, Sillard R, Leeb-Lundberg LM, Olde B. Lysophosphatidic acid binds to and activates GPR92, a G protein-coupled receptor highly expressed in gastrointestinal lymphocytes. J Pharmacol Exp Ther. 2006;318(2):619–28.
9. Pasternack SM, von Kügelgen I, Al Aboud K, Lee YA, Rüschendorf F, Voss K, Hillmer AM, Molderings GJ, Franz T, Ramirez A, et al. G protein-coupled receptor P2Y5 and its ligand LPA are involved in maintenance of human hair growth. Nat Genet. 2008;40(3):329–34.
10. Chun J, Hla T, Lynch KR, Spiegel S, Moolenaar WH. International Union of Basic and Clinical Pharmacology. LXXVIII. Lysophospholipid receptor nomenclature. Pharmacol Rev. 2010;62(4):579–87.
11. Mills GB, Moolenaar WH. The emerging role of lysophosphatidic acid in cancer. Nat Rev Cancer. 2003;3(8):582–91.
12. Stähle M, Veit C, Bachfischer U, Schierling K, Skripczynski B, Hall A, Gierschik P, Giehl K. Mechanisms in LPA-induced tumor cell migration: critical role of phosphorylated ERK. J Cell Sci. 2003;116(Pt 18):3835–46.
13. Yamada T, Sato K, Komachi M, Malchinkhuu E, Tobo M, Kimura T, Kuwabara A, Yanagita Y, Ikeya T, Tanahashi Y, et al. Lysophosphatidic acid (LPA) in malignant ascites stimulates motility of human pancreatic cancer cells through LPA1. J Biol Chem. 2004;279(8):6595–605.
14. Kanegasaki S, Nomura Y, Nitta N, Akiyama S, Tamatani T, Goshoh Y, Yoshida T, Sato T, Kikuchi Y. A novel optical assay system for the quantitative measurement of chemotaxis. J Immunol Methods. 2003;282(1-2):1–11.
15. Jang MH, Sougawa N, Tanaka T, Hirata T, Hiroi T, Tohya K, Guo Z, Umemoto E, Ebisuno Y, Yang BG, et al. CCR7 is critically important for migration of dendritic cells in intestinal lamina propria to mesenteric lymph nodes. J Immunol. 2006;176(2):803–10.
16. Nishio M, Watanabe K, Sasaki J, Taya C, Takasuga S, Iizuka R, Balla T, Yamazaki M, Watanabe H, Itoh R, et al. Control of cell polarity and motility by the PtdIns(3,4,5)P3 phosphatase SHIP1. Nat Cell Biol. 2007;9(1):36–44.
17. Ito A, Suganami T, Yamauchi A, Degawa-Yamauchi M, Tanaka M, Kouyama R, Kobayashi Y, Nitta N, Yasuda K, Hirata Y, et al. Role of CC Chemokine receptor 2 in bone marrow cells in the recruitment of macrophages into obese adipose tissue. J Biol Chem. 2008;283(51):35715 23.
18. Nishikimi A, Fukuhara H, Su W, Hongu T, Takasuga S, Mihara H, Cao Q, Sanematsu F, Kanai M, Hasegawa H, et al. Sequential regulation of DOCK2 dynamics by two phospholipids during neutrophil chemotaxis. Science. 2009;324(5925):384–7.
19. Uchida M, Oyanagi E, Miyachi M, Yamauchi A, Yano H. Relationship between macrophage differentiation and the chemotactic activity toward damaged myoblast cells. J Immunol Methods. 2013;393(1-2):61–9.
20. Yamauchi A, Degawa-Yamauchi M, Kuribayashi F, Kanegasaki S, Tsuchiya T. Systematic single cell analysis of migration and morphological changes of human neutrophils over stimulus concentration gradients. J Immunol Methods. 2014;404:59–70.
21. Kurose K, Ohue Y, Sato E, Yamauchi A, Eikawa S, Isobe M, Nishio Y, Uenaka A, Oka M, Nakayama E. Increase in activated Treg in TIL in lung cancer and in vitro depletion of Treg by ADCC using an antihuman CCR4 mAb (KM2760). J Thorac Oncol. 2015;10(1):74–83.
22. Ishii M, Egen JG, Klauschen F, Meier-Schellersheim M, Saeki Y, Vacher J, Proia RL, Germain RN. Sphingosine-1-phosphate mobilizes osteoclast precursors and regulates bone homeostasis. Nature. 2009;458(7237):524–8.
23. Nitta N, Tsuchiya T, Yamauchi A, Tamatani T, Kanegasaki S. Quantitative analysis of eosinophil chemotaxis tracked using a novel optical device - TAXIScan. J Immunol Methods. 2007;320(1-2):155–63.
24. Terashima Y, Onai N, Murai M, Enomoto M, Poonpiriya V, Hamada T, Motomura K, Suwa M, Ezaki T, Haga T, et al. Pivotal function for cytoplasmic protein FROUNT in CCR2-mediated monocyte chemotaxis. Nat Immunol. 2005;6(8):827–35.
25. Takamatsu H, Takegahara N, Nakagawa Y, Tomura M, Taniguchi M, Friedel RH, Rayburn H, Tessier-Lavigne M, Yoshida Y, Okuno T, et al. Semaphorins guide the entry of dendritic cells into the lymphatics by activating myosin II. Nat Immunol. 2010;11(7):594–600.
26. Yamauchi A, Hadjur C, Takahashi T, Suzuki I, Hirose K, Mahe YF. Human skin melanocyte migration towards stromal cell-derived factor-1 alpha demonstrated by optical real-time cell mobility assay: modulation of their chemotactic ability by alpha-melanocyte-stimulating hormone. Exp Dermatol. 2013;22(10):664–7.
27. Jongsma M, Matas-Rico E, Rzadkowski A, Jalink K, Moolenaar WH. LPA is a chemorepellent for B16 melanoma cells: action through the cAMP-elevating LPA5 receptor. PLoS One. 2011;6(12):e29260.
28. Ohta H, Sato K, Murata N, Damirin A, Malchinkhuu E, Kon J, Kimura T, Tobo M, Yamazaki Y, Watanabe T, et al. Ki16425, a subtype-selective antagonist for EDG-family lysophosphatidic acid receptors. Mol Pharmacol. 2003;64(4):994–1005.
29. BOYDEN S. The chemotactic effect of mixtures of antibody and antigen on polymorphonuclear leucocytes. J Exp Med. 1962;115:453–66.
30. Schuller HM, Al-Wadei HA, Majidi M. GABA B receptor is a novel drug target for pancreatic cancer. Cancer. 2008;112(4):767–78.
31. Schuller HM, Al-Wadei HA, Majidi M. Gamma-aminobutyric acid, a potential tumor suppressor for small airway-derived lung adenocarcinoma. Carcinogenesis. 2008;29(10):1979–85.
32. König J, Weiss G, Rossi D, Wankhammer K, Reinisch A, Kinzer M, Huppertz B, Pfeiffer D, Parolini O, Lang I. Placental mesenchymal stromal cells derived from blood vessels or avascular tissues: what is the better choice to support endothelial cell function? Stem Cells Dev. 2015;24(1):115–31.
33. Kestens C, Siersema PD, Offerhaus GJ, van Baal JW. BMP4 signaling is able to induce an epithelial-Mesenchymal transition-like phenotype in Barrett's esophagus and esophageal Adenocarcinoma through induction of SNAIL2. PLoS One. 2016;11(5):e0155754.
34. Hattori H, Subramanian KK, Sakai J, Jia Y, Li Y, Porter TF, Loison F, Sarraj B, Kasorn A, Jo H, et al. Small-molecule screen identifies reactive oxygen species as key regulators of neutrophil chemotaxis. Proc Natl Acad Sci U S A. 2010;107(8):3546–51.

A Phase I clinical trial of EUS-guided intratumoral injection of the oncolytic virus, HF10 for unresectable locally advanced pancreatic cancer

Yoshiki Hirooka[1*], Hideki Kasuya[2], Takuya Ishikawa[3], Hiroki Kawashima[3], Eizaburo Ohno[3], Itzel B. Villalobos[2], Yoshinori Naoe[2], Toru Ichinose[2], Nobuto Koyama[4], Maki Tanaka[4], Yasuhiro Kodera[5] and Hidemi Goto[3]

Abstract

Background: Prognosis of pancreatic cancer is poor with a 5-year survival rate of only 7%. Although several new chemotherapy treatments have shown promising results, all patients will eventually progress, and we need to develop newer chemotherapy treatments to improve response rates and overall survival (OS). HF10 is a spontaneously mutated oncolytic virus derived from a herpes simplex virus-1, and it has potential to show strong antitumor effect against malignancies without damaging normal tissue. We aimed to evaluate the safety and anti-tumor effectiveness in phase I dose-escalation trial of direct injection of HF10 into unresectable locally advanced pancreatic cancer under endoscopic ultrasound (EUS)-guidance in combination with erlotinib and gemcitabine administration. The mid-term results have been previously reported and here we report the final results of our study.

Methods: This was a single arm, open-label Phase I trial. HF10 was injected once every 2 weeks and continued up to four times in total unless dose-limiting toxicity (DLT) appears. A total of nine subjects in three Cohorts with dose-escalation were planned to be enrolled in this trial. The primary endpoint was the safety assessment and the secondary endpoint was the efficacy assessment.

Results: Twelve patients enrolled in this clinical trial, and ten subjects received this therapy. Five patients showed Grade III myelosuppression and two patients developed serious adverse events (AEs) (perforation of duodenum, hepatic dysfunction). However, all of these events were judged as AEs unrelated to HF10. Tumor responses were three partial responses (PR), four stable diseases (SD), and two progressive diseases (PD) out of nine subjects who completed the treatment. Target lesion responses were three PRs and six SDs. The median progression free survival (PFS) was 6. 3 months, whereas the median OS was 15.5 months. Two subjects from Cohort 1 and 2 showed downstaging and finally achieved surgical complete response (CR).

(Continued on next page)

* Correspondence: hirooka@med.nagoya-u.ac.jp
Annotation: Mid-term results of this study were presented in International Association of Pancreatology (IAP) meeting 2016 (Sendai, Japan) (Hirooka Y, Kawashima H, Ohno E, Kasuya H, Tanaka M, Goto H: Phase 1 dose-escalation clinical trial of EUS-guided injection of HF10 for unresectable locally advanced pancreatic cancer. *Pancreatology* 2016, 16(4, Supplement):S17).
[1]Department of Endoscopy, Nagoya University Hospital, 65 Tsuruma-cho, Showa-ku, Nagoya 466-8550, Japan
Full list of author information is available at the end of the article

(Continued from previous page)

Conclusions: HF10 direct injection under EUS-guidance in combination with erlotinib and gemcitabine was a safe treatment for locally advanced pancreatic cancer. Combination therapy of HF10 and chemotherapy should be explored further in large prospective studies.

Keywords: Pancreatic cancer, Oncolytic virus, HF10, EUS-guidance

Background

The number of death due to pancreatic cancer has been increasing and now it is the fourth leading cause of cancer mortality in the United States with a 5 year survival rate of 7% [1], which was similar in Japanese population [2]. Surgery offers the only chance for cure, but most of the patients present with advanced stage and only 15–20% of those are candidates for curative resection [3, 4]. Chemotherapy may play a more important role in the treatment of advanced or inoperable pancreatic cancer. Although the appearance of several new chemotherapy treatments has shown improving survival, all patients will eventually progress and die of the disease. Therefore, we need to develop novel anti-cancer treatments to achieve further improvement of prognosis.

Because of their distinctive characteristics in replication and antitumor immune responses, Oncolytic viruses (OVs) are considered to be a new option in cancer therapy. Most of the OVs developed in the past have been generated to increase the tumor selectivity and efficacy. However, in contrast to those artificially modified OV mutants, HF10 is a spontaneously mutated OV derived from a herpes simplex virus-1 (HSV-1). Genetically, HF10 naturally lacks the expression of *UL43*, *UL49.5*, *UL55*, *UL56*, and latency-associated transcripts, and overexpresses *UL53* and *UL54* [5]. Although the effect of these genetic changes are still under investigation, based on the previous studies, the characteristics of HF10 can be summarized into following five points: 1. high tumor selectivity, 2. high viral replication, 3. initiation of a cytopathic effect, 4. intermediation of potent bystander effect, and 5. strong antitumor effect against various malignancies [5]. In addition, it has been reported that lack of UL 56 expression may reduce the neuroinvasiveness [6]. Following these results, successful clinical trials with promising results have been reported in different cancer types including recurrent metastatic breast cancer [7, 8], recurrent head and neck squamous cell carcinoma (HNSCC) [9], unresectable pancreatic cancer [10], refractory and superficial cancers [11], and melanoma [12].

Up to now, OVs have not shown serious toxicities or any therapeutic resistance, contrary to chemotherapeutic drugs that may cause severe dose limiting toxicities (DLT). As OVs and chemotherapeutic drugs have different mechanisms of action each other, combination therapy is expected to increase the antitumor effect with limited side effects. Although the data on HF10 in preclinical and clinical trials suggest that therapeutic applications can be developed with a high safety margin, ideal combination therapies with either chemotherapy or immunotherapeutic agents still need more investigation [5]. In this study, we conducted the phase I dose-escalation trial of HF10 direct injection into unresectable locally advanced pancreatic cancer under EUS-guidance in combination with erlotinib and gemcitabine administration. We assessed the safety and antitumor effectiveness of a novel triple combination therapy. The mid-term results have been previously reported [13] and here we report the final results of our study.

Methods

Study design

This was a single arm, open-label Phase I trial. This study was registered in UMIN-CTR (UMIN000010150) and was approved by the Ethical Committee in our institute. Written informed consents to participate were obtained from all the patients in this study.

The following inclusion criteria were used for the selection of the patients: 1) Patients diagnosed with pancreatic cancer histopathologically through EUS-guided fine needle aspiration (EUS-FNA) and considered as locally advanced unresectable without distant metastasis (including non-regional lymph node metastasis) after discussion with surgical department based on NCCN Clinical Practice Guidelines in Oncology [14] (Additional file 1: Table S1); 2) Accessible for injection of HF10 under EUS-guidance; 3) At least one measurable lesion according to Response Evaluation Criteria in Solid Tumors (RECIST) criteria; 4) Eastern Cooperative Oncology Group (ECOG) performance status (PS) of 0–2; 5) Estimated life expectancy of more than 3 months; 6) Older than 20 years and younger than 80 years of age; 7) adequate bone marrow function (white blood cell count$\geq$4000/mm^3, neutrophil count$\geq$2000/mm^3, platelet count$\geq$100,000/mm^3); 8) Adequate renal function (creatinine clearance (Cockroft-Gault Equation)$\geq$60 ml/min); 9) Adequate liver function (serum total bilirubin$\leq$2 times the upper limits of normal (ULN), transaminases$\leq$1.5 times ULN); 10) Patients who provided written informed consent; 11) Positive HSV-1 antibody.

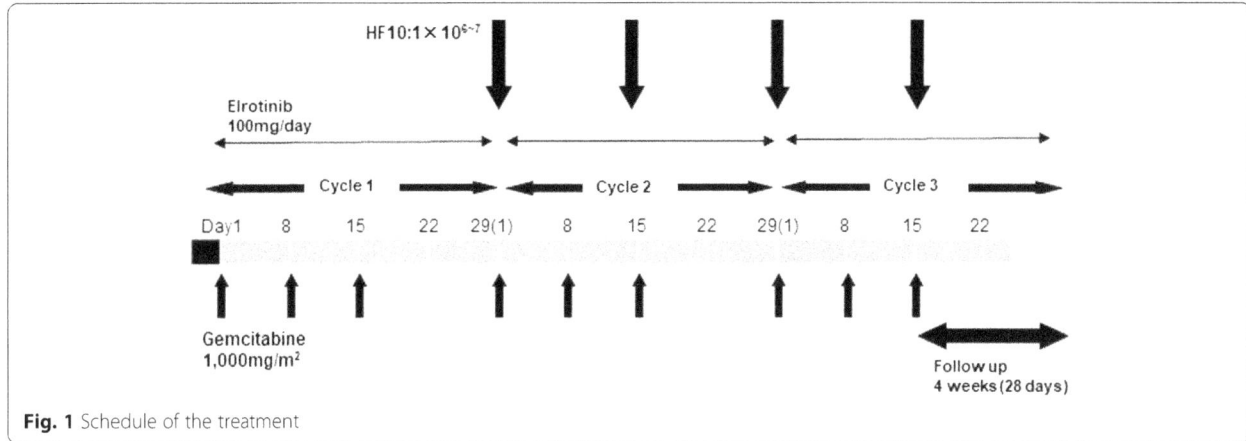

Fig. 1 Schedule of the treatment

The exclusion criteria were as follows: Bleeding diathesis; Ascites, pleural effusion, cardiac effusion to be treated; Active infection; Duplicated active cancers (synchronous duplicated cancer or metachronous cancer with less than 5 years of disease free period); Increased intracranial pressure to be treated due to brain metastases; pregnant or lactating women; Allergic to live vaccine; Use of anti HSV drugs; Implementation of immunotherapy for cancer; Positive HBs antigen, HCV antibody or HIV antibody; Adrenal insufficiency, hemodialysis, unilateral kidney.

Treatment

Following one cycle of erlotinib and gemcitabine therapy (gemcitabine 1000 mg/m2 weekly for 3 weeks, followed by a 1-week rest; erlotinib 100 mg orally, once daily), those judged tolerable for next cycle were final candidates. HF 10 injection was started at day 1 of cycle 2. The number of HF10 injection under EUS-guidance was to be four times in total (once every 2 weeks) unless DLT appears. DLT was defined as non-hematological toxicity higher than grade III according to the Common Terminology Criteria for Adverse Events, version 4.0 (CTCAE v4.0), febrile neutropenia

or thrombocytopenia requiring transfusion. Three Cohorts, a total of nine subjects were planned to be enrolled in this trial [Cohort 1 (1×10^6 pfu/day $\times 4$ times): three subjects, Cohort 2 (3×10^6 pfu/day x 4times): three subjects, Cohort 3 (1×10^7 pfu/day x 4times): three subjects] (Fig. 1). If there was no DLT in the first three cases of each Cohort, the trial was proceeded with the next Cohort until the maximum tolerated dose (MTD) was determined. If one out of three cases showed DLT, three additional cases were registered for the same Cohort. If there was no DLT in the additional three cases, the trial was proceeded with the next Cohort. If one of them showed DLT, the dose was not increased considering it exceeded the MTD. If two out of three cases showed DLT, no more cases were added.

Injection of HF10 was performed under EUS-guidance to deliver the virus into the tumor.

Assessments

The primary endpoint was the safety assessment (frequency and degree of toxicity). The adverse events (AEs) were graded according to the Common Terminology Criteria for Adverse Events, version 3.0 (CTCAE v3.0). A Safety Evaluation Committee was periodically held

Table 1 Patients profiles

Patient no.		Age	Contents (p.f.u) X Time	Injection site	Staging[a] (radiological)	Staging[a] (postoperative)
Cohort 1	HF-1-02	60s	1X10⁶X4	Pancreas head	III (T4N0M0)	NA
	HF-1-04	60s	1X10⁶X4	Pancreas head (uncinate process)	III (T4N0M0)	NA
	HF-1-05	60s	1X10⁶X4	Pancreas body	III (T4N0M0)	IIA (T3N0M0)
Cohort 2	HF-2-01	60s	3X10⁶X4	Pancreas body	III (T4N0M0)	NA
	HF-2-02	60s	3X10⁶X4	Pancreas head (uncinate process)	III (T4N0M0)	IIA (T3N0M0)
	HF-2-03	60s	3X10⁶X4	Pancreas body	III (T4N0M0)	NA
Cohort 3	HF-3-01	60s	1X10⁷X3	Pancreas body	III (T4N0M0)	NA
	HF-3-02	50s	1X10⁷X4	Pancreas head (uncinate process)	III (T4N0M0)	NA
	HF-3-03	60s	1X10⁷X4	Pancreas body	III (T4N0M0)	NA
	HF-3-04	60s	1X10⁷X4	Pancreas head	III (T4N0M0)	NA

[a]Based on NCCN Clinical Practice Guidelines in Oncology [13]

Table 2 Safety evaluation

Patient no.		Toxicity of HF10	DLT	Evaluation (CTCAE ver 4.0)
Cohort 1	HF-1-02	(−)	(−)	Grade III Neutrophil and Platlet count decrease, Duodenal stenosis, Perforative peritonitis
	HF-1-04	(−)	(−)	Grade II fever, Blood bilirubin increase (stent failure), Interstitial pneumonia (After treatment)
	HF-1-05	(−)	(−)	NA
Cohort 2	HF-2-01	(−)	(−)	Grade III Neutrophil decrease
	HF-2-02	(−)	(−)	Grade III Neutrophil decrease
	HF-2-03	(−)	(−)	Grade III Neutrophil decrease and Grade II ALT increase
Cohort 3	HF-3-01	(−)	(−)	Grade IV Hepatobiliary disorder
	HF-3-02	(−)	(−)	NA
	HF-3-03	(−)	(−)	NA
	HF-3-04	(−)	(−)	Grade III Neutrophil decrease

DLT dose-limiting toxicity

during the study and the correlation between HF 10 injection and AEs was discussed. The secondary endpoint was the efficacy assessment (complete response (CR), partial response (PR), stable disease (SD), and progressive disease (PD)), which was done by a computed tomography (CT) scan, which was performed at least once every 4 weeks according to the RECIST criteria. A CR was defined as the disappearance of all known disease determined by two observations not less than 3 weeks apart. A CR achieved after surgical approach was defined as surgical CR. A PR was defined as at least a 30% decrease in measurable disease by two observations not less than 3 weeks apart and no evidence of any new lesions or progression of any existing lesions. An inability to demonstrate a 30% decrease in tumor size or a 20%

increase in the size of one or more lesions, as well as no new lesions for more than 6 weeks, was defined as SD. A 20% increase in the size of one or more measurable lesions or the appearance of any new lesions was defined as PD. The progression free survival (PFS) was measured from the date of enrollment until the date of PD. The overall survival (OS) was calculated from the date of enrollment until the date of death.

Results

Safety assessment

From June 2013 to May 2015, 12 patients were enrolled in the study. Two cases were excluded prior to the HF10 injection due to interstitial pneumonia and lymph node metastases after one cycle of erlotinib and gemcitabine therapy. Ten subjects including one dropout subject received this therapy (Table 1). Five of ten subjects showed myelosuppression (Grade III) caused by chemotherapy. Two of ten subjects developed serious AEs. One case developed perforative peritonitis following duodenal stenosis. Another case developed Grade IV hepatic dysfunction 1 week after the third injection of HF10, and the treatment was discontinued at this point (Table 2). All of these events were judged as AEs unrelated to HF10. There was no complication related to EUS or EUS-guided injection of HF10.

Efficacy assessment

Nine subjects who completed four injections of HF10 were included for the efficacy assessment.

Overall responses were three PRs, four SDs, and two PDs. Target lesion responses were three PRs, six SDs out of nine subjects. Overall effective response (PR + SD) was 78%. The median PFS was 6.3 months, whereas the median OS was 15.5 months. Two subjects from Cohort 1 and 2 showed down staging, being reevaluated as resectable cancer, and finally achieved surgical CR (Table 3).

Table 3 Efficacy evaluation

Patient no.		Evaluation (RECIST ver 1.1)			Time to response (days)	Duration of response (days)	PFS (days)	OS (days)
		Target response	Overall response	Surgical response				
Cohort 1	HF-1-02	SD	PD				119	150
	HF-1-04	SD	PD				91	465
	HF-1-05	PR	PR	CR	48	288	335	611
Cohort 2	HF-2-01	SD	SD				663	1211
	HF-2-02	PR	PR	CR	13	444	456	1189
	HF-2-03	SD	SD				48	336
Cohort 3	HF-3-02	SD	SD				217	694
	HF-3-03	SD	SD				69	273
	HF-3-04	PR	PR		34	156	189	255

PFS progression free survival, *OS* overall survival, *PR* partial response, *SD* stable disease, *CR* complete response

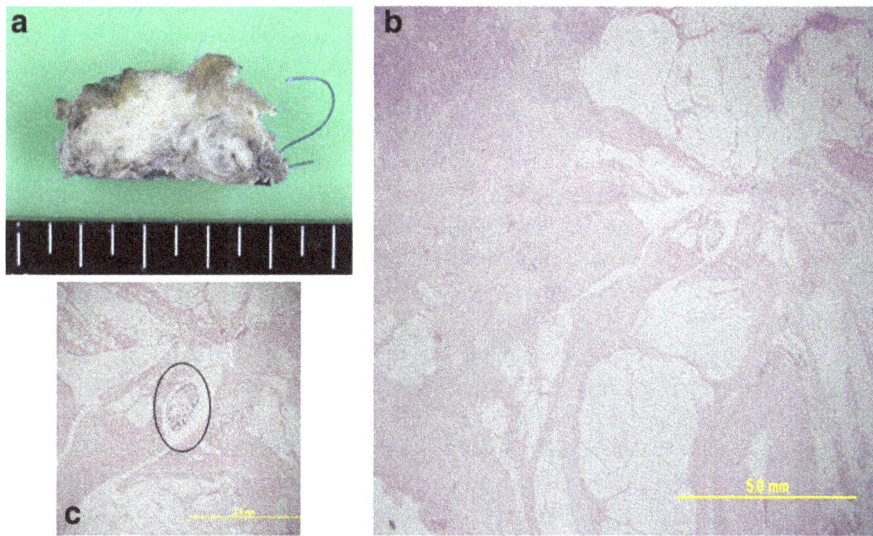

Fig. 2 a A cut surface of the pancreatic body showed a fibrotic tissue in the area where the tumor was located (HF-1-05). **b** On histological analysis, 99% of the cancer cells had disappeared and had been replaced with fibrotic tissue. **c** High-power photomicrograph revealed a minute residual cancer tissue (circle)

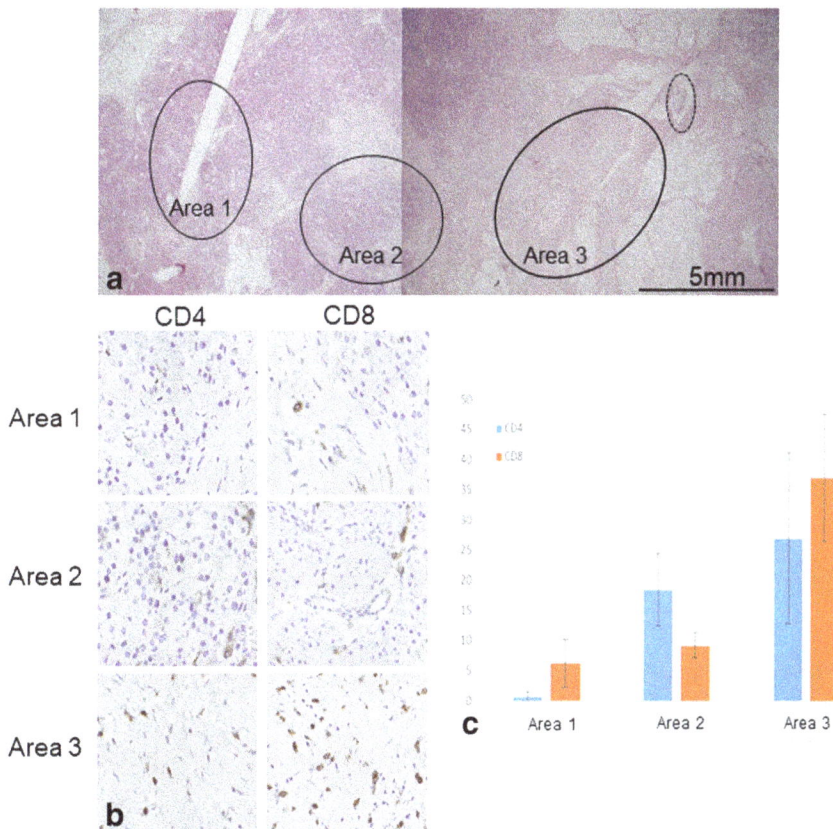

Fig. 3 Evaluation of CD4+ and CD8+ cells infiltration around the cancer tissue (HF-1-05). **a** Three areas in different distances (circle) from the residual cancer (dot-line circle) were evaluated. **b**, **c** Infiltration of CD4+ and CD8+ cells was significant in the fibrosis near the residual cancer tissue (area 3) and it became obscure as the areas receded from the cancer tissue

Cases with surgical CR

The first case was a 66 years old female in Cohort 1 who received HF10 of 1.0×10^6 pfu $\times 4$ times and had radiation therapy of 1.8 Gy $\times 28$ times after clinical trial. Distal pancreatectomy was performed 5 months after registration and the resected specimen showed 99% disappearance of the cancer cells in the tumor (Fig. 2). We examined the infiltration of CD4+ and CD8+ cells by immunostaining. Infiltration of CD4+ and CD8+ cells was significant in the fibrosis near the residual cancer cells and it became obscure as the areas receded from the cancer cells (Fig. 3). Unfortunately, she developed peritoneal dissemination 6 months after surgery and the survival time was 22 months. The second case was a 65 years old male in Cohort 2 who received HF10 of 3.0×10^6 pfu $\times 4$ times. This patient had radiation therapy of 1.8 Gy $\times 28$ times before clinical trial. The invasion to plexus of superior mesenteric artery had shown decrease in size after HF10 injection, and he underwent pancreaticoduodenectomy 7 months after registration. Resected specimen showed 90% disappearance of cancer cells (Fig. 4). On immunostaining, infiltration of CD8+ cells was detected alongside the cancer cells (Fig. 5). Although CT scan revealed the recurrence in mesenteric lymph nodes 6 months after the surgery, long term survival was obtained and the survival time was 39. 6 months.

Discussion

In this study, we performed a phase I dose-escalation trial of HF10 direct injection therapy for unresectable locally advanced pancreatic cancer under EUS-guidance in combination with erlotinib and gemcitabine administration, which was safe and effective with all doses (1×10^6, 3×10^6, or 1×10^7 pfu/day $\times 4$ times).

Since 1997, gemcitabine therapy has been the standard first-line treatment for patients with unresectable locally advanced or metastatic pancreatic cancer with a median survival rate of 4.4–5.6 months [15, 16]. Several combination treatments based on gemcitabine have been investigated; however, most have not significantly improved survival versus gemcitabine alone [17–29], except for the combination therapy with gemcitabine plus elrotinib, which showed a significant improvement in overall survival for 2 weeks in median [30]. More recently, FOL-FIRINOX therapy (leucovorin, fluorouracil, irinotecan and oxaliplatin) [31] and gemcitabine plus nab-paclitaxel therapy [32] have been approved for unresectable

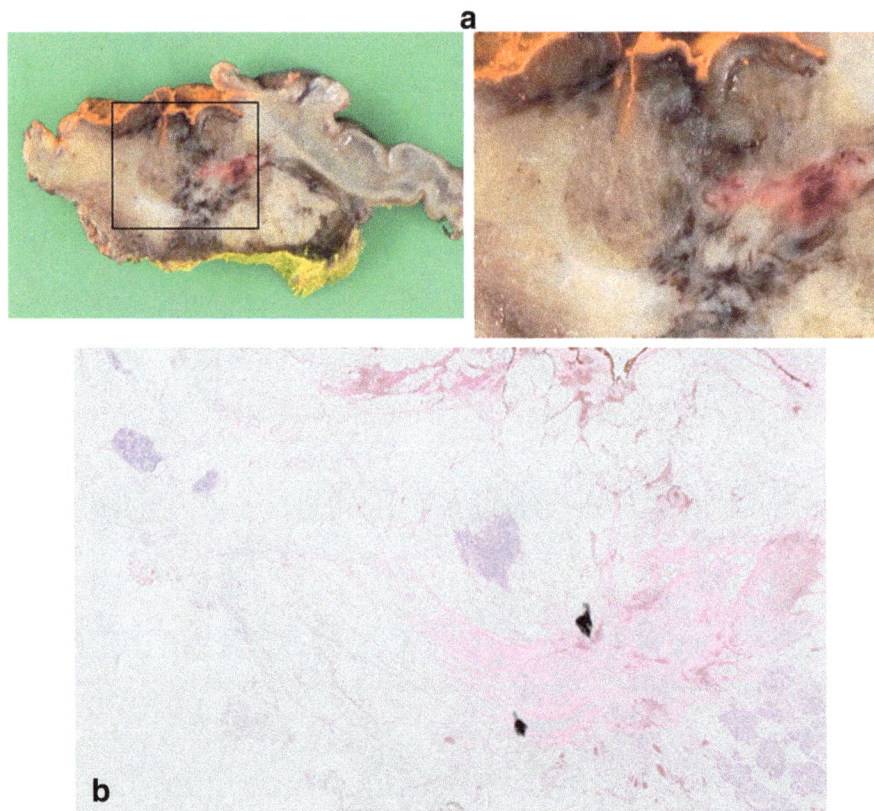

Fig. 4 a A cut surface of the pancreatic head of HF-2-02. The left image showed showed fibrosis in the middle and the right showed a magnified image. **b** Histopathological findings of the tumor in the pancreatic head showed 90% disappearance of cancer cells with fibrosis

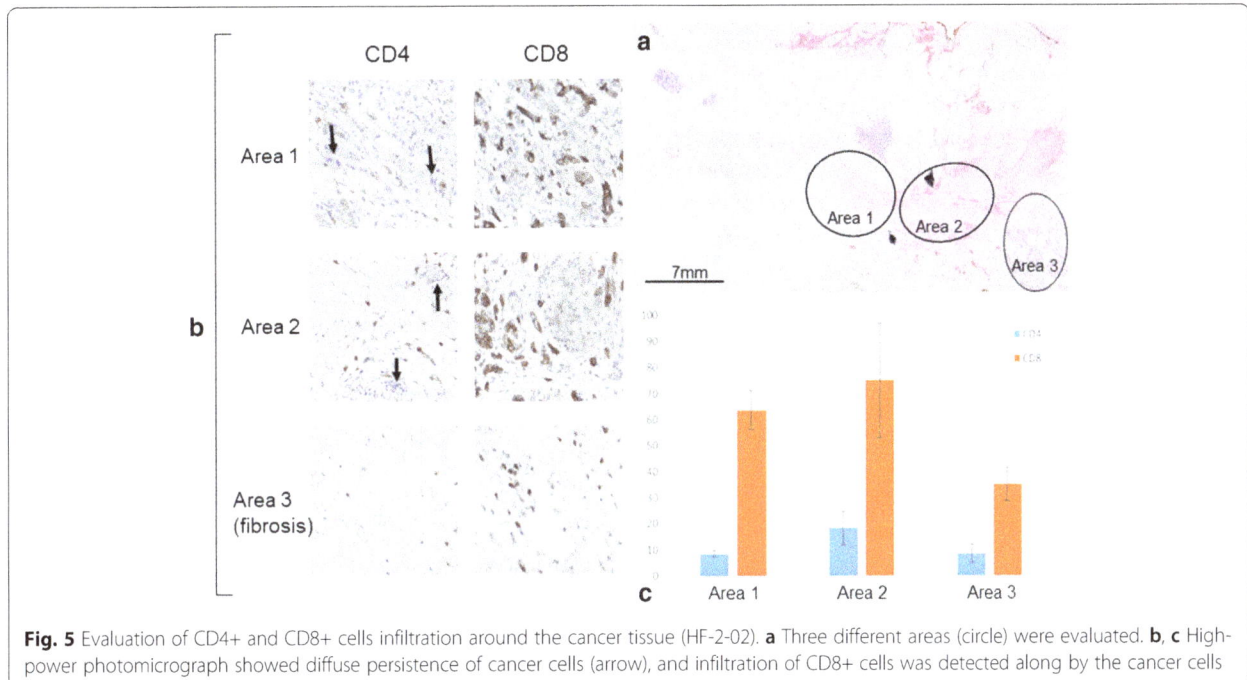

Fig. 5 Evaluation of CD4+ and CD8+ cells infiltration around the cancer tissue (HF-2-02). **a** Three different areas (circle) were evaluated. **b, c** High-power photomicrograph showed diffuse persistence of cancer cells (arrow), and infiltration of CD8+ cells was detected along by the cancer cells

pancreatic cancer in Japan. They have significantly improved survival and are now used as a first-line chemotherapy for unresectable pancreatic cancers. However, since the majority of patient eventually progress on these therapies, novel therapies are required.

HF10 has shown a promising antitumor effect with a high safety margin in the investigator-initiated clinical studies for pancreatic cancer [5]. Phase I clinical trial using HF10 in advanced pancreatic cancer was reported from the department of surgery II at Nagoya University in Japan [10]. They initiated pilot studies by injecting six patients with non-resectable pancreatic cancer with three doses of HF10 (1×10^5/two patients, 5×10^5/one patient, and 1×10^6/three patients). They observed some therapeutic potential based on tumor marker levels, survival, pathological findings and diagnostic radiography. The important thing is that there were no adverse side-effects in these patients. As gemcitabine is an anticancer drug which has been well investigated in combination with many OVs in different malignancies including pancreatic cancer [33–37], the combination of HF10 and gemcitabine can be an ideal therapy against pancreatic cancer to achieve a potent antitumor effect with minimal side effects. Given the results in a Japanese phase II pancreatic cancer trial using gemcitabine and erlotinib with acceptable tolerance and mild AEs [38], we have decided to combine HF10 with gemcitabine and erlotinib in our study. Five out of 10 patients showed Grade III myelosuppression and one patient showed interstitial pneumonia after treatment, but all of them recovered by discontinuing the treatment. Unfortunately, two patients developed serious AEs (perforative peritonitis and hepatic dysfunction). Regarding the perforative peritonitis of HF-1-02, the tumor radiologically showed direct invasion to the duodenum from the beginning. Eventually the tumor caused obstruction of the duodenum with increased pressure inside the lumen, which led to the perforation. As a result, all of the AEs occurred in our study were judged as AEs unrelated to HF10, and there was no increase in AEs according to the dose of HF10 escalating up to 1×10^7 pfu/day x 4times.

It is noteworthy that although the median PFS in our study was relatively short as 6.3 months, median OS was 15.5 months and two patients achieved long term survival over 3 years. Interestingly, the patient who achieved the longest survival did not have surgery and the best overall response was SD, suggesting the development of acquired immunity by this treatment. With regard to the histopathological findings, previous clinical studies have revealed that HF10 increased the number of CD4+, CD8 + and natural killer cells within the tumor, which may lead to the tumor growth reduction and prolonged survival rates [5, 7, 8]. In two cases who underwent surgery in our study, infiltration of CD4+ or CD8+ cells was well detected in the area nearby the residual cancer cells. It is considered that the anti-tumor effects of OVs are not only the direct cancer cell destruction but also the stimulation of anti-tumor immunity, and these results support the above hypothesis.

Conclusions

HF10 direct injection therapy for unresectable locally advanced pancreatic cancer under EUS-guidance in combination with erlotinib and gemcitabine administration was safe and demonstrated anti-tumor effectiveness with higher those than used in previous studies. HF10 combination therapy should be explored further in large prospective studies. In the near future, we plan to perform a clinical trial in combination of HF10 and gemcitabine with nab-paclitaxel treatment aiming at unresectable pancreatic cancers with or without metastases.

Abbreviations

AE: Adverse event; CR: Complete response; CT: Computed tomography; CTCAE: Common Terminology Criteria for Adverse Events; DLT: Dose limiting toxicity; ECOG: Eastern Cooperative Oncology Group; EUS: Endoscopic ultrasound; EUS-FNA: EUS-guided fine needle aspiration; HNSCC: Head and neck squamous cell carcinoma; HSV-1: Herpes simplex virus-1; MTD: maximum tolerated dose; OS: Overall survival; OV: Oncolytic virus; PD: Progressive disease; PFS: Progression free survival; PR: Partial response; PS: Performance status; RECIST: Response Evaluation Criteria in Solid Tumors; SD: Stable disease; ULN: Upper limits of normal

Acknowledgements

The authors wish to thank Dr. Yukihiro Nishiyama (Nagoya University) for the invention of HF10 and Ms. Kazue Kawamura (Cancer Immune Therapy Research Center, Nagoya University Graduate School of Medicine) for the data consolidation.

Funding

The authors declare that no funding was received for the research.

Adherence to CONSORT guidelines

This study adheres to CONSORT guideline and a complete CONSORT checklist has been submitted as an additional file.

Authors' contributions

Conception and design: HY, KH1 (Hideki Kasuya), IT1 (Takuya Ishikawa), VIB, NY. Development of methodology: HY, NY, IT2 (Toru Ichinose). Acquisition of data: KH2 (Hiroki Kawashima), IT2, KN, GH. Analysis and interpretation of data: OE, TM, KY. Writing, review, and/or revision of the manuscript: HY, KH1, IT1, KH2, OE, VIB, NY, IT2, KN, TM, KY, GH. Administrative, technical, or material support (i.e., reporting or organizing data, constructing databases): HY, IT2, NY, TM. Study supervision: KH1, KY, GH. All authors have read and finally approved the manuscript.

Competing interests

The authors declare that they have no competing interests.

Author details

¹Department of Endoscopy, Nagoya University Hospital, 65 Tsuruma-cho, Showa-ku, Nagoya 466-8550, Japan. ²Cancer Immune Therapy Research Center, Nagoya University Graduate School of Medicine, Nagoya, Japan. ³Department of Gastroenterology, Nagoya University Graduate School of Medicine, Nagoya, Japan. ⁴Takara Bio Inc., Otsu, Japan. ⁵Department of Surgery II, Nagoya University Graduate School of Medicine, Nagoya, Japan.

References

1. Siegel RL, Miller KD, Jemal A. Cancer statistics, 2016. CA Cancer J Clin. 2016; 66(1):7–30.
2. Furuse J, Gemma A, Ichikawa W, Okusaka T, Seki A, Ishii T. Postmarketing surveillance study of erlotinib plus gemcitabine for pancreatic cancer in Japan: POLARIS final analysis. Jpn J Clin Oncol. 2017;47(9):1–8.
3. Sener SF, Fremgen A, Menck HR, Winchester DP. Pancreatic cancer: a report of treatment and survival trends for 100,313 patients diagnosed from 1985-1995, using the National Cancer Database. J Am Coll Surg. 1999;189(1):1–7.
4. Myrehaug S, Sahgal A, Russo SM, Lo SS, Rosati LM, Mayr NA, Lock M, Small W Jr, Dorth JA, Ellis RJ, et al. Stereotactic body radiotherapy for pancreatic cancer: recent progress and future directions. Expert Rev Anticancer Ther. 2016;16(5):523–30.
5. Eissa IR, Naoe Y, Bustos-Villalobos I, Ichinose T, Tanaka M, Zhiwen W, Mukoyama N, Morimoto T, Miyajima N, Hitoki H, et al. Genomic signature of the natural oncolytic herpes simplex virus HF10 and its therapeutic role in preclinical and clinical trials. Front Oncol. 2017;7:149.
6. Koshizuka T, Goshima F, Takakuwa H, Nozawa N, Daikoku T, Koiwai O, Nishiyama Y. Identification and characterization of the UL56 gene product of herpes simplex virus type 2. J Virol. 2002;76(13):6718–28.
7. Kimata H, Imai T, Kikumori T, Teshigahara O, Nagasaka T, Goshima F, Nishiyama Y, Nakao A. Pilot study of oncolytic viral therapy using mutant herpes simplex virus (HF10) against recurrent metastatic breast cancer. Ann Surg Oncol. 2006;13(8):1078–84.
8. Nakao A, Kimata H, Imai T, Kikumori T, Teshigahara O, Nagasaka T, Goshima F, Nishiyama Y. Intratumoral injection of herpes simplex virus HF10 in recurrent breast cancer. Ann Oncol. 2004;15(6):988–9.
9. Fujimoto Y, Mizuno T, Sugiura S, Goshima F, Kohno S, Nakashima T, Nishiyama Y. Intratumoral injection of herpes simplex virus HF10 in recurrent head and neck squamous cell carcinoma. Acta Otolaryngol. 2006; 126(10):1115–7.
10. Nakao A, Kasuya H, Sahin TT, Nomura N, Kanzaki A, Misawa M, Shirota T, Yamada S, Fujii T, Sugimoto H, et al. A phase I dose-escalation clinical trial of intraoperative direct intratumoral injection of HF10 oncolytic virus in non-resectable patients with advanced pancreatic cancer. Cancer Gene Ther. 2011;18(3):167–75.
11. Ferris RL, Gross ND, Nemunaitis JJ, Andtbacka RHI, Argiris A, Ohr J, Vetto JT, Senzer NN, Bedell C, Ungerleider RS, et al. Phase I trial of intratumoral therapy using HF10, an oncolytic HSV-1, demonstrates safety in HSV plus /HSV- patients with refractory and superficial cancers. J Clin Oncol. 2014; 32(15 Suppl):6082.
12. Andtbacka RHI, Ross MI, Agarwala SS, Taylor MH, Vetto JT, Neves RI, Daud A, Khong HT, Ungerleider RS, Boran A, et al. Preliminary results from phase II study of combination treatment with HF10, a replication competent HSV-1 oncolytic virus, and ipilimumab in patients with stage IIIb, IIIc, or IV unresectable or metastatic melanoma. J Clin Oncol. 2016;34(15 Suppl):9543.
13. Hirooka Y, Kawashima H, Ohno E, Kasuya H, Tanaka M, Goto H. Phase 1 dose-escalation clinical trial of EUS-guided injection of HF10 for unresectable locally advanced pancreatic cancer. Pancreatology. 2016;16(4, Supplement):S17.
14. Tempero MA, Malafa MP, Al-Hawary M, Asbun H, Bain A, Behrman SW, Benson AB 3rd, Binder E, Cardin DB, Cha C, et al. Pancreatic adenocarcinoma, version 2.2017, NCCN clinical practice guidelines in oncology. J Natl Compr Cancer Netw. 2017;15(8):1028–61.
15. Burris HA 3rd, Moore MJ, Andersen J, Green MR, Rothenberg ML, Modiano MR, Cripps MC, Portenoy RK, Storniolo AM, Tarassoff P, et al. Improvements in survival and clinical benefit with gemcitabine as first-line therapy for patients with advanced pancreas cancer: a randomized trial. J Clin Oncol. 1997;15(6):2403–13.
16. Katopodis O, Souglakos J, Stathopoulos E, Christopoulou A, Kontopodis E, Kotsakis A, Kalbakis K, Kentepozidis N, Polyzos A, Hatzidaki D, et al. Frontline treatment with gemcitabine, oxaliplatin and erlotinib for the treatment of advanced or metastatic pancreatic cancer: a multicenter phase II study of the Hellenic Oncology Research Group (HORG). Cancer Chemother Pharmacol. 2014;74(2):333–40.
17. Berlin JD, Catalano P, Thomas JP, Kugler JW, Haller DG, Benson AB 3rd. Phase III study of gemcitabine in combination with fluorouracil versus gemcitabine alone in patients with advanced pancreatic carcinoma: Eastern Cooperative Oncology Group Trial E2297. J Clin Oncol. 2002;20(15):3270–5.
18. Colucci G, Giuliani F, Gebbia V, Biglietto M, Rabitti P, Uomo G, Cigolari S, Testa A, Maiello E, Lopez M. Gemcitabine alone or with cisplatin for the

treatment of patients with locally advanced and/or metastatic pancreatic carcinoma: a prospective, randomized phase III study of the Gruppo Oncologia dell'Italia Meridionale. Cancer. 2002;94(4):902–10.

19. Abou-Alfa GK, Letourneau R, Harker G, Modiano M, Hurwitz H, Tchekmedyian NS, Feit K, Ackerman J, De Jager RL, Eckhardt SG, et al. Randomized phase III study of exatecan and gemcitabine compared with gemcitabine alone in untreated advanced pancreatic cancer. J Clin Oncol. 2006;24(27):4441–7.

20. Bramhall SR, Rosemurgy A, Brown PD, Bowry C, Buckels JA, Marimastat Pancreatic Cancer Study G. Marimastat as first-line therapy for patients with unresectable pancreatic cancer: a randomized trial. J Clin Oncol. 2001;19(15): 3447–55.

21. Heinemann V, Quietzsch D, Gieseler F, Gonnermann M, Schonekas H, Rost A, Neuhaus H, Haag C, Clemens M, Heinrich B, et al. Randomized phase III trial of gemcitabine plus cisplatin compared with gemcitabine alone in advanced pancreatic cancer. J Clin Oncol. 2006;24(24):3946–52.

22. Herrmann R, Bodoky G, Ruhstaller T, Glimelius B, Bajetta E, Schuller J, Saletti P, Bauer J, Figer A, Pestalozzi B, et al. Gemcitabine plus capecitabine compared with gemcitabine alone in advanced pancreatic cancer: a randomized, multicenter, phase III trial of the Swiss Group for Clinical Cancer Research and the Central European Cooperative Oncology Group. J Clin Oncol. 2007;25(16):2212–7.

23. Kindler HL. Pancreatic cancer: an update. Curr Oncol Rep. 2007;9(3):170–6.

24. Louvet C, Labianca R, Hammel P, Lledo G, Zampino MG, Andre T, Zaniboni A, Ducreux M, Aitini E, Taieb J, et al. Gemcitabine in combination with oxaliplatin compared with gemcitabine alone in locally advanced or metastatic pancreatic cancer: results of a GERCOR and GISCAD phase III trial. J Clin Oncol. 2005;23(15):3509–16.

25. Moore MJ, Hamm J, Dancey J, Eisenberg PD, Dagenais M, Fields A, Hagan K, Greenberg B, Colwell B, Zee B, et al. Comparison of gemcitabine versus the matrix metalloproteinase inhibitor BAY 12-9566 in patients with advanced or metastatic adenocarcinoma of the pancreas: a phase III trial of the National Cancer Institute of Canada Clinical Trials Group. J Clin Oncol. 2003; 21(17):3296–302.

26. Oettle H, Richards D, Ramanathan RK, van Laethem JL, Peeters M, Fuchs M, Zimmermann A, John W, Von Hoff D, Arning M, et al. A phase III trial of pemetrexed plus gemcitabine versus gemcitabine in patients with unresectable or metastatic pancreatic cancer. Ann Oncol. 2005;16(10): 1639–45.

27. Rocha Lima CM, Green MR, Rotche R, Miller WH Jr, Jeffrey GM, Cisar LA, Morganti A, Orlando N, Gruia G, Miller LL. Irinotecan plus gemcitabine results in no survival advantage compared with gemcitabine monotherapy in patients with locally advanced or metastatic pancreatic cancer despite increased tumor response rate. J Clin Oncol. 2004;22(18):3776–83.

28. Stathopoulos GP, Syrigos K, Aravantinos G, Polyzos A, Papakotoulas P, Fountzilas G, Potamianou A, Ziras N, Boukovinas J, Varthalitis J, et al. A multicenter phase III trial comparing irinotecan-gemcitabine (IG) with gemcitabine (G) monotherapy as first-line treatment in patients with locally advanced or metastatic pancreatic cancer. Br J Cancer. 2006;95(5):587–92.

29. Van Cutsem E, van de Velde H, Karasek P, Oettle H, Vervenne WL, Szawlowski A, Schoffski P, Post S, Verslype C, Neumann H, et al. Phase III trial of gemcitabine plus tipifarnib compared with gemcitabine plus placebo in advanced pancreatic cancer. J Clin Oncol. 2004;22(8):1430–8.

30. Moore MJ, Goldstein D, Hamm J, Figer A, Hecht JR, Gallinger S, Au HJ, Murawa P, Walde D, Wolff RA, et al. Erlotinib plus gemcitabine compared with gemcitabine alone in patients with advanced pancreatic cancer: a phase III trial of the National Cancer Institute of Canada Clinical Trials Group. J Clin Oncol. 2007;25(15):1960–6.

31. Conroy T, Desseigne F, Ychou M, Bouche O, Guimbaud R, Becouarn Y, Adenis A, Raoul JL, Gourgou-Bourgade S, de la Fouchardiere C, et al. FOLFIRINOX versus gemcitabine for metastatic pancreatic cancer. N Engl J Med. 2011;364(19):1817–25.

32. Von Hoff DD, Ervin T, Arena FP, Chiorean EG, Infante J, Moore M, Seay T, Tjulandin SA, Ma WW, Saleh MN, et al. Increased survival in pancreatic cancer with nab-paclitaxel plus gemcitabine. N Engl J Med. 2013;369(18): 1691–703.

33. Bhattacharyya M, Francis J, Eddouadi A, Lemoine NR, Hallden G. An oncolytic adenovirus defective in pRb-binding (dl922-947) can efficiently eliminate pancreatic cancer cells and tumors in vivo in combination with 5-FU or gemcitabine. Cancer Gene Ther. 2011;18(10):734–43.

34. Cherubini G, Kallin C, Mozetic A, Hammaren-Busch K, Muller H, Lemoine NR, Hallden G. The oncolytic adenovirus AdDeltaDelta enhances selective cancer cell killing in combination with DNA-damaging drugs in pancreatic cancer models. Gene Ther. 2011;18(12):1157–65.

35. Kangasniemi L, Parviainen S, Pisto T, Koskinen M, Jokinen M, Kiviluoto T, Cerullo V, Jalonen H, Koski A, Kangasniemi A, et al. Effects of capsid-modified oncolytic adenoviruses and their combinations with gemcitabine or silica gel on pancreatic cancer. Int J Cancer. 2012;131(1):253–63.

36. Leitner S, Sweeney K, Oberg D, Davies D, Miranda E, Lemoine NR, Hallden G. Oncolytic adenoviral mutants with E1B19K gene deletions enhance gemcitabine-induced apoptosis in pancreatic carcinoma cells and anti-tumor efficacy in vivo. Clin Cancer Res. 2009;15(5):1730–40.

37. Onimaru M, Ohuchida K, Nagai E, Mizumoto K, Egami T, Cui L, Sato N, Uchino J, Takayama K, Hashizume M, et al. Combination with low-dose gemcitabine and hTERT-promoter-dependent conditionally replicative adenovirus enhances cytotoxicity through their crosstalk mechanisms in pancreatic cancer. Cancer Lett. 2010;294(2):178–86.

38. Okusaka T, Furuse J, Funakoshi A, Ioka T, Yamao K, Ohkawa S, Boku N, Komatsu Y, Nakamori S, Iguchi H, et al. Phase II study of erlotinib plus gemcitabine in Japanese patients with unresectable pancreatic cancer. Cancer Sci. 2011;102(2):425–31.

Inhibition of Six1 affects tumour invasion and the expression of cancer stem cell markers in pancreatic cancer

Tristan Lerbs[1], Savita Bisht[2], Sebastian Schölch[3], Mathieu Pecqueux[3], Glen Kristiansen[4], Martin Schneider[1], Bianca T. Hofmann[5], Thilo Welsch[3], Christoph Reissfelder[3], Nuh N. Rahbari[3], Johannes Fritzmann[3], Peter Brossart[2], Jürgen Weitz[3], Georg Feldmann[2†] and Christoph Kahlert[1,3*†]

Abstract

Background: Epithelial-to-mesenchymal transition (EMT) and cancer stem cells (CSC) contribute to tumour progression and metastasis. Assessment of transcription factors involved in these two mechanisms can help to identify new targets for an oncological therapy. In this study, we focused on the evaluation of the transcription factor Six1 (Sine oculis 1). This protein is involved in embryologic development and its contribution to carcinogenesis has been described in several studies.

Methods: Immunohistochemistry against Six1 was performed on a tissue microarray containing specimens of primary pancreatic ductal adenocarcinomas (PDAC) of 139 patients. Nuclear and cytoplasmic expression was evaluated and correlated to histopathological parameters. Expression of Six1 was inhibited transiently by siRNA in Panc1 and BxPc3 cells and stably by shRNA in Panc1 cells. Expression analysis of CDH1 and Vimentin mRNA was performed and cell motility was tested in a migration assay. Panc1 cells transfected with Six1 shRNA or scrambled shRNA were injected subcutaneously into nude mice. Tumour growth was observed for four weeks. Afterwards, tumours were stained against Six1, CD24 and CD44.

Results: Six1 was overexpressed in the cytoplasm and cellular nuclei in malignant tissues ($p < 0.0001$). No correlation to histopathological parameters could be detected. Six1 down-regulation decreased pancreatic cancer cell motility in vitro. CDH1 and vimentin expression was decreased after inhibition of the expression of Six1. Pancreatic tumours with impaired expression of Six1 showed significantly delayed growth and displayed loss of the CD24[+]/CD44[+] phenotype.

Conclusion: We show that Six1 is overexpressed in human PDAC and that its inhibition results in a decreased tumour progression in vitro and in vivo. Therefore, targeting Six1 might be a novel therapeutic approach in patients with pancreatic cancer.

Keywords: Six1, Pancreatic cancer, Epithelial-mesenchymal transition, Cancer stem cells

* Correspondence: christoph.kahlert.079@googlemail.com
†Equal contributors
[1]Department of General, Visceral and Transplantation Surgery, Im Neuenheimer Feld 110, 69120 Heidelberg, Germany
[3]Department of Gastrointestinal, Thoracic and Vascular Surgery, Medizinische Fakultät Carl Gustav Carus, Technische Universität Dresden, Fetscherstr. 74, 01307 Dresden, Germany
Full list of author information is available at the end of the article

Background

Pancreatic ductal adenocarcinoma (PDAC) is a highly malignant tumour with a poor prognosis. Despite its low prevalence, it is the fourth leading cause of cancer-related death in western countries [1]. Pancreatic cancer spreads rapidly and is highly resistant to chemotherapy. These features are determined by several biological features, which are considered to be hallmarks of tumour development and dissemination [2]. Among those fundamental cornerstones, epithelial-to-mesenchymal transition (EMT) plays a crucial role in tumour progression. By adopting a more mesenchymal phenotype, cells increase motility, augment invasiveness und enhance chemoresistance [3]. EMT is strongly connected to the concept of cancer stem cells (CSC) [4]. In this model, CSC represent only a minor fraction of a tumour but are hypothesized to be crucially involved in its progression [5]. They can divide infinitely and are strongly resistant to chemotherapeutics. Therefore, they can survive chemotherapy and form recurrent disease [2]. Brabletz et al. described a model, in which migrating CSC are responsible for tumour dissemination whereas the epithelial non-CSC form is responsible for the growth of a single tumour [4]. In good accordance with this assumption, Martin et al. showed that EMT augments self-renewal capability [6].

In this study we focused on the embryologic transcription factor Six1 (Sine Oculis 1). It contributes to organogenesis by inducing proliferation, migration and survival [7–9]. In tumour biology, however, Six1 exerts pro-tumourigenic functions by regulating EMT-related mechanisms [10]. The role of Six1 in carcinogenesis has already been studied in several malignancies including breast cancer [11, 12], cervical cancer [13, 14] ovarian cancer and hepatocellular cancer [15, 16]. Recently, our group has shown that overexpression of SIX1 is an independent prognostic marker in stage I - III colorectal cancer [17]. Moreover, Li et al. [18] and Jin et al. showed an overexpression of Six1 in PDAC in their recent studies. In the study by Jin et al. Six1 was also an independent prognostic marker in pancreatic cancer [19]. Additionally, Ono et al. showed that Six1 promotes EMT by activating ZEB1 [20]. The purpose of the present study was to evaluate the impact of Six1 expression on CSC- and EMT-phenotypes in PDAC. To this end, we analysed a tissue microarray including 139 patients. Furthermore, we assessed the impact of Six1 on EMT markers and migration in vitro in Panc1 and BxPc3 cells. Finally, we investigated the impact of Six1 on tumour growth in vivo in a xenograft model.

Methods

Patients

The Medical Ethical Committees of the University of Bonn has approved the use of the patient tissue samples and clinic-pathological information in this study (Antragsnummer 13–091). Written informed consent was obtained from each patient prior to this study. The study cohort included 139 patients who underwent tumour resection at the University Hospital of Bonn between 1998 and 2009. The analysis was performed retrospectively and it was not possible to deduce patient identity from patient data. Cores derived from cancer tissue as well as from adjacent non-affected normal pancreatic parenchyma were analyzed.

Immunohistochemistry

Immunohistochemical staining of human tissue microarray samples was performed as described previously [21]. Likewise, immunohistochemical staining on whole tissue specimens from xenograft samples was conducted. 2 μm sections of formalin-fixed, paraffin-embedded tumour specimens were cut and mounted on SUPERFROST® PLUS microscope slides (Menzel, Germany). After overnight incubation at 37 °C, samples were dewaxed with xylol, rehydrated in a graded series of ethanol and subjected to heat-induced antigen retrieval (Dako REAL™ Target Retrieval Solution, pH 6.00, DAKO Denmark A/S) in a pressure cooker for 15 min. Nonspecific binding was blocked using an Avidin/Biotin Blocking Kit (Vector Laboratories, Inc., Burlingame, CA, USA). After antigen retrieval, slides were placed in an automated staining machine (DAKO Automatic Stainer) and incubated with the primary antibody for 30 min. Whole tissue specimens from xenografts specimens were additionally incubated with primary antibodies against CD44 (Rabbit monoclonal, ab151037, abcam, United Kingdom) and CD24 (Rabbit monoclonal, ab17982, Abcam, United Kingdom) for 30 min. Incubation with primary antibodies was followed by the biotinylated secondary antibody (DAKO REAL™ Biotinylated Secondary Antibody Anti -Rabbit, part of the DAKO REAL™ Detection System Peroxidase/AEC, Rabbit/Mouse, Code K5003, DAKO, Denmark) for 20 min. Afterwards, endogenous peroxidase was inhibited (DAKO REAL™ Peroxidase blocking solution, DAKO, Denmark) for 5 min followed by incubation with DAKO REAL™ streptavidin peroxidase (HRP) solution (part of DAKO REAL™ Detection System Peroxidase/AEC, Rabbit/Mouse, Code K5003, DAKO, Denmark) for 20 min. Finally, the specimens were visualised with DAKO REAL™ AEC/H2O2 Substrate Solution (part of DAKO REAL™ Detection System Peroxidase/ AEC, Rabbit/Mouse, Code K5003, DAKO, Denmark) and counterstained with haematoxylin. Two independent researchers (CK and TL) estimated the expression of SIX1 on a blind basis. A multi-head microscope was used and consensus was reached for each slide. The staining intensity in cytoplasm was classified as absent: 0, weak or intermediate: 1 and strong: 2. For cell nucleus staining, the percentage of positive cells was assessed: absent: 0, 0–25%: 1, 25–50%: 2, 50–75%: 3, > 75%: 4.

Cell lines and transfection

Panc1 and BxPc3 cell lines were purchased from the American Type Culture Collection (ATCC, Manassas, VA 20108, USA). Tumour cells were maintained in RPMI-1640 (Sigma, St. Louis, MO), supplemented with 10% (v/v) fetal calf serum (FCS), 100 U/ml penicillin and 100 μg/ml streptomycin in a humidified atmosphere of 5% CO_2 at 37 °C. The anti-Six1 shRNA plasmid (Mission® shRNA bacterial glycerol stock, SHCLNG-NM_005982, Sigma, USA) or an empty control vector (pLKO.1-puro, SHC001, Sigma, USA) were transfected using calcium phosphate-mediated transfection[285] (Pro-Fection® Mammalian, Cat. No. E1200, Promega, Germany) according to the manufacturer's protocol. Twenty-four hours after transfection, the cells were passaged 1:15 in appropriate medium containing 1 μg/ml puromycin for puromycin selection. Transfection efficiency was determined by quantitative RT-PCR (qPCR). A transient siRNA transfection [22] was performed using Lipofectamine 2000 [23] (invitrogen, USA) according to the manufacturer's specifications. An anti-Six1 siRNA from Sigma (Additional file 1: Table S1) and a negative control siRNA (AllStars, Qiagen, Netherlands) were purchased. Per 1200 pmol of siRNA, 30 μl of Lipofectamine 2000 were used for transfection. Afterwards, cells were incubated for 24 h and transfection efficiency was determined using quantitative RT-PCR (qPCR).

RNA extraction and quantitative RT-PCR [24, 25]

Total RNA from Panc1 and BxPc3 cells was extracted with the miRNeasy Mini Kit (Qiagen, Hilden, Germany) following the manual's instructions. RNA concentration was determined by a spectrophotometer (Nano Drop® 1000, Thermo Scientific, Germany) and reversely transcribed using the miScript Reverse Transcription Kit (Qiagen, Hilden, Germany). Five nanogram of the resulting cDNA was further subjected to qPCR (SYBR Green PCR Kit, Qiagen, Hilden, Germany) in a Roche Light Cycler™ (Roche Diagnostics GmbH, Mannheim, Germany). Ready specific primer pairs were purchased from Qiagen. Samples were normalized to GAPDH RNA and fold change of expression was calculated according to the $2^{-\Delta\Delta ct}$ method as previously described [26].

Cell migration assay

The migration assay was performed using 24 well migration chambers (ThinCerts™, 8 μm pore, Greiner Bio-One, 1780 Wemmel, Belgium). Panc1 and BxPc3 cells were starved overnight. Subsequently, 20.000 cells were plated in each migration chamber in 300 μl serum-free medium. Subsequently, the migration chambers were placed on 24 well plates containing medium with 10% (v/v) fetal calf serum. After an incubation for 24 h, Panc1 and BxPc3 cells at the bottom of the migration chamber were stained with 4′, 6-diamidino-2-phenylin-dole (DAPI). 20 representative figures of each migration membrane were taken using a fluorescent microscope and the number of migrated cells of each assay was counted. All assays were performed in triplicates.

Xenograft model

The study was approved by the regional authority for Nature, Environment and Consumer protection of the Land of North Rine-Westphalia (84–02.04.2015.A038). We used two groups each containing five mice (Athymic Nude Mouse, Crl:NU(NCr)-Foxn1^{nu}, Charles River, VA, USA). 2.5×10^6 cells were injected in each flank. Tumour growth and mice weight were assessed weekly for four weeks. After four weeks, the mice were euthanasized. Tumour samples were fixed in formalin and embedded in paraffin for further immunohistochemical analyses.

Statistical analysis

The software package GraphPad Prism, version 6 (GraphPad Software, La Jolla, CA, USA) was used for all calculations. Pearson's r test was applied to analyze the correlation between the expression of Six1 and pathological parameters. Differences in expression of Six1 in the PDAC cohort, Panc1 and BxPc3 cells, differences in migration and differences in tumour growth in vivo were assessed using the Student's t-test. The p values of all statistical tests were 2-sided, and $p \leq 0.05$ was considered to indicate a statistically significant result.

Results

Expression of Six1 in pancreatic ductal adenocarcinoma and its histopathological correlation

Patient characteristics and clinical specimens

Tissue samples from 139 patients suffering from primary pancreatic cancer were evaluated by IHC, out of these, sufficient material and data for final analysis were available in 137 cases. Of those 137 patients the median age was 66 years (36–85). 74 patients were male, 59 female. The UICC tumour stage at time of tumour resection was I in 2 cases, II in 9 cases, III in 123 cases and IV in 3 cases. 98 patients had positive lymph node metastasis (pN1), 38 patients were free of lymph node metastasis (pN0) and in 1 patient lymph node status was not known. Tumour grading was I in 1 case, II in 59 cases and III in 54 cases. In 23 cases grading could not be exactly determined. Characteristics of the cohort are shown in Table 1.

Table 1 Correlation of Six1 expression in cytoplasm to histopathological parameters

Parameter	Six1 expression in malignant tissue					Six1 expression in benign tissue				
	Number	No	Weak	Strong	p-value	Number	No	Weak	Strong	p-value
Total	137	50 (36,5%)	66 (48,2%)	21 (15,3%)		105	91 (86,7%)	14 (13,3%)	0	<0,0001
Age										
< Median	68 (49,6%)	26 (34,8%)	31	11	0,844	47 (44,8%)	38 (80,9%)	9 (19,1%)	0	0,253
≥ Median	69 (50,4%)	24 (34,8%)	35 (50,7%)	10 (14,5%)		58 (55,2%)	53 (91, 4%)	5 (8,6%)	0	
Sex[a]					0,591					0,902
Male	74 (56,5%)	27 (36,5%)	32 (43, 2%)	15 (20,3%)		56 (53,3%)	49 (87,5%)	(12,5%)	0	
Female	57 (43,5%)	19 (33,3%)	32 (56,01%)	6 (10,5%)		45 (46,7%)	39 (85,7%)	6 (14,3%)	0	
Tumor size[b]					1,000					0,428
pT1	2 (1,5%)	1 (50,0%)	1 (50,0%)	0		2 (1,9%)	2 (100%)	0	0	
pT2	9 (6,7%)	3 (33,3%)	5 (55,5%)	1 (11,1%)		8 (7,6%)	7 (87,5%)	1 (12,5%)	0	
pT3	121 (89,6%)	42 (34,7%)	59 (48,8%)	20 (16,5%)		90 (85,7%)	79 (87,8%)	11 (12,2%)	0	
pT4	3 (2,2%)	2 (66,7%)	1 (33,3%)	0		3 (2,9%)	3 (100%)	0	0	
Lymph node metastasis[c]					0,290					0,959
N0	38 (27,9%)	4 (10,5%)	19 (50,0%)	15 (39,5%)		31 (29,5%)	28 (90,3%)	3 (9,7%)	0	
N1	98 (72,1%)	34 (34,7%)	47 (48,0%)	17 (17,3%)		74 (70,5%)	63 (85,1%)	11 (14,9%)	0	
Grading					0,950					0,715
G1	1 (0,7%)	0	1 (100,0%)	0		1 (1,0%)	1 (100%)	0	0	
G2	59 (43,1%)	21 (35,6%)	28 (47,5%)	10 (16,9%)		44 (41,9%)	38 (86,4%)	6 (13,6%)	0	
G3	54 (39,4%)	18 (33,3%)	28 (51,2%)	8 (14,8%)		45 (42,9%)	38 (84,4%)	7 (15,6%)	0	
Gx	23 (14,4%)	11 (47,8%)	9 (39,1%)	3 (13,0%)		15 (14,3%)	14 (93,3%)	1 (6,7%)	0	

[a]sex was known in 131 malignant and 101 benign specimens. [b]Tumor size was known 135 malignant and 103 benign specimens. [c]Lymph node metastasis was only known in 136 malignant specimens

Expression of Six1 in human pancreatic ductal adenocarcinoma

We assessed Six1 expression in tissue samples derived from 139 patients with primary PDAC. In 137 out of 139 patients, cancer tissue could be evaluated and from 105 out of 139 patients, normal pancreatic parenchyma could be assessed. Evaluation was performed separately for Six1 expression in cytoplasm and nuclei, respectively (Fig. 1). 63.5 of the malignant specimens showed an expression of Six1 in the cytoplasm, whereas only 13.3% cases of benign tissue were positive for Six1 expression in the cytoplasm ($p < 0.0001$). In detail, 50 malignant tumours were negative, 66 PDAC samples showed a weak expression of Six1 and 21 tumour specimens had a high expression of Six1. In contrast, 91 specimens representing benign tissue were negative and only 14 samples displayed a weak expression of Six1 (Table 1). A positive nuclear expression of Six1 was observed in 40.8% (± 4.2) of cancer cells (0 = 81 cases; 1 = 31 cases; 2 = 17 cases, 3 = 4 cases, 4 = 4 cases). On the contrary, only 11.4% (± 3.1) of benign pancreatic tissue specimens displayed a positive expression of Six1 in the nucleus (0 = 93 cases; 1 = 10 cases, 2 = 2 cases). Further analysis between the expression of Six1 (cytoplasm and nucleus) and clinical and histopathological data revealed no significant association of those parameters: tumour stage ($p = 1.00$ and 0.40, respectively), lymph node status (0.29 and 0.48, respectively), tumour grading (0.95 and 0.19, respectively) (Table 1 and Additional file 1: Table S1).

Inhibition of Six1 impairs cell migration in vitro

Expression of Six1 was inhibited transiently by siRNA in Panc1 cells and BxPc3 cells. This resulted in a decreased expression of Six1 mRNA by 86% in Panc1 cells and by 48% in BxPc3 cells in comparison to controls (Fig. 2a, b). Furthermore, Six1 was stably downregulated in Panc1 cells using shRNA. This resulted in a decreased expression of Six1 by 64.5% when compared to control with scramble shRNA (Fig. 2a). Intriguingly, both approaches lead to a decreased transcription of E-Cadherin mRNA in siRNA-transfected (– 53.2%, $p = 0.005$) and shRNA-transfected (– 85.2%, $p < 0.0001$) Panc1 cells (Fig. 2c). Likewise, we observed a decreased expression of CDH1 mRNA in BxPc3 cells, when Six1 siRNA was transfected (−30%, $p = 0.03$) (Fig. 2d). Furthermore, we investigated the expression of vimentin in both cell lines. There was a slight, but not significant decrease in siRNA-transfected and shRNA- Panc1 cells (Fig. 2e). However, BxPC3 transfected with siRNA against Six1 showed a

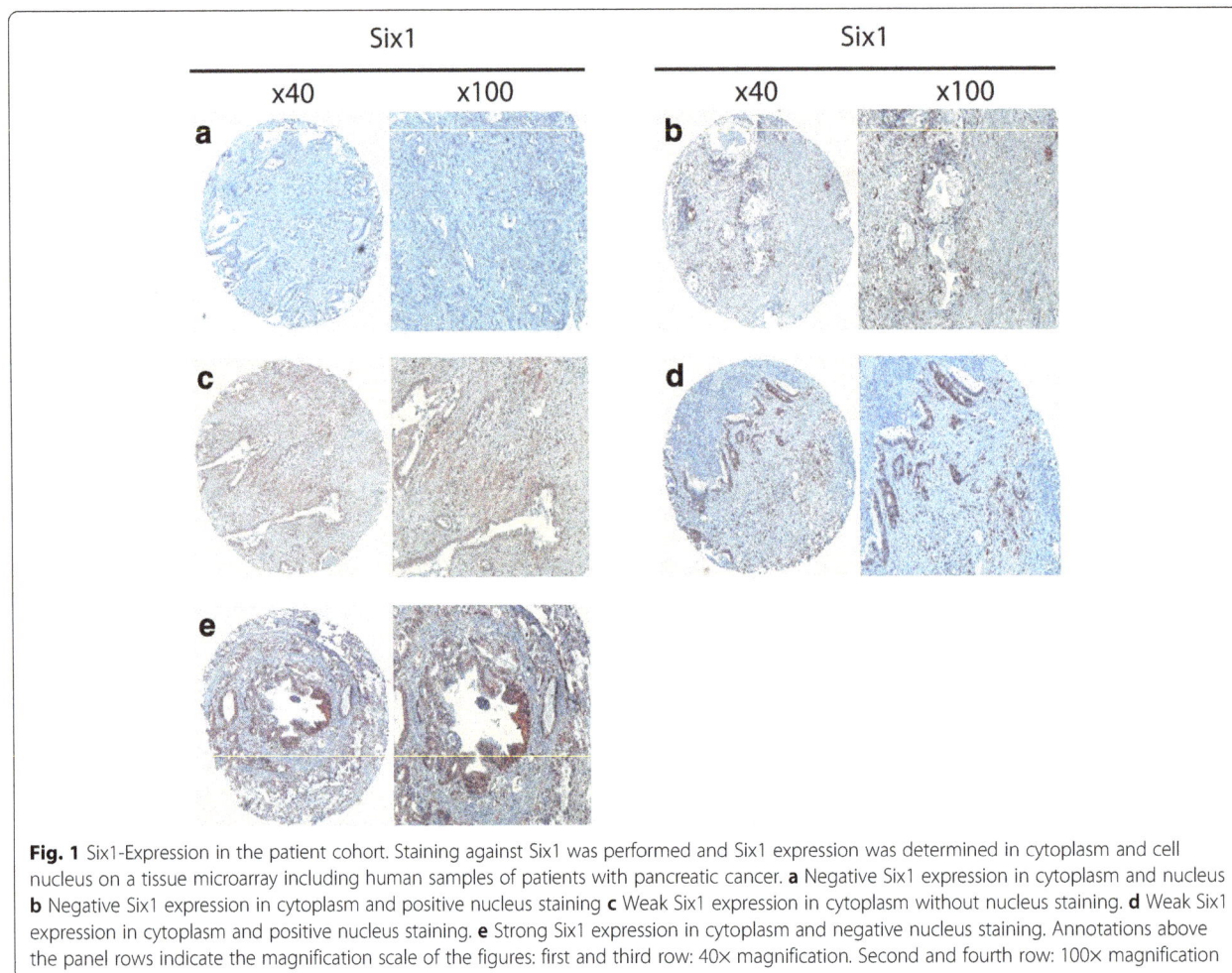

Fig. 1 Six1-Expression in the patient cohort. Staining against Six1 was performed and Six1 expression was determined in cytoplasm and cell nucleus on a tissue microarray including human samples of patients with pancreatic cancer. **a** Negative Six1 expression in cytoplasm and nucleus **b** Negative Six1 expression in cytoplasm and positive nucleus staining **c** Weak Six1 expression in cytoplasm without nucleus staining. **d** Weak Six1 expression in cytoplasm and positive nucleus staining. **e** Strong Six1 expression in cytoplasm and negative nucleus staining. Annotations above the panel rows indicate the magnification scale of the figures: first and third row: 40× magnification. Second and fourth row: 100× magnification

significantly declined expression of vimentin by 58.6% (p = 0.04) (Fig. 2f).

To assess the impact of Six1 inhibition on cell motility, we performed migration assays with Panc1 and BxPc3 cells, which had been transfected with siRNA against Six1 or control. Inhibition of Six1 reduced migration in Panc1 cells by 37% (p = 0.008) and in BxPc3 cells by 24.2% (p = 0.031) (Fig. 2g, h, Additional file 2: Fig. S1).

Effects of Six1 down regulation in Panc1 cells in vivo

We assessed the effect of Six1 inhibition in Panc1 cells in vivo in a xenograft model. For this analysis, shRNA-transfected Panc1 cells were used, showing a stably decreased expression of Six1. After injection of tumour cells into nude mice (2.5×10^6 cells/mouse), body weight and tumour growth were observed for four weeks (Fig. 3a–c). The body weight did not show any difference between these two groups during the observation time. In the beginning, the average tumour volume was 47.65 mm^3 (±19.34) in the control group (Panc1^{shctrl}) and 47.00 mm^3 (±15.90) in the group with Six1-shRNA (Panc1^{shSix1}). After two weeks, the tumour volume had increased to 86.78 mm^3 (±33.93) in the

control group and had declined to 39.84 mm^3 (±18.54) in Panc1^{shSix1}group (p = 0.0018). At time of euthanasia, the average tumour volume was 124.13 mm^3 (±46.59) in the Panc1^{shctrl} group and 50.22 mm^3 (±29.76) in Panc1^{shSix1} (p = 0.0008). After euthanasia, tumour samples of both groups were immunostained against Six1. As expected, tumours from the Panc1^{shctrl} group showed a higher expression of Six1 than tumours from the Panc1^{shSix1} group (Fig. 3d). Interestingly, in the tumour specimens of the Panc1^{shctrl} group, we observed an increased expression of Six1 at the invasive edge where EMT plays an important role for tumour invasion. Moreover, we evaluated the expression of CD44 and CD24 in those murine tumour samples to assess the co-expression of EMT markers and surrogate markers associated with a CSC phenotype [27]. Four out of five control tumours were CD44$^+$/CD24$^+$ whereas all Six1-downregulated tumours lost that phenotype and were CD44$^-$/CD24$^+$ (Fig. 3d, e, and f and Additional file 3: Table S2).

Discussion

Pancreatic cancer (PDAC) is one of the most aggressive types of tumours. For the last decade, its tumour biology

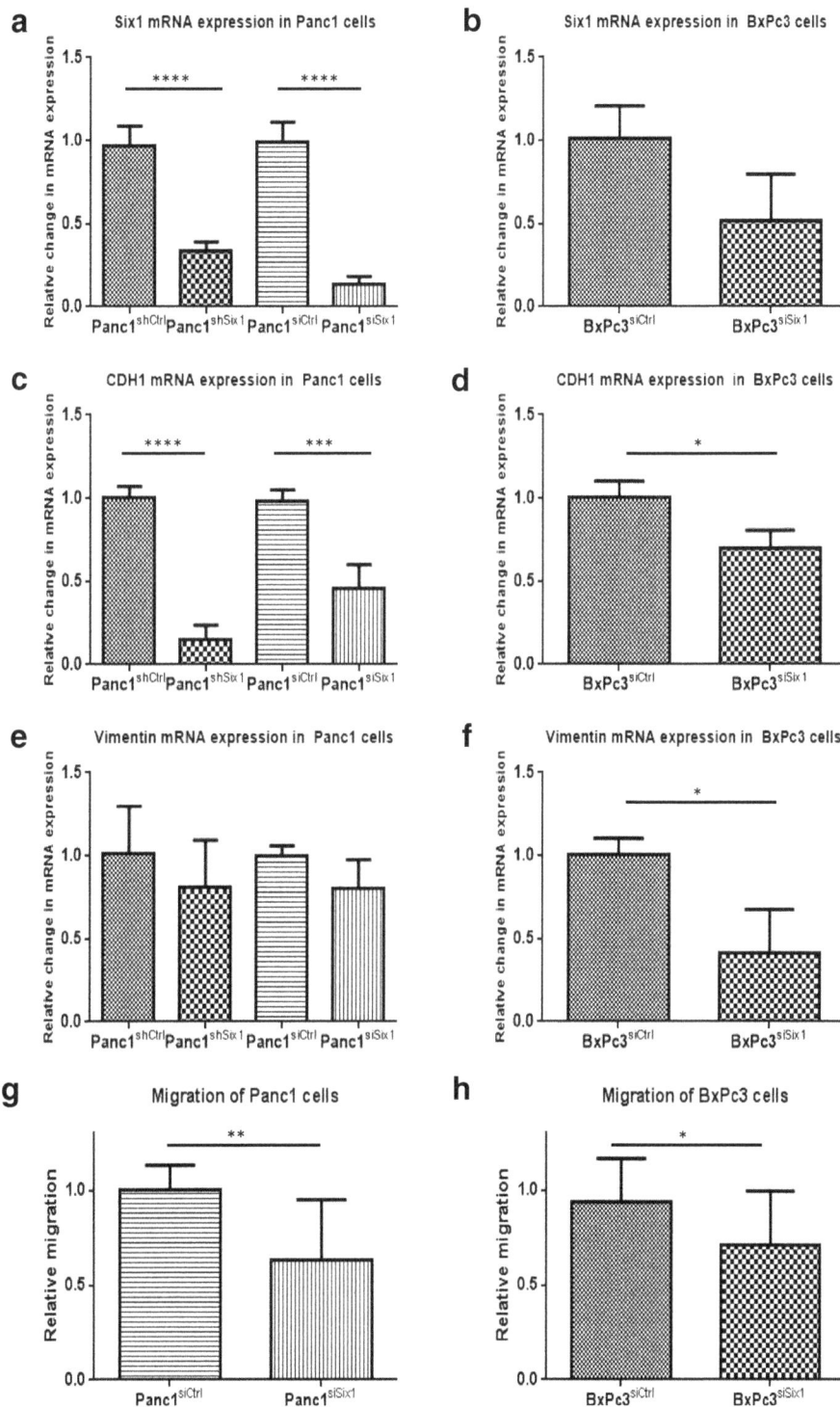

Fig. 2 Expression of Six1, CDH1 and vimentin in Panc1 and BxPc3 cells. **a** Six1 inhibition by shRNA or siRNA decreases Six1 expression in Panc1 cells in comparison to control (scramble shRNA or siRNA). **b** Six1 inhibition siRNA decreases Six1 expression in BxPc3 cells in comparison to scramble siRNA. (C) CDH1 expression in Panc1 cells is reduced after Six1 downregulation. **d** CDH1 expression in BcPc3 is decreased after Six1 downregulation. **e** Vimentin expression in Panc1 cells is not altered by Six1 downregulation. **f** Vimentin expression in BxPc3 cells is decreased by downregulation of Six1. **g** Downregulation of Six1 impairs migration of Panc1 cells. **h** Downregulation of Six1 impairs migration of BxPc3 cells

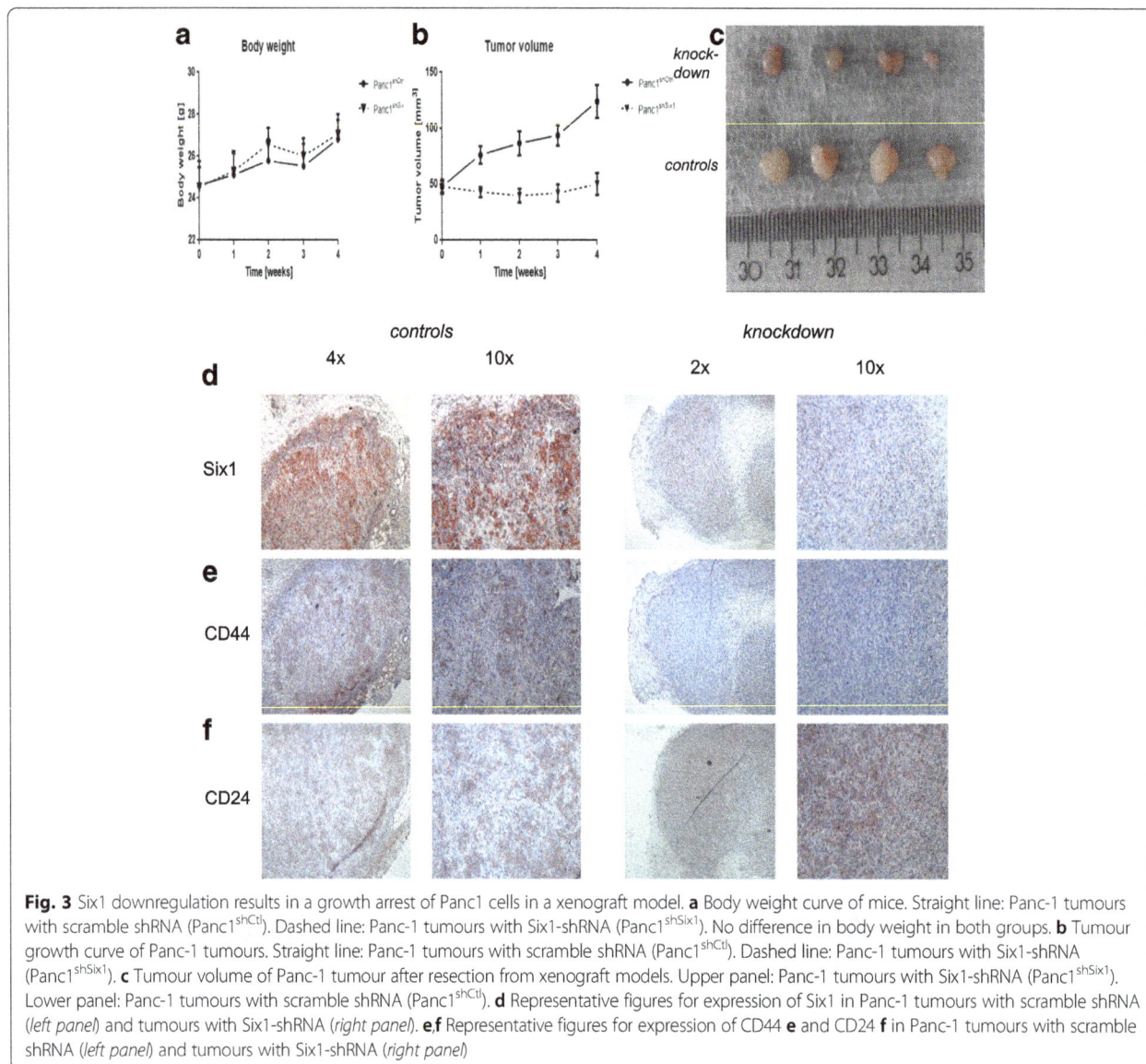

Fig. 3 Six1 downregulation results in a growth arrest of Panc1 cells in a xenograft model. **a** Body weight curve of mice. Straight line: Panc-1 tumours with scramble shRNA (Panc1^{shCtl}). Dashed line: Panc-1 tumours with Six1-shRNA (Panc1^{shSix1}). No difference in body weight in both groups. **b** Tumour growth curve of Panc-1 tumours. Straight line: Panc-1 tumours with scramble shRNA (Panc1^{shCtl}). Dashed line: Panc-1 tumours with Six1-shRNA (Panc1^{shSix1}). **c** Tumour volume of Panc-1 tumour after resection from xenograft models. Upper panel: Panc-1 tumours with Six1-shRNA (Panc1^{shSix1}). Lower panel: Panc-1 tumours with scramble shRNA (Panc1^{shCtl}). **d** Representative figures for expression of Six1 in Panc-1 tumours with scramble shRNA (*left panel*) and tumours with Six1-shRNA (*right panel*). **e,f** Representative figures for expression of CD44 **e** and CD24 **f** in Panc-1 tumours with scramble shRNA (*left panel*) and tumours with Six1-shRNA (*right panel*)

has been more and more elucidated, revealing the important role of EMT in tumour progression. Therefore, in this study, we focused on Six1, which originally has been described as an EMT regulator under physiological conditions in numerous types of tissue. However, its role in carcinogenesis has also become more evident recently [11, 12, 17]. In PDAC, two studies have investigated the role of Six1 so far [18, 19]. They demonstrated that overexpression of Six1 is associated with tumour stage, lymph node status and grading. Furthermore, Li et al. [18] showed that increased expression of Six1 is an independent prognostic marker for survival in pancreatic cancer. Our cohort consisted of 139 patients suffering from primary PDAC who were operated on at the university hospital in Bonn between 1998 and 2009. To our knowledge, this is the largest cohort of patients with

PDAC in which the expression of Six1 has been investigated to date. In 137 malignant and 105 benign samples, Six1 expression was assessed. In accordance with the two previous studies, we observed an overexpression of Six1 in cancer cells compared to healthy tissue. In contrast, we did not find a significant correlation between the expression of Six1 and any clinical or histopathological data. These controversial observations may be explained by the different clinical characteristics of our cohort in comparison to the previous studies: in our analysis, almost all tumours were diagnosed as stage pT3, grading G2 or G3 and lymph node status pN1. On the contrary, the population of Jin et al. was more heterogenous and tumours were in a less advanced stage. Taking into account the very homogenous characteristics of our cohort, statistical analysis would require a much higher number of participants to find a significant correlation.

EMT has been described as one of the hallmarks of cancer [2]. It increases motility and invasiveness. In line with this hallmark, we demonstrated that decreased expression of Six1 results in an impaired motility of Panc1 and BxPc3 cells. Several proteins were proposed as surrogate markers of EMT. CDH1 is a protein involved in cell-cell-contacts, thereby often used as marker for epithelial character [28]. Vimentin is an intermediate filament used as a surrogate for mesenchymal differentiation [29]. Under the assumption that Six1 induces a more mesenchymal phenotype, one would conjecture that Six1 down-regulation results in an increased expression of CDH1 and a decreased expression of vimentin. Intriguingly, in our study we were able to show by several independent experiments that decreased expression of Six1 induces a declined transcription of CDH1 in Panc1 and in BxPc3 cells. Moreover, reduced expression of Six1 slightly affected the expression of vimentin in Panc1, but showed a decreased regulation of Vimentin in BxPc3 cells. To some extent, these data are diametrically opposed to the assumed results. It is unlikely that the decreased expression of CDH1 is an arbitrary result of our transfection method or of the used siRNA. We performed our experiments in two different cell lines. Moreover, the expression of Six1 was reduced significantly by siRNA and by shRNA in comparison to scramble shRNA or control siRNA, respectively. In the light of this, our results underscore that both, CDH1 and Vimentin, are rather surrogate markers for EMT. There exists no definite and unique EMT marker. Cells undergoing EMT exhibit rather a dynamic phenotype, where epithelial and mesenchymal features occur in the same time. This is part of the EMT-MET (mesenchymal-to-epithelial transition) axis which regulates the phenotype of a pro-invasive (mesenchymal) state and an epithelial phenotype. Both types of differentiation are important for tumour spread: the mesenchymal state is important for tumour invasion whereas the epithelial state is required for the colonisation and formation of metastasis in distant organs. Such biphasic effects have also been observed for other EMT-related transcription factors, such as TWIST1 [30]. This transcription factor can induce the expression of miR-424, potentially facilitating earlier, but repressing later stages of metastasis by regulating an EMT-MET axis [30]. It remains speculative but our data may indicate that inhibition of Six1 may affect the EMT-MET axis by regulating both mesenchymal and epithelial genes. However, a relative preponderance of mesenchymal processes versus epithelial processes may shift the balance towards a pro-migratory phenotype, which may explain the results of our migration assays.

Finally, we investigated the impact of Six1 in Panc1 cells in a xenograft model. In this experiment we could observe that tumour growth was impaired significantly when the expression of Six1 was decreased in stable transfected clones by shRNA. These data are in good accordance with the assumption that the inhibition of EMT-related transcription factors results in a diminished tumour growth [31]. To further elucidate those findings, we evaluated the expression of cancer stem cell (CSC) markers in the murine xenograft tumours. Ford et al. have described that Six1 increases the population of CSCs in breast cancer [32]. Conclusively, we hypothesized that decreased expression of Six1 would also result in a reduced number of tumour cells with a CSC-phenotype. We therefore analysed the expression of CD24 and CD44 since Li et al. [27] had identified CD24$^+$/CD44$^+$/ESA$^+$ cells as pancreatic cancer stem cells. In our experiment, control tumours displayed a significantly stronger expression CD24$^+$/CD44$^+$ cells than tumours with down-regulation of Six1. The latter were characterised by cells with a CD24$^+$/CD44$^-$ phenotype, which represents cells with less CSC features. These findings may suggest that decreased expression of Six1 impairs fundamental CSC functions which also results in a less aggressive and less invasive phenotype. Although this result is in good accordance with biological hypotheses and findings in breast cancer, further studies would certainly be warranted to better characterize the effects of Six1 on CSC induction in PDAC in vitro and in vivo.

Conclusion

In conclusion, in the largest cohort of patients studied so far, we confirm the results of previous reports that Six1 is overexpressed in PDAC. Furthermore, we show that inhibition of Six1 leads to decreased cell motility in Panc1 and BxPc3 cells. These results are in good accordance with the hypothesis that Six1 induces EMT. Interestingly, CDH1 mRNA expression was also decreased by impaired expression of Six1 which deserves further investigation in following studies and may reflect a biphasic effect of Six1 on the EMT-MET axis. Moreover, our data show that stable inhibition of Six1 decreases tumour growth in a xenograft model. This is associated with a decreased expression of CSC-markers in the tumour tissue. Overall, our results provide further evidence that Six1 co-promotes tumour progression in pancreatic cancer. Therefore, targeting Six1 might be a novel promising therapeutic approach in patients with pancreatic cancer.

Abbreviations

CSC: Cancer stem cells; EMT: Epithelial-mesenchymal transition; PDAC: Pancreatic ductal adenocarcinoma

Acknowledgements

GF was supported in part by the European Community's Seventh Framework Program [FP7-2007-2013] under grant agreement HEALTH-F2-2011-256986, by the German Cancer Foundation (Deutsche Krebshilfe) grant number 109929, as well as by the Center of Integrated Oncology (CIO) Cologne-Bonn.

Competing interests

We have read and understood BMC Cancer poly on declaration of interests and declare that we have no competing interests.

Author's contributions

Conception and design: TL, GF, CK, Development of methodology: TL, CK, GF, SB, BTH, Acquisition of data: TL, CK, GF, GK, MP, BTH, SS, NNR, TW, CR, MS, Analysis and interpretation of data (e. g. statistical analysis, biostatistics, computational analysis): TL, CK, GF, SB; Writing, review and/or revision of the manuscript: TL, CK, GF, SB, TW, CR, JF; Study supervision: CK, JW, GF, PB. All authors read and approved the final manuscript.

Author details

[1]Department of General, Visceral and Transplantation Surgery, Im Neuenheimer Feld 110, 69120 Heidelberg, Germany. [2]Department of Internal Medicine 3, Center of Integrated Oncology (CIO) Cologne-Bonn, University Hospital of Bonn, Bonn, Germany. [3]Department of Gastrointestinal, Thoracic and Vascular Surgery, Medizinische Fakultät Carl Gustav Carus, Technische Universität Dresden, Fetscherstr. 74, 01307 Dresden, Germany. [4]Department of Pathology, Center of Integrated Oncology Cologne-Bonn, University Hospital of Bonn, Bonn, Germany. [5]Department of General, Visceral and Thoracic Surgery, University Medical Center Hamburg-Eppendorf, Martinistrasse 52, 20246 Hamburg, Germany.

References

1. Siegel RL, Miller KD, Jemal A. Cancer statistics, 2015. CA Cancer J Clin. 2015;65(1):5–29.
2. Hanahan D, Weinberg RA. Hallmarks of cancer: the next generation. Cell. 2011;144(5):646–74.
3. Brabletz T, Hlubek F, Spaderna S, Schmalhofer O, Hiendlmeyer E, Jung A, Kirchner T. Invasion and metastasis in colorectal cancer: epithelial-mesenchymal transition, mesenchymal-epithelial transition, stem cells and beta-catenin. Cells Tissues Organs. 2005;179(1–2):56–65.
4. Brabletz T. To differentiate or not–routes towards metastasis. Nat Rev Cancer. 2012;12(6):425–36.
5. Al-Hajj M, Wicha MS, Benito-Hernandez A, Morrison SJ, Clarke MF. Prospective identification of tumorigenic breast cancer cells. Proc Natl Acad Sci U S A. 2003;100(7):3983–8.
6. Martin A, Cano A. Tumorigenesis: Twist1 links EMT to self-renewal. Nat Cell Biol. 2010;12(10):924–5.
7. Solnica-Krezel L. Conserved patterns of cell movements during vertebrate gastrulation. Curr Biol. 2005;15(6):R213–28.
8. Tucker RP. Neural crest cells: a model for invasive behavior. Int J Biochem Cell Biol. 2004;36(2):173–7.
9. Nawshad A, LaGamba D, Hay ED. Transforming growth factor beta (TGFbeta) signalling in palatal growth, apoptosis and epithelial mesenchymal transformation (EMT). Arch Oral Biol. 2004;49(9):675–89.
10. Sherr CJ, DePinho RA. Cellular senescence: Minireview mitotic clock or culture shock? Cell. 2000;102(4):407–10.
11. Ford HL, Kabingu EN, Bump EA, Mutter GL, Pardee AB. Abrogation of the G2 cell cycle checkpoint associated with overexpression of HSIX1: a possible mechanism of breast carcinogenesis. Proc Natl Acad Sci. 1998;95(21):12608–13.
12. Micalizzi DS, Christensen KL, Jedlicka P, Coletta RD, Baron AE, Harrell JC, Horwitz KB, Billheimer D, Heichman KA, Welm AL, et al. The Six1 homeoprotein induces human mammary carcinoma cells to undergo epithelial-mesenchymal transition and metastasis in mice through increasing TGF-beta signaling. J Clin Invest. 2009;119(9):2678–90.
13. Tan J, Zhang C, Qian J. Expression and significance of Six1 and Ezrin in cervical cancer tissue. Tumor Biol. 2011;32(6):1241–7.
14. Zheng XH, Liang PH, Guo JX, Zheng YR, Han J, Yu LL, Zhou YG, Li L. Expression and Clinical Implications of Homeobox Gene Six1 in Cervical Cancer Cell Lines and Cervical Epithelial Tissues. Int J Gynecol Cancer. 2010;20(9):1587–92.
15. Ng KT, Lee TK, Cheng Q, Wo JY, Sun CK, Guo DY, Lim ZX, Lo CM, Poon RT, Fan ST, et al. Suppression of tumorigenesis and metastasis of hepatocellular carcinoma by shRNA interference targeting on homeoprotein Six1. Int J Cancer. 2010;127(4):859–72.
16. Behbakht K, Qamar L, Aldridge CS, Coletta RD, Davidson SA, Thorburn A, Ford HL. Six1 overexpression in ovarian carcinoma causes resistance to TRAIL-mediated apoptosis and is associated with poor survival. Cancer Res. 2007;67(7):3036–42.
17. Kahlert C, Lerbs T, Pecqueux M, Herpel E, Hoffmeister M, Jansen L, Brenner H, Chang-Claude J, Bläker H, Kloor M, et al. Overexpression of SIX1 is an independent prognostic marker in stage I–III colorectal cancer. Int J Cancer. 2015;137(9):2104–13.
18. Li Z, Tian T, Lv F, Chang Y, Wang X, Zhang L, Li X, Li L, Ma W, Wu J, et al. Six1 promotes proliferation of pancreatic cancer cells via Upregulation of Cyclin D1 expression. PLoS ONE. 2013;8(3):e59203.
19. Jin A, Xu Y, Liu S, Jin T, Li Z, Jin H, Lin L, Lin Z. Sineoculis homeobox homolog 1 protein overexpression as an independent biomarker for pancreatic ductal adenocarcinoma. Exp Mol Pathol. 2014;96(1):54–60.
20. Ono H, Imoto I, Kozaki K, Tsuda H, Matsui T, Kurasawa Y, Muramatsu T, Sugihara K, Inazawa J. SIX1 promotes epithelial-mesenchymal transition in colorectal cancer through ZEB1 activation. Oncogene. 2012;31(47):4923–34.
21. Kahlert C, Gaitzsch E, Steinert G, Mogler C, Herpel E, Hoffmeister M, Jansen L, Benner A, Brenner H, Chang-Claude J, et al. Expression analysis of aldehyde dehydrogenase 1A1 (ALDH1A1) in colon and rectal cancer in association with prognosis and response to chemotherapy. Ann Surg Oncol. 2012;19(13):4193–201.
22. Hamilton AJ. A species of small antisense RNA in posttranscriptional Gene silencing in plants. Science. 1999;286(5441):950–2.
23. Holmen S, Vanbrocklin M, Eversole R, Stapleton S, Ginsberg L. Efficient lipid-mediated transfection of DNA into primary rat hepatocytes. In Vitro Cell Dev Biol Anim. 1995;31(5):347–51.
24. Mullis K, Faloona F, Scharf S, Saiki R, Horn G, Erlich H. Specific enzymatic amplification of DNA in vitro: the polymerase chain reaction. Cold Spring Harb Symp Quant Biol. 1986;1986(51):263–73.
25. Mullis K. Specific enzymatic amplification of DNA in vitro: the polymerase chain reaction. Cold Spring Harb Symp Quant Biol. 1986;1986(51):263–73.
26. Pfaffl MW. A new mathematical model for relative quantification in real-time RT-PCR. Nucleic Acids Res. 2001;29(9):e45.
27. Li C, Heidt DG, Dalerba P, Burant CF, Zhang L, Adsay V, Wicha M, Clarke MF, Simeone DM. Identification of pancreatic cancer stem cells. Cancer Res. 2007;67(3):1030–7.
28. Yilmaz M, Christofori G. EMT, the cytoskeleton, and cancer cell invasion. Cancer Metastasis Rev. 2009;28(1–2):15–33.
29. Huang RY, Guilford P, Thiery JP. Early events in cell adhesion and polarity during epithelial-mesenchymal transition. J Cell Sci. 2012;125(Pt 19):4417–22.
30. Drasin DJ, Guarnieri AL, Neelakantan D, Kim J, Cabrera JH, Wang C-A, Zaberezhnyy V, Gasparini P, Cascione L, Huebner K, et al. TWIST1-induced miR-424 reversibly drives Mesenchymal programming while inhibiting tumor initiation. Cancer Res. 2015;75(9):1908–21.
31. Micalizzi DS, Farabaugh SM, Ford HL. Epithelial-mesenchymal transition in cancer: parallels between normal development and tumor progression. J Mammary Gland Biol Neoplasia. 2010;15(2):117–34.
32. McCoy EL, Iwanaga R, Jedlicka P, Abbey NS, Chodosh LA, Heichman KA, Welm AL, Ford HL. Six1 expands the mouse mammary epithelial stem/progenitor cell pool and induces mammary tumors that undergo epithelial-mesenchymal transition. J Clin Invest. 2009;119(9):2663–77.

Loss of PDPK1 abrogates resistance to gemcitabine in label-retaining pancreatic cancer cells

Dandan Li[1†], John E. Mullinax[2†], Taylor Aiken[3,4], Hongwu Xin[5], Gordon Wiegand[6], Andrew Anderson[7], Snorri Thorgeirsson[8], Itzhak Avital[9] and Udo Rudloff[1*] [iD]

Abstract

Background: Label-retaining cancer cells (LRCC) have been proposed as a model of slowly cycling cancer stem cells (CSC) which mediate resistance to chemotherapy, tumor recurrence, and metastasis. The molecular mechanisms of chemoresistance in LRCC remain to-date incompletely understood. This study aims to identify molecular targets in LRCC that can be exploited to overcome resistance to gemcitabine, a standard chemotherapy agent for the treatment of pancreas cancer.

Methods: LRCC were isolated following Cy5-dUTP staining by flow cytometry from pancreatic cancer cell lines. Gene expression profiles obtained from LRCC, non-LRCC (NLRCC), and bulk tumor cells were used to generate differentially regulated pathway networks. Loss of upregulated targets in LRCC on gemcitabine sensitivity was assessed via RNAi experiments and pharmacological inhibition. Expression patterns of PDPK1, one of the upregulated targets in LRCC, was studied in patients' tumor samples and correlated with pathological variables and clinical outcome.

Results: LRCC are significantly more resistant to gemcitabine than the bulk tumor cell population. Non-canonical EGF (epidermal growth factor)-mediated signal transduction emerged as the top upregulated network in LRCC compared to non-LRCC, and knock down of EGF signaling effectors PDPK1 (3-phosphoinositide dependent protein kinase-1), BMX (BMX non-receptor tyrosine kinase), and NTRK2 (neurotrophic receptor tyrosine kinase 2) or treatment with PDPK1 inhibitors increased growth inhibition and induction of apoptosis in response to gemcitabine. Knockdown of PDPK1 preferentially increased growth inhibition and reduced resistance to induction of apoptosis upon gemcitabine treatment in the LRCC vs non-LRCC population. These findings are accompanied by lower expression levels of PDPK1 in tumors compared to matched uninvolved pancreas in surgical resection specimens and a negative association of membranous localization on IHC with high nuclear grade ($p < 0.01$).

Conclusion: Pancreatic cancer cell-derived LRCC are relatively resistant to gemcitabine and harbor a unique transcriptomic profile compared to bulk tumor cells. PDPK1, one of the members of an upregulated EGF-signaling network in LRCC, mediates resistance to gemcitabine, is found to be dysregulated in pancreas cancer specimens, and might be an attractive molecular target for combination therapy studies.

Keywords: Pancreatic cancer, Cancer stem cell, Label-retaining cancer cells (LRCC), PDPK1, Chemoresistance

* Correspondence: rudloffu@mail.nih.gov
†Dandan Li and John E. Mullinax contributed equally to this work.
[1]Rare Tumor Initiative, Cancer for Cancer Research, National Cancer Institute, Building 10, Room 2B-38E, Bethesda, MD, USA
Full list of author information is available at the end of the article

Background

Pancreatic ductal adenocarcinoma (PDAC) is an especially lethal disease with 53,070 new cases diagnosed last year and 41,780 deaths due to disease [1]. Its 5-year survival rate of 5–8% has not substantially changed over the last three decades and the American Association for Cancer Research (AACR) estimates pancreas cancer to rank second in cancer-related mortality in the U. S by the year 2020 [2]. Despite recent significant advances in the knowledge of the underlying molecular mechanisms in PDAC, meaningful long term survival remains elusive [3]. More than 80% of patients present with locally advanced or distant metastatic disease at time of diagnosis, which precludes operative extirpation and, therefore the only modality associated with longer term survival. These patients are thus relegated to palliative systemic therapies with the best combination of conventional cytotoxic chemotherapy for advanced pancreas cancer conferring a median survival estimate of less than 1 year [4, 5]. Given the dismal long term survival for the vast majority of patients with this disease, new therapeutic approaches in treatment of this disease are needed.

The cancer stem cell (CSC) theory holds that: 1) cancer arises from cells with dysregulated self-renewal mechanisms; and, 2) cancer is comprised of a heterogeneous mass of cells, a small fraction of which consists of stem-like progenitor cells that drive tumor growth and metastasis [6, 7]. The theory itself is a progression of Knudson's two-hit hypothesis of carcinogenesis (initiation and promotion), though the origin of the cell lineage involved with initiation and promotion of neoplastic growth is different. A detailed pancreas cancer-specific stem cell phenotype-genotype association remains elusive, which is, in part, due to the different standards of definition and isolation of such cells but also due to an increased recognition of the inherent heterogeneity of the CSC fraction [8–12] While many groups have described cancer stem cells from multiple tissue sources using a variety of methods, these reported methods rely on cell surface moieties as a surrogate for the identification of these stem cells, but do not necessarily isolate CSCs in a manner reflective of their proposed function and hierarchy [12–15].

Almost 40 years ago 'mutational selection' in cancer was described and followed 3 years later by the first description of label retaining cells (LRC) and the 'immortal strand hypothesis' [16, 17]. Label-retaining cells (LRC) are associated with populations of cells enriched with adult tissue stem cells [18–21]. Many solid organ cancers develop in tissues found to harbor LRC and it is increasingly recognized that slowly cycling LRCC exhibit cancer stem cell and pluripotency traits representing a distinct subpopulation of the heterogeneous CSC pool [5, 22–26]. The clinical importance of the LRCC subpopulation has recently been demonstrated in a sentinel report of repopulation of residual tumors post-chemotherapy treatment with new cancer cells from this pool of cells [27]. Other reports have linked slowly cycling LRCC to disseminated tumor cells (DTC), relapse, and metastasis in cancer patients [28, 29]. Recently, we demonstrated that label-retaining cancer cells (LRCC) undergo asymmetric cell division, and represent a unique subpopulation of tumor-initiating stem-like cells with pluripotency gene expression profiles [20]. While early reports described fixed cells, which precluded downstream analysis, we recently published on such a method for the isolation of live tissue-derived LRC allowing for future assays dependent on live functioning cells. Using these methods it was shown that LRC do, in fact, undergo asymmetric cell division with non-random chromosomal cosegregation (ACD-NRCC) [20, 30].

The identification of LRCs in PDAC [i.e. pancreatic cancer-derived label retaining cancer cells (LRCC)] would offer a unique opportunity to study features of cancer stemness, in particular with regard to identifying vulnerabilities of this cell population knowledge which has remained elusive for the design of more effective therapies in pancreas cancer and drug development in general. Despite the ability to potentially impact sentinel events in cancer recurrence and progression, there is significant paucity in the understanding of selective molecular mechanisms in LRCC.

In the following report, we compare the transcriptome of LRCC and non-LRRC in pancreas cancer cell lines and identify perturbations unique to LRCC. Targeting one of the genes selectively upregulated in LRCC, 3-phosphoinositide dependent protein kinase-1 (PDPK1), we demonstrate that the phenotype resistance to chemotherapy in pancreatic cancer LRCC can be abrogated as a potentially novel treatment avenue against this difficult to treat cell population possibly guiding novel combination therapies in this lethal disease.

Methods
Cell culture

The cell lines MiaPaCa2 (ATCC, Manassas, VA, Cat. # ATCC-CRL-1420), Panc-1 (ATCC, Manassas, VA, Cat. # ATCC-CRL-1469), and were grown in DMEM medium supplemented with 10% FBS, 1% PenStrep, and 1% 200 mM L-glutamine (Gibco, Grand Island, NY). The Nor-P1 (Riken BioResource Research Center, Japan, Cat.# RBRC-RCB2139) cell line was grown in RPMI 1640 medium supplemented with 10% FBS, 1% PenStrep, and 1% 200 mM L-glutamine (Gibco, Grand Island, NY). Hereafter these media are considered "standard" media. Serum free media contained all elements with the exception of FBS and antibiotic free media contained all elements with the exception of PenStrep.

Isolation of label retaining cancer cells

Cells were cultured in standard media until 80% confluency. One cell cycle before labeling, the media was changed to serum free media. Prior to labeling, the cells were lifted with 0.25% Trypsin (Gibco, Grand Island, NY) and resuspended in R-buffer (Invitrogen, Grand Island, NY) at a concentration of 5×10^6 cells/100uL. Cy5-dUTP (GE Healthcare, Piscataway, NJ) was added at a concentration of $12uL/5 \times 10^6$ cells. The cells were transfected using the Invitrogen Neon Transfection System using 1200 V for 20 milliseconds and 2 pulses. Immediately following transfection, the cells were placed in antibiotic free media and grown at 37 °C with 5% CO_2 for one cell cycle. Following this brief culture, the cells were again lifted and sorted for Cy5-dUTP purity using a BD FACSAria II instrument (BD Biosciences, San Jose, CA). The Cy5-dUTP$^+$ fraction was placed back into culture and expanded for 8 cell cycles, splitting cells at 70% confluency. Subsequently, the cells were sorted using a BD FACSAria II instrument (BD Biosciences, San Jose, CA). The Cy5-dUTP$^+$ cells represent the label retaining cancer cells and the Cy5-dUTP$^-$ cells represent the non-label retaining cancer cells. Cells were used immediately for downstream analyses.

Gene expression analysis

Total RNA was isolated using Arcturus PicoPure RNA Isolation Kit (LifeTechnologies, Carlsbad, CA). The quality and quantity of RNA was assessed using the Agilent 2100 Bioanalyzer (Agilent Technologies, Wilmington, DE) and only total RNA with a RIN > 8 was amplified using the Illumina TotalPrep RNA Amplification Kit (Life Technologies, Carlsbad, CA). Following amplification of 200 ng total RNA, the biotin-cRNA was loaded onto an Illumina HT-12v4 BeadChip and data was obtained using the Illumina iScan device (Illumina, San Diego, CA). Raw data was exported from Illumina GenomeStudio to Agilent GeneSpring GX v11 for downstream expression analysis. Pathway analysis was performed using Ingenuity Pathway Analysis software. Results were validated using TaqMan qRT-PCR with primers specific to the microarray sequences which were obtained from Genecopoeia (Rockville, MD).

Cell cycle analysis

Live cells were fixed using 70% EtOH following FACS sorting. The cells were washed twice using PBS and resuspended in 1 mL of staining solution which contained 10 ml of 0.1% (v/v) Triton X-100 (Sigma) in PBS, 2 mg DNase-free RNase A (Sigma), and 200 µl of 1 mg/ml PI (Sigma). Cells were incubated at 37 °C for 30 min and then immediately analyzed using the BD FACSAria II instrument.

Cell proliferation and apoptosis assay

The IC50 dose of gemcitabine hydrochloride (Gemzar® Eli Lilly, Indianapolis, IN) was calculated for each cell line using the CellTiter-Glo® assay (Promega, Madison, WI), after exposure to a serial dilution of drug in a 96 well plate format for 72 h. Live cells were plated following FACS at a concentration of 3000 cells/well in 100uL standard media. Following incubation for 24 h at 37 °C with 5% CO_2, the media was changed to standard media with the addition of the IC50 dose of gemcitabine hydrochloride for the given cell line. After 72 h cell proliferation was assessed using the CellTiter-Glo® assay with levels of untreated cells normalized to 100%. Additionally, apoptosis was evaluated at the same time using the Caspase-Glo®3/7 assay (Promega, Madison, WI).

Exposure to gemcitabine following siRNA transfection

Cells were plated at a concentration of 3000 cells/well in 100uL media containing antibiotic free media with the addition of 0.3 µL RNAi Max transfection agent (Life Technologies, Carlsbad, CA) and 2 µL of 1 µM siRNA (GeneSolution, Qiagen, Valencia, CA) reconstituted in RNase free water. Following transfection for 48 h, cells were then exposed to gemcitabine hydrochloride for 72 h and final cell viability and apoptosis were measured using the CellTiter-Glo® assay and Caspase-Glo®3/7 assay, respectively. Data analysis was performed using GraphPad Prism6 software. Drug response curves were created using a four-parameter equation fitting technique.

Tissue microarray (TMA) composition

De-identified cancer tissues were confirmed to be pancreatic ductal adenocarcinomas based on pathology slide review at the National Cancer Institute. The analytic dataset included 144 specimens from the Iowa, Hawaii and Los Angeles Surveillance, Epidemiology, and End Results (SEER) Residual Tumor Registries pancreatic cancer tissue microarray (TMA) [31]. An additional commercial TMA (Biomax) with 40 matched tumor and normal pancreatic tissue specimens was used to compare PDK1 expression between tumor specimens and normal pancreatic tissue.

Immunoblot and immunofluorescence analysis

Cancer cells were lysed with M-PER® Mammalian Protein Extraction Reagent (Cat#78501, ThermoScientific, Waltham, USA) plus Halt™ protease & phosphatase inhibitor cocktail (Cat#1861284, ThermoScientific, Waltham, USA). Protein concentration was determined via BCA analysis kit (ThermoScientific, Waltham, USA). For immunoblotting, proteins were transferred from 4 to

20% SDS/Polyacrylamide gels to nitrocellulose blotting papers via the iBlot®2 Gel Transfer Device (LifeTechnologies, Carlsbad, CA). The phospho-PDPK1 Ser241 antibody (Cat#3438), the phospho-AKT Ser473 antibody (Cat#9271), the AKT antibody (Cat#9272) and β-Actin antibody (Cat#4970, all Cell Signaling, Danvers, USA) were applied and bands were visualized via the Odyssey luminescence scanner (Li-Cor, Lincoln, USA). For immunofluorescence analysis, approximately 50,000 were centrifuged onto a glass slide with Rotofix 32 A centrifuge (Hettich Lab Technology, Tuttlingen, Germany) and fixed in 4% paraformaldehyde at 4 °C overnight. Cells were permeabilized in 0.25% TritonX-100 and blocked with 5% normal goat serum in PBS at room temperature in a humidified chamber for 2 h. Slides were incubated anti-phosphatidylinositol 3,4,5-trisphosphate (PIP3) (Cat#Z-P345, Echelon Biosciences Inc., Salt Lake City, UT) monoclonal antibodies. Alexa Fluor® 488 goat anti-mouse IgG (H + L) secondary antibody was then applied for 1 h at room temperature. Slides were mounted with Vectashield/DAPI (Vector Laboratories, Burlingame, CA). Images were captured using a Zeiss LSM 510 UV confocal microscope (Zeiss, Thornwood, NY).

Immunohistochemistry and statistical analysis

Immunohistochemical staining for PDPK1 (HPA027376; Sigma Aldrich, St. Louis, MO) was performed by NDBio, Baltimore, MD. PDPK1 expression was evaluated semi-quantitatively for expression levels via a four-tier scale (0 = negative; 1 = background; 2 = positive; 3 = strongly positive) and for cellular localization as having cytoplasmic PDPK1 expression, membrane PDPK1 expression, or a combination of both patterns. Evaluation of staining was carried out in a blinded fashion with respect to outcome and stage.

Statistical analysis

Matched tumor and normal pancreatic tissues were compared using Wilcoxon matched-pairs signed rank test. Product-limit survival estimates were plotted using the Kaplan-Meier method with significance determined by log-rank test. Comparison of staining pattern (cytoplasmic vs membrane) with respect to histologic grade was performed using Fisher's exact test.

Results

Pancreas cancer label retaining cancer cell (LRCC) isolation

Label retaining cancer cells (LRCC) were isolated from the cell lines MiaPaCa2, Panc-1, and Nor-P1 following culture for a period equal to eight doubling times (Fig. 1). Following this expansion, approximately 0.4% of the cells would be mathematically expected to retain the label

assuming symmetric division. The proportion of LRCC exceeded that which would be expected mathematically (0.4%) with 3.07, 4.30, and 3.55% measured LRCC fraction isolated for MiaPaCa2, Panc-1, and Nor-P1, respectively ($p = 0.0119$). This significant increase in the observed compared to the expected proportion of LRCC is consistent with previous observations of ours and others of non-stoichiometric division of genetic material during cell division suggestive of known asymmetric cell divisions of pluripotent cells with stemness features [20, 30].

Responses to gemcitabine differ in LRCC and bulk cell population

LRCC, non-label retaining cancer cells (NLRCC), and unsorted cells were exposed to the previously determined GI50 of gemcitabine of bulk cells of 33 nM (MiaPaCa2), 3 μM (Panc-1) and 3.3 nM (Nor-P1) for a period equal to two doubling times. After normalizing vehicle-treated cells (VTC) to 100%, relative proliferation after exposure to gemcitabine GI50 of the LRRC fraction was 103.7% for cell line MiaPaCa2, 88.5% for Panc-1, and 99.7% for Nor-P1, whereas survival in the NLRCC fractions decreased to 71.3, 56.6, and 80% compared to vehicle-treated cells (LRCC vs non-LRCC populations in MiaPaCa2 ($p < 0.001$), Panc-1 ($p < 0.01$), and Nor-P1 ($p < 0.05$) cells), following treatment with gemcitabine, respectively (Fig. 2a). In line with the genotoxic activity of gemcitabine, we examined levels of apoptosis in LRCC and non-LRCC populations as a possible mechanism of action for the observed difference in response to gemcitabine. Activated caspase 3/7 activity in the LRCC fraction of MiaPaCa2, Panc-1, and Nor-P1 was measured as 109.4, 127.7, and 181.5% compared to vehicle-treated control whereas apoptosis in the NLRCC fraction upon gemcitabine treatment increased to 126.6% ($p < 0.05$), 160.0% ($p < 0.01$), and 207.4% ($p < 0.01$), respectively (Fig. 2b). Apoptosis levels of LRCC and NLRCC subpopulations were normalized to caspase 3/7 levels of vehicle-treated cells.

Resistance to gemcitabine is an indigenous feature of LRCC

Next, we evaluated the possibility that resistance to gemcitabine might have been a consequence of an increased proportion of LRCC induced by gemcitabine treatment. It has been shown previously that cytotoxic chemotherapy, including gemcitabine in Panc1 cells, can induce stem cell fractions, as measured by side population fraction or by cell surface marker CD133 positive cell populations in pancreas cancer [32, 33]. Cy5+ labelled cells were expanded for a time period equal to six doubling times, and then treated with the GI50 dose of gemcitabine for two doubling times prior to sorting for LRCC and NLRCC. In the case of

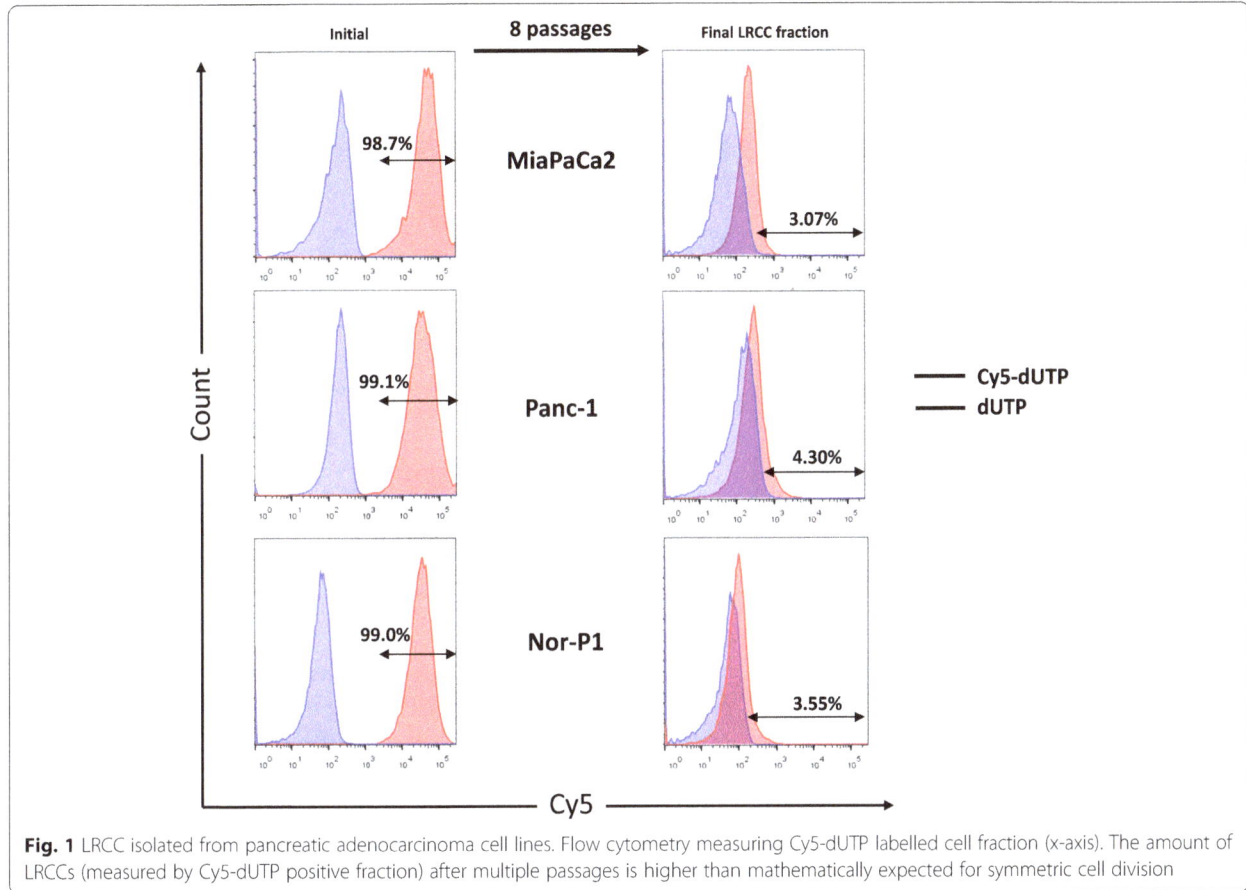

Fig. 1 LRCC isolated from pancreatic adenocarcinoma cell lines. Flow cytometry measuring Cy5-dUTP labelled cell fraction (x-axis). The amount of LRCCs (measured by Cy5-dUTP positive fraction) after multiple passages is higher than mathematically expected for symmetric cell division

MiaPaCa2 and Panc-1, the average LRCC percentages after gemcitabine exposure was no different than without gemcitabine exposure (2.0% vs. 3.7%, $p = 0.0746$) (Fig. 3a).

In order to test the possibility that LRCC are quiescent relative to NLRCC and consequent decreased number of cell divisions confers resistance to gemcitabine therapy, cell cycle analysis of Cy5$^+$ labelled cells were performed using a propidium iodide (PI) method. FACS analysis of PI staining revealed no difference in S-phase between LRCC and NLRCC of the average of the three cell lines (27.45% vs. 27.05%, $p = 0.9247$, Fig. 3b). Finally, to evaluate if gemcitabine resulted in slowed division of LRCC relative to NLRCC, cell cycle analysis was performed following gemcitabine exposure. Following exposure to GI50 gemcitabine concentrations there was also no difference in S-phase between LRCC and NLRCC (26.05% vs. 28.35%, $p = 0.8006$, Fig. 3c), nor was there any difference between the proportion of LRCC in S-phase which had been exposed to gemcitabine (26.05%) compared to the proportion of LRCC in S-phase (27.45%, $p = 0.8893$) of vehicle treated cells (Fig. 3d). These findings suggest mechanisms of resistance to gemcitabine are an indigenous feature of LRCC, not due to alterations in cell cycle progression or proliferation, and, at least initially, not associated with expansion of the LRCC fraction.

Gene expression analysis

We next pursued possible intrinsic mechanisms of resistance inherent to the LRCC population by using a global comparative gene expression approach between the two cell populations. Unsupervised cluster analysis of gene expression levels of the LRCC, NLRCC and bulk cell fractions revealed that the LRCC and bulk fractions were more similar to each other than the NLRCC fraction for the cell lines Panc-1 and MiaPaCa2 on hierarchical clustering analysis visualized as dendrograms (data not shown). In each of the cell lines, the LRCC and NLRCC had the greatest distance between them by IPA dendrogram measurements considering both lengths of branches as well as the splits.

Probes representing genes up-regulated and down-regulated > 2.0-fold change in the LRCC fraction compared to the NLRCC fraction were identified. A Venn diagram analysis was constructed including all cell lines, which allowed for identification of the genes commonly up- or down-regulated common to all three lines. There were 383 probes up-regulated more than 2.0-fold change in the LRCC compared to the NLRCC and 432 probes down-regulated more than 2.0-fold change in the LRCC compared to the NLRCC.

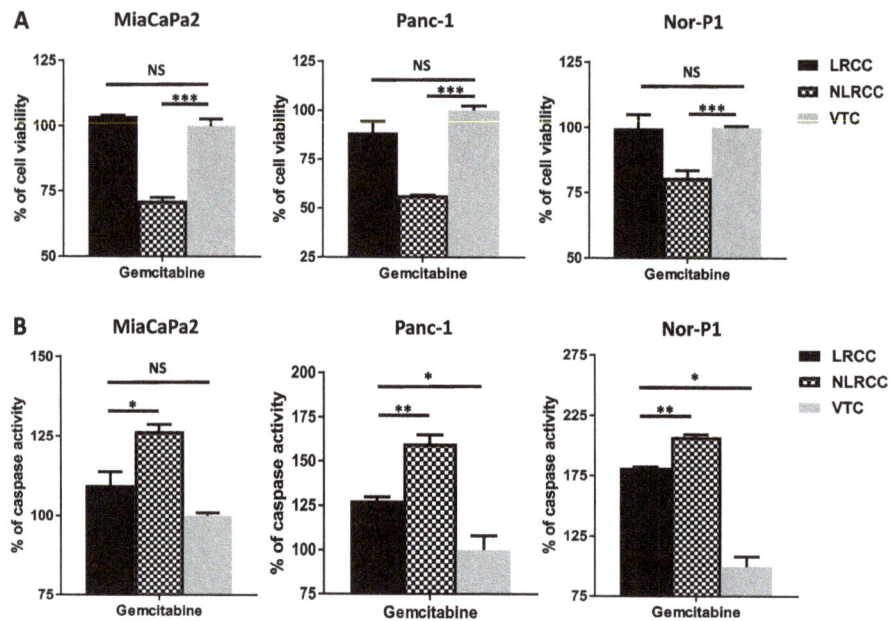

Fig. 2 Responses in LRCC and NLRCC differ following exposure to gemcitabine. **a** LRCC resistance as measured by cell proliferation assay (normalized to vehicle-treated cells (VTC) after treatment with gemcitabine (GI50) for two doubling times in MiaPaCa2, Panc-1, and Nor-P1 cells (*$p < 0.05$, **$p < 0.01$, ***$p < 0.001$; paired t-test). **b** Activated caspase 3/7 assay measures reduced apoptosis in LRCC population upon exposure to gemcitabine compared to NLRCC

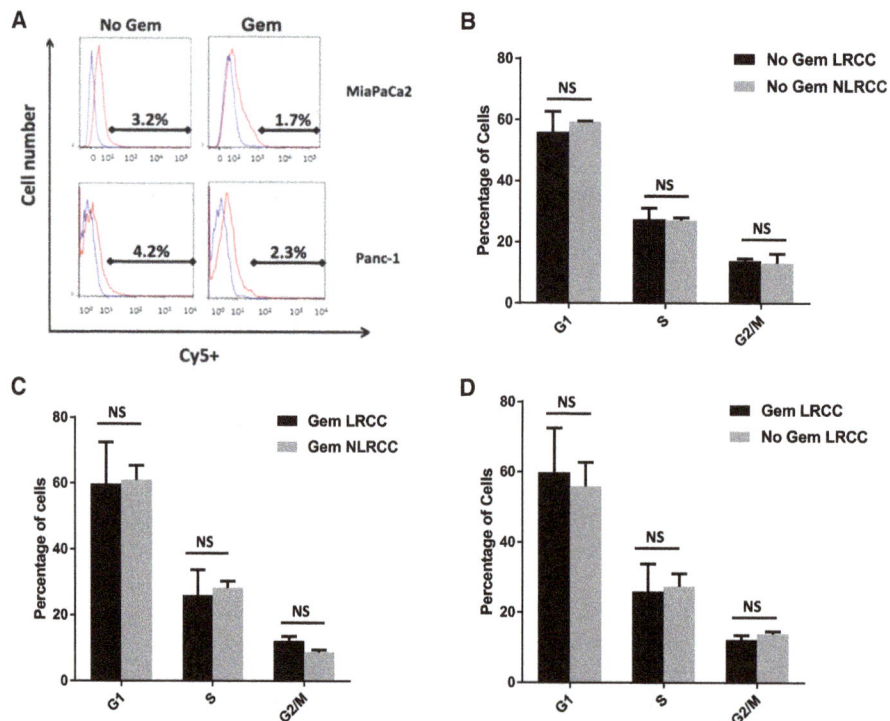

Fig. 3 LRCC resistance is not due to increased proportion of the LRCC fraction or increased quiescence following exposure to gemcitabine. **a** Flow cytometry measuring Cy5-dUTP labelled cells (x-axis) are shown. Gemcitabine (at GI50 for individual cell line) was administered after 6 doubling times and measurements were taken after a total of 8 cycles. **b** Cell cycle distribution of LRCC and NLRCC cells without gemcitabine treatment, average of two cell lines of ≥2 independent experiments per cell line are shown. **c** Cell cycle distribution of gemcitabine treated LRCC and NLRCC cells, average of two cell lines of ≥2 independent experiments per cell line are shown. **d** Cell cycle distribution of gemcitabine treated and untreated LRCC cells, average of two cell lines of ≥2 independent experiments per cell line are shown

Pathway analysis of the up-regulated genes revealed enrichment of interactions around the EGF ligand mediated and related pathways as the top enriched network (Fig. 4a). Three kinases and a synthase were identified in this network—NOS2A (nitric oxide synthase 2; iNOS, Entrez ID 4843), NTRK2 (neurotrophic receptor tyrosine kinase 2; TrkB, Entrez ID 4915), PDPK1 (PDK1, Entrez ID 5170), and BMX (BMX non-receptor tyrosine kinase; ETK, Entrez ID 660). The average fold change of up-regulation in the LRCC compared to NLRCC across the three cell lines for each gene was 6.62, 2.74, 7.22, and 5.12 for NOS2A, NTRK2, PDPK1, and BMX, respectively). Validation of the microarray data using qRT-PCR confirmed expression fold change > 2.0 (LRCC vs. NLRCC) for each gene (NOS2A = 5.6, NTRK2 = 7.2, PDPK1 = 2.4, BMX = 2.8) initially observed on the microarray study (Fig. 4b).

Response to gemcitabine following siRNA knockdown of target genes

Next, to study whether these upregulated genes in the LRCC population are involved in mediation of response to gemcitabine, full drug-response curves of gemcitabine with and without silencing of the four tyrosine kinases overexpressed in the LRCC fraction were generated. First, four sequences for each target gene were tested for effective silencing of target genes confirmed by qRT-PCR in all cell lines and the two sequences inducing the most efficient loss of mRNA expression (≥88%) were selected for further studies (Fig. 5a, Additional file 1: Figure S1A and Additional file 1: Figure S1C). The reduction of knock-down of PDPK1 was also confirmed by Western Blot in all three cell lines (Additional file 1: Figure S1B). Drug response curves with gemcitabine in

MiaPaCa2, Panc-1, and Nor-P1 cells (Fig. 5a and Additional file 1: Figure S1C) showed increased sensitivities to gemcitabine with IC50s greater than up to 10-fold lower compared to scrambled siRNA control upon silencing of BMX, NTRK2, and PDPK1. In line with reduced proliferation, silencing of the 3 genes in MiaPaCa2, Panc-1, and Nor-P1 cells significantly increased apoptosis upon treatment with gemcitabine (Fig. 5b). In contrast, silencing of iNOS gene did not affect gemcitabine drug response.

Next, we investigated whether pharmacological inhibition could phenocopy above sensitization findings induced by siRNA silencing and selected PDPK1 as a major regulator for the activation of AGC kinases (serine/threonine kinases of the protein kinase A, G, and C family) and canonical AKT signaling in cancer cells. To show that LRCC also harbor increased PDPK1 activity, we first compared phospho-PDPK1 in the LRCC vs NLRCC fractions of the three cell lines next (Fig. 6a). In line with increased phospho-levels of PDPK1, levels of the upstream activator of PDPK1, phosphatidylinositol 3,4,5-trisphosphate (PIP3), required for membrane lipid binding and activation of PDPK1 for canonical AKT (AKT Serine/Threonine Kinase 1) activation was also significantly increased in LRCC vs NLRCC in all three cell lines (Fig. 6b). Next, we determined drug response profiles to the PDPK1 small molecule inhibitors BX795 and AR-12 in the three cell lines and selected concentrations of BX795 and AR-12 for gemcitabine combination studies which did not affect proliferation (Additional file 2: Figure S2). The addition of PDPK1 blockade increased the growth inhibitory effect of gemcitabine (Fig. 6c). In addition, the addition of the PDPK1 inhibitors to gemcitabine significantly increased the induction of apoptosis (Fig. 6d).

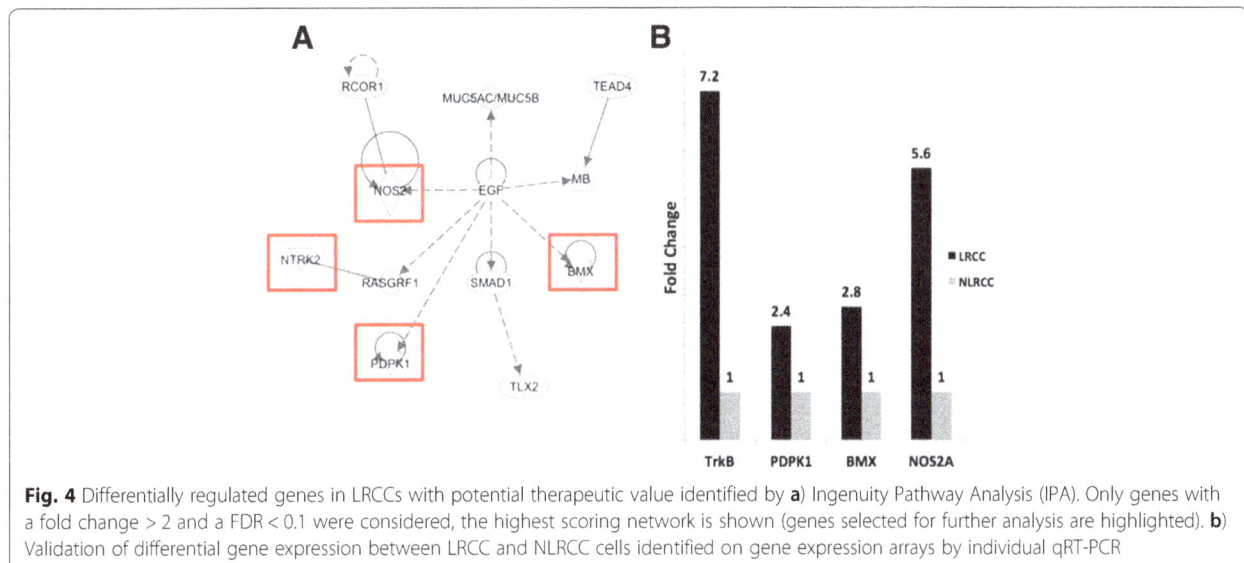

Fig. 4 Differentially regulated genes in LRCCs with potential therapeutic value identified by **a**) Ingenuity Pathway Analysis (IPA). Only genes with a fold change > 2 and a FDR < 0.1 were considered, the highest scoring network is shown (genes selected for further analysis are highlighted). **b**) Validation of differential gene expression between LRCC and NLRCC cells identified on gene expression arrays by individual qRT-PCR

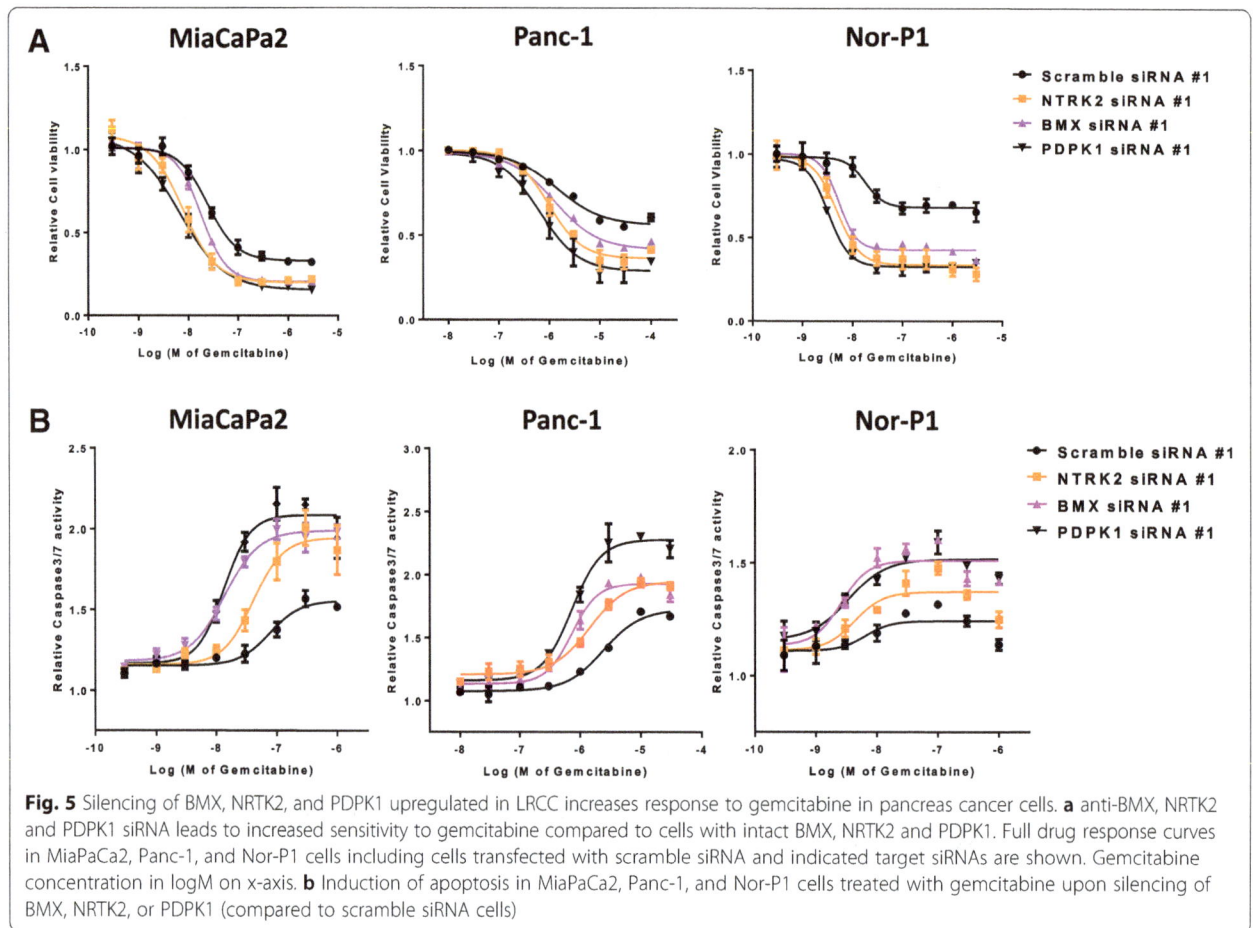

Fig. 5 Silencing of BMX, NRTK2, and PDPK1 upregulated in LRCC increases response to gemcitabine in pancreas cancer cells. **a** anti-BMX, NRTK2 and PDPK1 siRNA leads to increased sensitivity to gemcitabine compared to cells with intact BMX, NRTK2 and PDPK1. Full drug response curves in MiaPaCa2, Panc-1, and Nor-P1 cells including cells transfected with scramble siRNA and indicated target siRNAs are shown. Gemcitabine concentration in logM on x-axis. **b** Induction of apoptosis in MiaPaCa2, Panc-1, and Nor-P1 cells treated with gemcitabine upon silencing of BMX, NRTK2, or PDPK1 (compared to scramble siRNA cells)

PDPK1/PDK1 knockdown abrogates resistance to apoptosis in LRCC

To provide support that knockdown of kinases with elevated expression levels in the slowly cycling LRCC fraction was indeed involved in the altered gemcitabine drug phenotype, we studied the impact of PDPK1 silencing in the individual LRCC and NLRCC cell subpopulation on cell growth and induction of apoptosis upon gemcitabine exposure in the three cell lines next. Following FACS of Cy5$^+$ cells to separate LRCC and NLRCC, both cell populations were individually transfected with anti-PDPK1 siRNA. Equal knockdown in both cell populations was confirmed by qRT-PCR and viability and caspase levels of untreated cells transfected with scramble siRNA was set to 100%. In the absence of gemcitabine treatment there was minimal impact of loss of PDKP1 on cell viability or apoptosis levels in untreated cells when compared to cells transfected with scramble siRNA (Fig. 7a and b). In cells treated with gemcitabine, loss of PDPK1 affected growth of LRCC proportionally significantly more than the NLRCC fraction (% change compared to vehicle control cells of LRCC transfected with scramble siRNA vs PDPK1 siRNA: 80.23% vs 43.32% in MiaPaCa2, 92.28% vs 45.17% in Panc-1, and 77.88% vs 26.57% in

Nor-P1) (Fig. 7a). Similarly, upon loss of PDPK1 gemcitabine, apoptosis levels more in LRCC compared to NLRCC (% change compared to vehicle control transfected with scramble siRNA vs PDPK1 siRNA: 105.64% vs 177.69% in MiaPaCa2, 97.32% vs 144.63% in Panc-1, and 110.26% vs 145.36% in Nor-P1) (Fig. 7b). In summary, these findings suggest PDPK1 signaling to be essential in LRCC for the mediation of gemcitabine resistance.

PDPK1 is dysregulated in pancreatic cancer

To examine if correlative tissue studies on PDPK1 expression in clinical specimens support a role of this enzyme in pancreas cancer biology, we first examined levels of total PDPK1 expression in tumor versus matched normal, uninvolved pancreas tissue via IHC on a total of 40 pancreas cancer specimens. Significantly reduced PDPK1 levels were seen in the tumor specimens with a ≥ 5-fold reduction of the number of cases staining 2+ and a concomitant increase in the number of cases who lost PDPK1 or stained weakly positive in the tumors (Wilcoxon matched-pairs signed rank test; $p < 0.0001$) (Fig. 8a and b). We then examined association between PDPK1 expression levels and pathological variables and

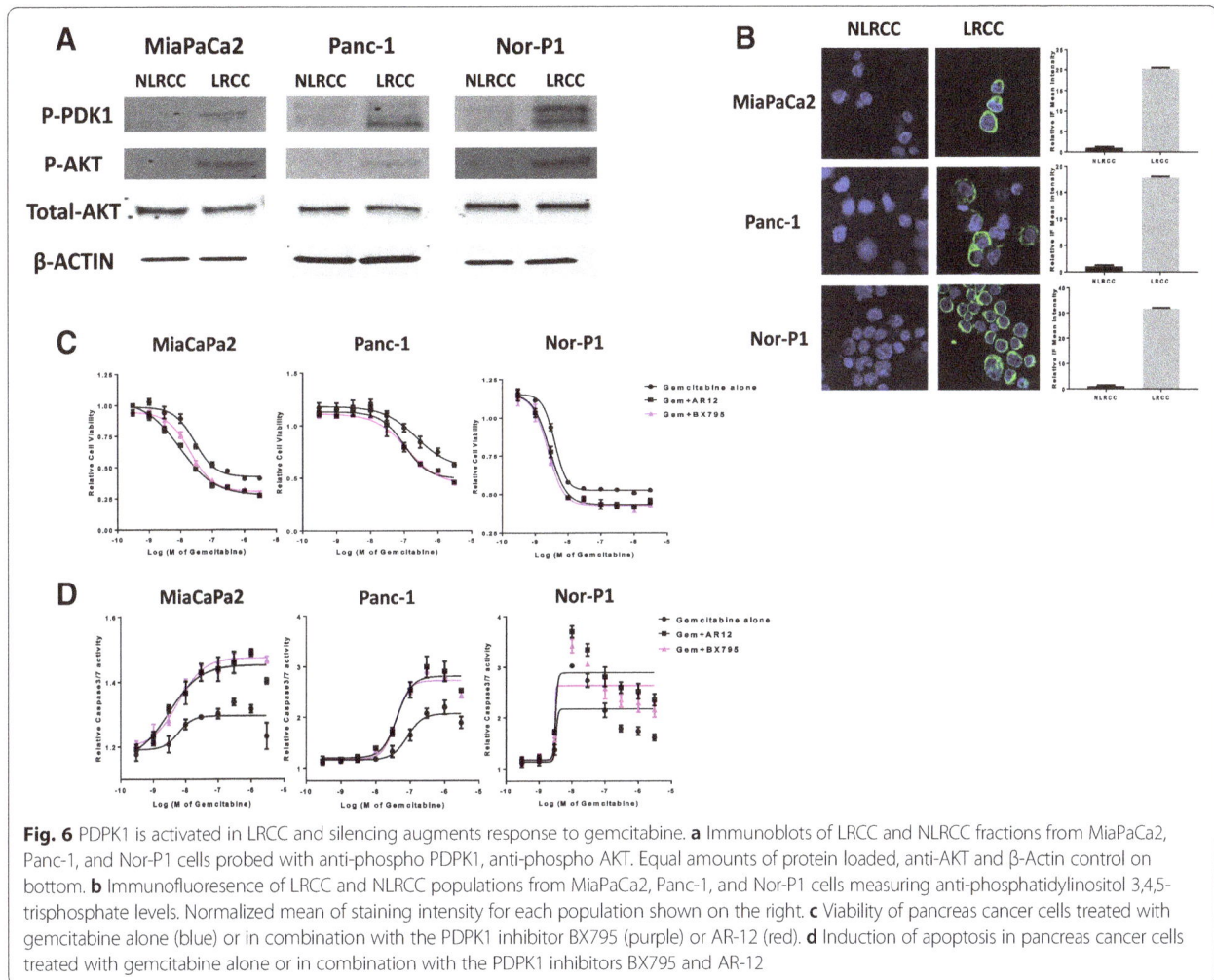

Fig. 6 PDPK1 is activated in LRCC and silencing augments response to gemcitabine. **a** Immunoblots of LRCC and NLRCC fractions from MiaPaCa2, Panc-1, and Nor-P1 cells probed with anti-phospho PDPK1, anti-phospho AKT. Equal amounts of protein loaded, anti-AKT and β-Actin control on bottom. **b** Immunofluoresence of LRCC and NLRCC populations from MiaPaCa2, Panc-1, and Nor-P1 cells measuring anti-phosphatidylinositol 3,4,5-trisphosphate levels. Normalized mean of staining intensity for each population shown on the right. **c** Viability of pancreas cancer cells treated with gemcitabine alone (blue) or in combination with the PDPK1 inhibitor BX795 (purple) or AR-12 (red). **d** Induction of apoptosis in pancreas cancer cells treated with gemcitabine alone or in combination with the PDPK1 inhibitors BX795 and AR-12

clinical outcome including overall survival. There was no association of overall expression with survival or correlation with one of the pathological variables nuclear grade, differentiation, or involvement of locoregional lymph nodes. Since a majority of studies on the potential role of PI3K-PDPK1-AKT signal transduction in a number of malignancies, including pancreas cancer, found that activation state measured as phosphorylation rather than amplification or overall expression levels to be clinically significant, we re-examined staining pattern of PDPK1 for membranous vs cytoplasmic staining. For PDPK1 to be activated by phosphatidylinositol (3,4,5)-trisphosphate (PIP3) generated by PI3K, its N-terminal pleckstrin homology domain provides a lipid-anchoring part to direct PDPK1 to PI3K-generated PIP3, recruiting the enzyme to the plasma membrane. Using membrane recruitment as a measure of PDPK1 activation, we compared membranous versus cytoplasmic staining patterns with nuclear grade distribution, lymph node involvement, and survival. Only ~ 15% of cases showed membranous staining. Membranous staining was negatively

correlated with high nuclear grade ($p = 0.0029$, Fig. 8c) and there was a trend towards improved survival in patients who showed membranous PDPK1 staining in their surgical or biopsy specimens (Fig. 8d). Membranous staining was not associated with overall expression levels. These observed associations of perturbations of PDPK1 expression patterns in patients' specimens suggest that PDPK1 regulation might be involved in pancreatic carcinogenesis and pancreas cancer biology.

Discussion

Conventional treatment with systemic cytotoxic chemotherapeutics, which non-specifically targets rapidly dividing cells, is ideally replaced, or supplemented, by therapy that targets the cells driving recurrence and metastasis—the primary causes of most cancer-related death for patients afflicted by pancreas cancer [3]. Here we demonstrate that by inhibiting genes overexpressed in label-retaining cancer cells, an in vitro model of slowly cycling cells and subpopulation of CSC, can improve response to the standard cytotoxic chemotherapy with gemcitabine.

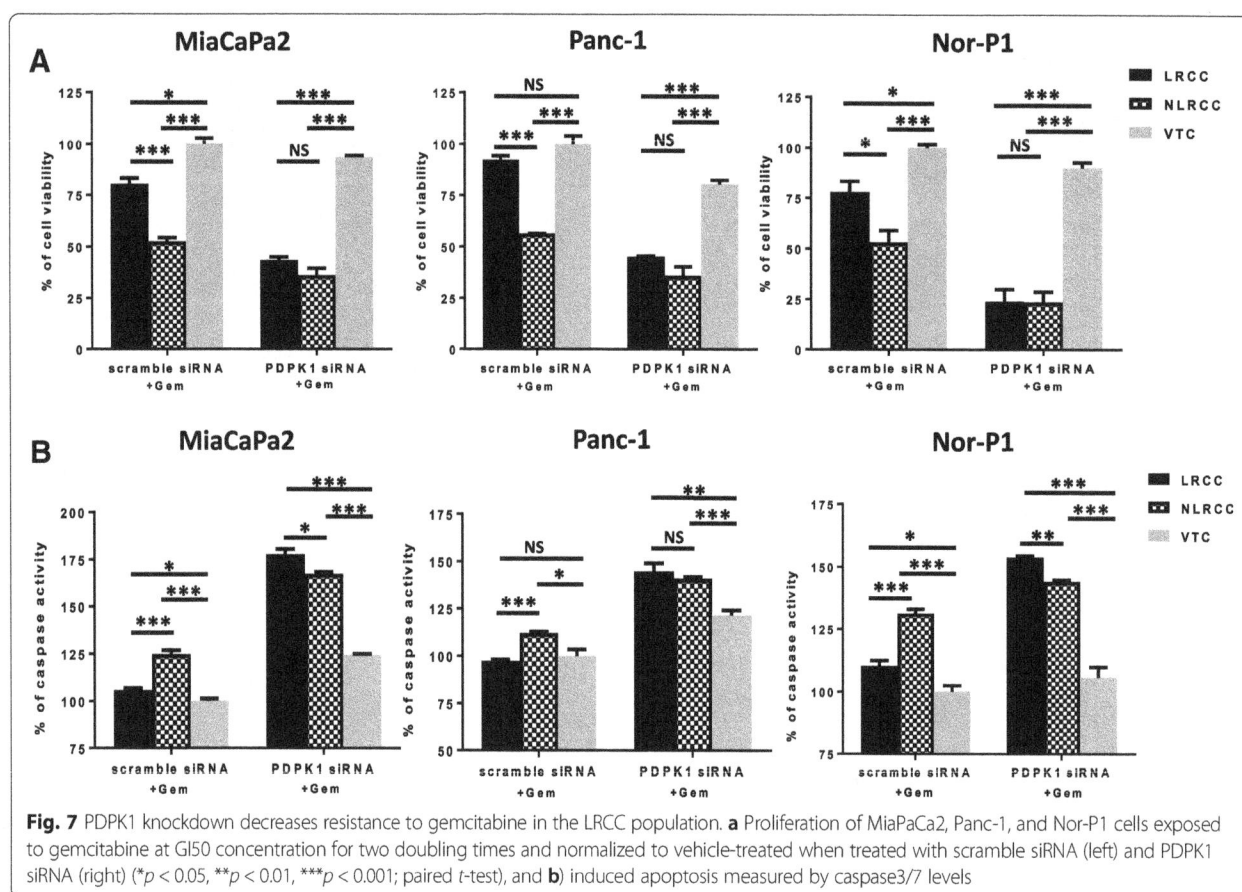

Fig. 7 PDPK1 knockdown decreases resistance to gemcitabine in the LRCC population. **a** Proliferation of MiaPaCa2, Panc-1, and Nor-P1 cells exposed to gemcitabine at GI50 concentration for two doubling times and normalized to vehicle-treated when treated with scramble siRNA (left) and PDPK1 siRNA (right) (*$p < 0.05$, **$p < 0.01$, ***$p < 0.001$; paired t-test), and **b**) induced apoptosis measured by caspase3/7 levels

The rationale of manipulating sub-populations of malignant cells within a tumor, in particular sub-populations involved in chemoresistance and metastasis, has recently been shown in elegant murine models of breast and pancreas cancer, and could have important implications in the treatment of patients with cancer [34–36].

While the identification of cancer stem cells in the literature is largely based on cell surface phenotype [12–14, 37–39], previous work from our group and others has shown that identification of a population of cells based on proposed function and hierarchy within a tumor is possible [19, 40]. Our group has previously shown that LRCC undergo asymmetric cell division with non-random chromosomal cosegregation (ACD-NRCC), which is consistent with the carcinogenesis (initiation and promotion) portion of the cancer stem cell theory [18, 20, 41]. Further, LRCC have been shown to be more tumorigenic, which is consistent with the tumor progression (tumor growth and metastasis) portion of the cancer stem cell theory [18, 25]. More recently, there have been more reports on LRCC mediating chemoresistance, early tumor recurrence, and metastasis [29, 42, 43]. However, there has been only one report on slowly cycling cells in pancreas cancer using the label DiI, and a surprising paucity on intracellular signaling features

unique to LRCC governing chemoresistance or tumor initiation [44]. In this report we aimed to assess the possible clinical significance of the LRCC population in terms of response to gemcitabine, one of the standard therapies for patients with pancreas cancer. Deriving LRCC from different pancreatic cancer cell lines we first showed that LRCC are, in fact, resistant to this'therapeutic' agent and that decreased rates of apoptosis upon gemcitabine treatment contributed to gemcitabine resistance phenotype of LRCC. One of the initially vexing findings was the decreased reduction of NLRCC growth after gemcitabine administration without a concomitant increase in the LRCC cells. We attributed this to the relative short treatment course of two doubling times possibly too short to detect differences considering the small number of LRCC but also possibly to a to-date incompletely understood interplay between LRCC and non-cancer stem cells along the concept of the 'stem cell niche'. We speculate that LRCC might feed resistance signals to the bulk population but as viability and growth of NLRCC decreases as a consequence of the cytotoxic treatment ultimately also the pool of stem cells or LRCC is afflicted. Tumor resistance has then developed when stem cells recreate the niche, a biological function our presented in vitro LRCC model with limited gemcitabine

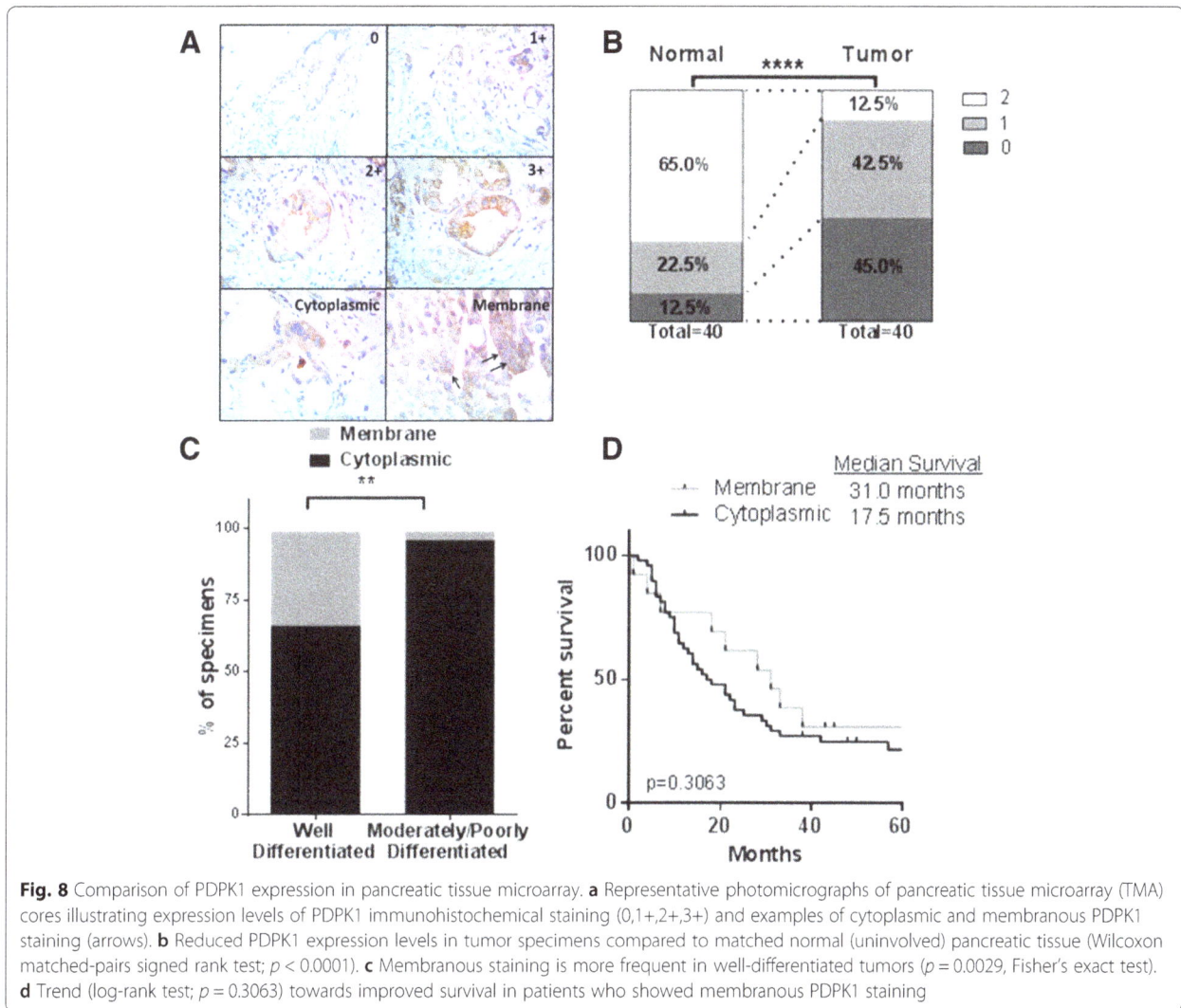

Fig. 8 Comparison of PDPK1 expression in pancreatic tissue microarray. **a** Representative photomicrographs of pancreatic tissue microarray (TMA) cores illustrating expression levels of PDPK1 immunohistochemical staining (0,1+,2+,3+) and examples of cytoplasmic and membranous PDPK1 staining (arrows). **b** Reduced PDPK1 expression levels in tumor specimens compared to matched normal (uninvolved) pancreatic tissue (Wilcoxon matched-pairs signed rank test; $p < 0.0001$). **c** Membranous staining is more frequent in well-differentiated tumors ($p = 0.0029$, Fisher's exact test). **d** Trend (log-rank test; $p = 0.3063$) towards improved survival in patients who showed membranous PDPK1 staining

exposure times was not able to measure. Such dynamic interplay between non-cancer stem cells and cancer stem cells has now been observed in a number of in vitro models and early paracrine signaling cues involved in this crosstalk involve HIFα (hypoxia inducible factors' α subunits), sonic hedgehog, TGFβ1 (transforming growth factor beta 1), and nodal/activin to name some described from pancreatic cancer stem cell niche models or, importantly, prostaglandin E2-induced repopulation of the tumor following chemotherapy treatment from the slowly cycling CSC as shown in patient-derived xenotransplanted bladder cancer [27, 45, 46].

In order to investigate differences between the two cell populations and possibly home in on mechanisms of action governing inherent chemoresistance features of the LRCC sub-population, we compared transcriptomic profiles of LRCC to the NLRCC population and identified a top-ranking network by IPA enriched for EGF ligand signaling. Of note, this network is different from the

canonical erb receptor tyrosine kinase signal transduction cascades focusing on immediate EGFR (epidermal growth factor receptor) or HER2 (human epidermal growth factor receptor 2) downstream signaling studied in many cancers and more similar to finding from our prior work identifying EGF and MET-mediated signaling as top regulators of cell fate and lineage specific progenitor cell differentiation in the liver [41]. Studies by Takebe and Jeanes et al. in breast and other solid tumors on cell differentiation and stemness have also reported on an intimate role of a more extended, non-canonical erb signaling network and cancer stemness [47, 48]. We selected three kinases of the network for further loss-of-function studies and showed that NTRK2/TrkB, PDPK1/PDK1, and BMX/ETK were involved in regulation of gemcitabine sensitivity. Individual knockdown of PDPK1/PDK1 in both the LRCC and NLRCC subpopulations demonstrated that PDPK1/PDK1 inhibition lowered resistance to gemcitabine preferentially in the

LRCC population and less in the NLRCC cells. Loss of PDPK1 had minimal impact on growth and apoptosis rates of untreated cells suggesting an essential role of this regulator in the LRCC population. Along these lines, recent work has PDPK1 also been implicated in the regulation of self-renewal, cellular transformation, and stemness in several diseases including cancer. Of importance, this work identified downstream signaling cascades regulated by PDPK1 outside the canonical receptor tyrosine kinase, PI3K and AKT-cascade PDKP1 was first described. These include phospholipase C, protein kinase C, or Hippo signaling governing stemness features through crosstalk with WNT [wingless-type MMTV (mouse mammary tumor virus) integration site] or β-catenin signaling [49–52].

In pancreas cancer, Eser et al. have shown that PDK1 is an essential effector of KRAS, and that an intact PDK1/PI3K axis is an essential tumor initiating event in cooperation with KRAS for increased cell plasticity, acinar-to-ductal metaplasia (ADM), and pancreatic ductal adenocarcinoma (PDAC) formation [53]. The pro-tumor function of an intact PI3K/PDPK1 axis reported by Eser and colleagues appears to be at odds with our findings of decreased PDPK1 expression levels in tumor tissues, and the associations of membranous localization with well-differentiated tumors and a trend towards improved clinical outcome. PDPK1 signals in a PI3K-depedent manner activating AKT, S6K (ribosomal protein S6 kinase), and SGK (serum/glucocorticoid regulated kinase) but can also activate PKC and p90RSK independent of PI3K and PIP3-mediated activation. PKC (protein kinase C) and p90RSK (p90 ribosomal S6 kinase) were found activated by alternative RAS-mediated signaling pathways independent of PDPK1 in the study by Eser et al. suggesting a non-essential role of PDPK1 in these tumors [53]. Additionally, downstream PDPK1 canonical signaling measured by phospho-AKT and phospho-GSK3β (S9) levels was lower in the evolved pancreas cancers compared to pre-cursor ADM and PanIN lesions also raising the possibility of the more involved cancers having become independent of the PDPK1 signaling axis and more driven by signal transduction perturbations of additional pathways acquired during the later stages of pancreas cancer progression [53]. Such a hypothesis appears to be in line with the decreased PDPK1 expression levels in the tumor vs matched clinical specimens on tissue microarray staining. While correlative tissue studies with phospho-AKT measures have shown the more commonly found negative correlation between increased AKT activation and clinical outcome, it is possible that there is a subset of pancreas cancer, similar to studies in non-small cell lung cancer, where phospho-AKT levels as a measure of EGFR-PI3K-AKT signaling have been shown to be associated with improved outcome [54–57]. It is intriguing to speculate that the hypothesis of a greater dependency on PDPK1 signaling in the early tumor-initiating events of ADM and PanIN formation, as seen in the transgenic animal studies, versus a later loss of addiction to canonical PDPK1 signaling and overtake by PDPK1 independent oncogenic events is commensurate with the cancer stem cell hallmark of tumor initiation by this cell population [12, 53]. Irrespective of possible differences in PDPK1 function in early vs late or primary vs metastatic tumors as a possible explanation of the observed PDPK1 expression pattern on our cancer tissue microarrays, the association of the heterogeneous PDPK1 expression pattern with important clinicopathological outcomes appears to be in line with the intratumoral heterogeneity of this regulator found to be overexpressed and activated in the LRCC vs NLRCC subpopulations where it is essential for chemoresistance.

On a preclinical level, PDPK1 has shown to confer oncogenic signaling and CSC renewal. The other targets derived from the differential gene expression screen in LRCC vs NLRCC have also been previously linked to stemness. The Tec kinase BMX non-receptor tyrosine kinase (BMX) has been shown a tumor promoting role in gliolastoma multiforme through mediation of self-renewal and growth, and the neurotrophic tyrosine receptor kinase 2 (NRTK2) in precursor growth and differentiation [14, 58, 59]. On the other hand, the gene expression differences identified in our in vitro model of cancer stemness, LRCC vs NRLCC, showed limited overlap with other in vitro models comparing gene expression and pathway alterations between stem cell and non-cancer stem cell fractions. For example, similar IPA network analysis comparing 3D spheroid Panc1 cells, originally described as the invasive Panc1 cell population, versus 2D monolayer cells resembling non-cancer stem cells identified as the top differentially regulated network genes involved in DNA damage repair [60]. When comparing side population versus non-side population bulk cells from patient-derived xenograft models an extensive network enriched with transcription factors of pluripotency, cell differentiation, and EMT (epithelial-mesenchymal transition) can be identified [61]. Whether these differences are due to the different platforms or due to the increasingly recognized heterogeneity of different CSC population is currently not known. The two currently available drug discovery studies performed in pancreas cancer stem cell in vitro models using either a reporter line for the 26S proteasome activity of pancreas cancer cells or a 3D pancreatic carcinoma spheroid model yielded drug activities in the 3D CSC model with inhibition of phosphoinositide 3-kinase signaling, however there was an underrepresentation of selective PDPK1 inhibitors [62, 63].

This study is not without its limitations. First, the isolation of LRCC requires the assumption that all cells within the Cy5+ labeled population are expanding at the same rate. Since long term cultured cell lines were used, this assumption is based on the clonality and homogeneity of these lines. While cells were synchronized via transfer to serum-free media 24 h prior to labeling we cannot rule out that present clonal subpopulation with different growth rates in the used pancreas cancer cell lines increased the NLRCC subpopulation. However, we believe this fraction to be small. Second, the apoptosis experiments upon administration of gemcitabine were based on the concentration of the drug for 50% of maximal inhibition of cell proliferation, GI50, after two doubling times (determined individually for each cell line). This includes experiments on induction of apoptosis upon silencing of the genes found to be overexpressed in the LRCC population. We cannot rule out that the impact on induction of apoptosis, or silencing of PDPK1 on gemcitabine drug response, might have been higher or lower either in the LRCC or NLRCC populations when other concentrations were used. For the presented in vitro comparisons, it was necessary to establish a consistent cutoff point that allowed for comparisons including downstream evaluation (i.e. qRT-PCR, cell cycle analysis, FACS) without complete mortality of the cells after gemcitabine exposure.

Conclusion

In summary, we present in LRCC, an in vitro model of slowly cycling pancreatic cancer stem cells implicated in chemoresistance and tumor recurrence, the discovery of novel targets involved in response to gemcitabine treatment, one of the standard chemotherapy approaches used for pancreas cancer in the clinic. For decades, chemotherapy regimens have been based on the cell cycle differential that exists between normal and malignant tissue. Given the continued and unchanged dismal prognosis for patients with pancreas cancer this rationale has proven not specific enough and not sufficiently efficacious. Here, we have shown that LRCC harbor distinct transcriptomic profiles involved in mediation of chemoresistance and that targeting essential regulators of this program in LRCC can sensitize pancreas cancer cells. These findings offer novel hypotheses for the derivation of effective combination therapy approaches in a disease void of impactful interventions.

Additional files

Additional file 1: Figure S1. Confirmation of silencing of BMX, NRTK2, and PDPK1 mediated by siRNA (set 1- #1) knockdown. A) Expression level of BMX, NRTK2 and PDPK1 in in MiaPaCa2, Panc-1, and Nor-P1 cells when scramble siRNA or anti- BMX, NRTK2 and PDPK1 siRNA (set 1- #1) are present. B) Protein level of BMX, NRTK2 and PDPK1 of the three cell lines in immunoblotting. C) anti-BMX, NRTK2 and PDPK1 siRNA (set 2- #2) leads to increased sensitivity to gemcitabine compared to cells with intact BMX, NRTK2 and PDPK1. Full drug response curves in MiaPaCa2, Panc-1, and Nor-P1 cells including cells transfected with scramble siRNA and indicated target siRNAs (set 2- #2) are shown.

Additional file 2: Figure S2. Full drug response curves of the PDPK1 inhibitor BX795 (purple, A) or AR-12 (red, B) in MiaPaCa2, Panc-1, and Nor-P1 cells.

Abbreviations

ACD-NRCC: Asymmetric cell division with non-random chromosomal cosegregation; ADM: Acinar-to-ductal metaplasia; AGC Kinases: serine/threonine kinases of the protein kinase A, G, and C family; AKT: AKT Serine/Threonine Kinase 1; BMX: BMX non-receptor tyrosine kinase; CSC: Cycling cancer stem cells; EGF: Epidermal growth factor; EGFR: Epidermal growth factor receptor; EMT: Epithelial-mesenchymal transition; HER2: Human epidermal growth factor receptor 2 (receptor tyrosine-protein kinase erbB-2); HIFα: Hypoxia inducible factors' α subunits; LRC: Label retaining cells; LRCC: Label-retaining cancer cells; NOS2A: NOS2 nitric oxide synthase 2; NTRK2: Neurotrophic receptor tyrosine kinase 2; P90RSK: p90 ribosomal S6 kinase; PDAC: Pancreatic ductal adenocarcinoma; PDPK1 (PDK1): 3-phosphoinositide dependent protein kinase-1; PI: Propidium iodide; PIP3: Phosphatidylinositol 3,4,5-trisphosphate; PKC: Protein kinase C; S6K: Ribosomal Protein S6 Kinase; SGK: Serum/glucocorticoid regulated kinase; TGFβ: Transforming growth factor beta; TMA: Tissue microarray; WNT: Wingless-type MMTV (mouse mammary tumor virus) integration site

Funding

This study was supported, in part, by the Intramural Research Program (IRP) of the NIH, National Cancer Institute, Center for Cancer Research (ZIA BC 011267) and donations from 'Running for Rachel' and the Pomerenk family via the Rachel Guss and Bob Pomerenk Pancreas Cancer Research Fellowship to NCI. The funding body had no role in the design of the study and collection, analysis, and interpretation of data or in writing of the manuscript. The study was conducted within the mission of the IRP and designed, conducted, analyzed, and summarized as listed under Authors Contributions. The opinions expressed in this article are the author's own and do not reflect the view of the National Institutes of Health, the Department of Health and Human Services, or the United States government.

Authors' contributions

The study was designed by ST, IA and UR. DL, JM and GW were involved in isolation of LRCC, determination of LRCC fractions, and cell cycle analysis of LRCC. DL and JM conducted all the in-vitro drug response experiments, cell viability, apoptosis, siRNA silencing, and immuno-blotting experiments. Gene expression microarrays, analysis and bioinformatics were conducted by HW, JM and AA. Tissue microarray analysis was conducted by TA and DL, who together with JM compiled all the figures. The manuscript was written by DL, JM and UR and approved by all co-authors.

Competing interests

The authors declare that they have no competing interests.

Author details

[1]Rare Tumor Initiative, Cancer for Cancer Research, National Cancer Institute, Building 10, Room 2B-38E, Bethesda, MD, USA. [2]Sarcoma Department, Moffitt Cancer Center, Tampa, FL, USA. [3]Thoracic & GI Oncology Branch, Center for Cancer Research, National Cancer Institute, Bethesda, MD, USA. [4]Department of Surgery, University of Wisconsin School of Medicine and Public Health, Madison, WI, USA. [5]Laboratory of Oncology, Center for Molecular Medicine and Department of Molecular Biology and Biochemistry, School of Basic Medicine, Yangtze University, Jingzhou, Hubei, China. [6]Flow Cytometry Core, Hollings Cancer Center, Medical University of South Carolina, Charleston, SC, USA. [7]Gilead Sciences, Foster City, CA, USA. [8]Laboratory of Experimental

Carcinogenesis, Center for Cancer Research, National Cancer Institute, NIH, Bethesda, USA. ⁹St. Peter's Hospital, Rutgers University, Robert Wood Johnson School of Medicine, New Brunswick, NJ, USA.

References

1. Siegel RL, Miller KD, Jemal A. Cancer statistics, 2016. CA Cancer J Clin. 2016; 66:7–30.

2. Rahib L, Smith BD, Aizenberg R, et al. Projecting cancer incidence and deaths to 2030: the unexpected burden of thyroid, liver, and pancreas cancers in the United States. Cancer Res. 2014;74:2913–21.

3. Ma J, Jemal A. The rise and fall of cancer mortality in the USA: why does pancreatic cancer not follow the trend? Future Oncol. 2013;9:917–9.

4. Conroy T, Desseigne F, Ychou M, et al. FOLFIRINOX versus gemcitabine for metastatic pancreatic cancer. N Engl J Med. 2011;364:1817–25.

5. Von Hoff DD, Ervin T, Arena FP, et al. Increased survival in pancreatic cancer with nab-paclitaxel plus gemcitabine. N Engl J Med. 2013;369:1691–703.

6. McDermott SP, Wicha MS. Targeting breast cancer stem cells. Mol Oncol. 2010;4:404–19.

7. Kreso A, Dick JE. Evolution of the cancer stem cell model. Cell Stem Cell. 2014;14:275–91.

8. Li C, Heidt DG, Dalerba P, et al. Identification of pancreatic cancer stem cells. Cancer Res. 2007;67:1030–7.

9. Yachida S, Jones S, Bozic I, et al. Distant metastasis occurs late during the genetic evolution of pancreatic cancer. Nature. 2010;467:1114–7.

10. Waclaw B, Bozic I, Pittman ME, et al. A spatial model predicts that dispersal and cell turnover limit intratumour heterogeneity. Nature. 2015;525:261–4.

11. Vicente-Duenas C, Romero-Camarero I, Cobaleda C, et al. Function of oncogenes in cancer development: a changing paradigm. EMBO J. 2013;32: 1502–13.

12. Hermann PC, Huber SL, Herrler T, et al. Distinct populations of cancer stem cells determine tumor growth and metastatic activity in human pancreatic cancer. Cell Stem Cell. 2007;1:313–23.

13. Al-Hajj M, Wicha MS, Benito-Hernandez A, et al. Prospective identification of tumorigenic breast cancer cells. Proc Natl Acad Sci U S A. 2003;100:3983–8.

14. Bartkowska K, Paquin A, Gauthier AS, et al. Trk signaling regulates neural precursor cell proliferation and differentiation during cortical development. Development. 2007;134:4369–80.

15. Shah AN, Summy JM, Zhang J, et al. Development and characterization of gemcitabine-resistant pancreatic tumor cells. Ann Surg Oncol. 2007;14: 3629–37.

16. Cairns J. Mutation selection and the natural history of Cancer. Nature. 1975; 255:197–200.

17. Potten CS, Hume WJ, Reid P, et al. The segregation of DNA in epithelial stem cells. Cell. 1978;15:899–906.

18. Xin HW, Ambe CM, Hari DM, et al. Label-retaining liver cancer cells are relatively resistant to sorafenib. Gut. 2013;62:1777–86.

19. Hari D, Xin H-W, Jaiswal K, et al. Isolation of live label-retaining cells and cells undergoing asymmetric cell division via nonrandom chromosomal Cosegregation from human cancers. Stem Cells Dev. 2011;20(10):1649-58.

20. Xin HW, Hari DM, Mullinax JE, et al. Tumor-initiating label-retaining cancer cells in human gastrointestinal cancers undergo asymmetric cell division. Stem Cells. 2012;30:591–8.

21. Schillert A, Trumpp A, Sprick MR. Label retaining cells in cancer--the dormant root of evil? Cancer Lett. 2013;341:73–9.

22. Deleyrolle LP, Harding A, Cato K, et al. Evidence for label-retaining tumour-initiating cells in human glioblastoma. Brain. 2011;134:1331–43.

23. Moore N, Houghton J, Lyle S. Slow-cycling therapy-resistant cancer cells. Stem Cells Dev. 2012;21:1822–30.

24. Xin HW, Ambe CM, Miller TC, et al. Liver label retaining Cancer cells are relatively resistant to the reported anti-Cancer stem cell drug metformin. J Cancer. 2016;7:1142–51.

25. Perego M, Maurer M, Wang JX, et al. A slow-cycling subpopulation of melanoma cells with highly invasive properties. Oncogene. 2018;37:302–12.

26. Zhang D, Jeter C, Gong S, et al. Histone 2B-GFP label-retaining prostate luminal cells possess progenitor cell properties and are intrinsically resistant to castration. Stem Cell Reports. 2018;10:228–42.

27. Kurtova AV, Xiao J, Mo Q, et al. Blocking PGE2-induced tumour repopulation abrogates bladder cancer chemoresistance. Nature. 2015;517:209–13.

28. Balic M, Lin H, Young L, et al. Most early disseminated cancer cells detected in bone marrow of breast cancer patients have a putative breast cancer stem cell phenotype. Clin Cancer Res. 2006;12:5615–21.

29. Morgan TM, Lange PH, Porter MP, et al. Disseminated tumor cells in prostate cancer patients after radical prostatectomy and without evidence of disease predicts biochemical recurrence. Clin Cancer Res. 2009;15:677–83.

30. Pine SR, Ryan BM, Varticovski L, et al. Microenvironmental modulation of asymmetric cell division in human lung cancer cells. Proc Natl Acad Sci U S A. 2010;107:2195–200.

31. Takikita M, Altekruse S, Lynch CF, et al. Associations between selected biomarkers and prognosis in a population-based pancreatic Cancer tissue microarray. Cancer Res. 2009;69:2950–5.

32. Cabarcas SM, Mathews LA, Farrar WL. The cancer stem cell niche--there goes the neighborhood? Int J Cancer. 2011;129:2315–27.

33. Van den Broeck A, Gremeaux L, Topal B, et al. Human pancreatic adenocarcinoma contains a side population resistant to gemcitabine. BMC Cancer. 2012;12:354.

34. Polyak K, Weinberg RA. Transitions between epithelial and mesenchymal states: acquisition of malignant and stem cell traits. Nat Rev Cancer. 2009;9:265–73.

35. Zheng X, Carstens JL, Kim J, et al. Epithelial-to-mesenchymal transition is dispensable for metastasis but induces chemoresistance in pancreatic cancer. Nature. 2015;527:525–30.

36. Fischer KR, Durrans A, Lee S, et al. Epithelial-to-mesenchymal transition is not required for lung metastasis but contributes to chemoresistance. Nature. 2015;527:472–6.

37. Dontu G, Al-Hajj M, Abdallah W, et al. Stem cells in normal breast development and breast Cancer. Cell Prolif. 2003;36:59–72.

38. Korkaya H, Paulson A, Charafe-Jauffret E, et al. Regulation of mammary stem/progenitor cells by PTEN/Akt/beta-catenin signaling. PLoS Biol. 2009;7: e1000121.

39. Lapidot T, Sirard C, Vormoor J, et al. A cell initiating human acute myeloid Leukaemia after transplantation into SCID mice. Nature. 1994;367:645–8.

40. Moore N, Lyle S. Quiescent, slow-cycling stem cell populations in cancer: a review of the evidence and discussion of significance. J Oncol. 2011;2011.

41. Kitade M, Factor VM, Andersen JB, et al. Specific fate decisions in adult hepatic progenitor cells driven by MET and EGFR signaling. Genes Dev. 2013;27:1706–17.

42. Fillmore CM, Kuperwasser C. Human breast cancer cell lines contain stem-like cells that self-renew, give rise to phenotypically diverse progeny and survive chemotherapy. Breast Cancer Res. 2008;10:R25.

43. Roesch A, Fukunaga-Kalabis M, Schmidt EC, et al. A temporarily distinct subpopulation of slow-cycling melanoma cells is required for continuous tumor growth. Cell. 2010;141:583–94.

44. Dembinski JL, Krauss S. Characterization and functional analysis of a slow cycling stem cell-like subpopulation in pancreas adenocarcinoma. Clin Exp Metastasis. 2009;26:611–23.

45. Sainz B, Alcala S, Garcia E, et al. Microenvironmental hCAP-18/LL-37 promotes pancreatic ductal adenocarcinoma by activating its cancer stem cell compartment. Gut. 2015;64:1921–35.

46. Carnero A, Lleonart M. The hypoxic microenvironment: a determinant of cancer stem cell evolution. Inside the Cell. 2016;1:96–105.

47. Takebe N, Warren RQ, Ivy SP. Breast cancer growth and metastasis: interplay between cancer stem cells, embryonic signaling pathways and epithelial-to-mesenchymal transition. Breast Cancer Res. 2011;13:211.

48. Jeanes A, Gottardi CJ, Yap AS. Cadherins and cancer: how does cadherin dysfunction promote tumor progression? Oncogene. 2008;27:6920–9.

49. Cunningham JT, Ruggero D. New connections between old pathways: PDK1 signaling promotes cellular transformation through PLK1-dependent MYC stabilization. Cancer Discov. 2013;3:1099–102.

50. Tan J, Li Z, Lee PL, et al. PDK1 signaling toward PLK1-MYC activation confers oncogenic transformation, tumor-initiating cell activation, and resistance to mTOR-targeted therapy. Cancer Discov. 2013;3:1156–71.

51. Shahbazian D, Roux PP, Mieulet V, et al. The mTOR/PI3K and MAPK pathways converge on eIF4B to control its phosphorylation and activity. EMBO J. 2006;25:2781–91.

52. Fan R, Kim NG, Gumbiner BM. Regulation of hippo pathway by mitogenic growth factors via phosphoinositide 3-kinase and phosphoinositide-dependent kinase-1. Proc Natl Acad Sci U S A. 2013;110:2569–74.

53. Eser S, Reiff N, Messer M, et al. Selective requirement of PI3K/PDK1 signaling for Kras oncogene-driven pancreatic cell plasticity and cancer. Cancer Cell. 2013;23:406–20.

54. Cicenas J. The potential role of Akt phosphorylation in human cancers. Int J Biol Markers. 2008;23:1–9.

55. Shah A, Swain WA, Richardson D, et al. Phospho-Akt expression is associated with a favorable outcome in non-small cell lung cancer. Clin Cancer Res. 2005;11:2930–6.

56. Schlieman MG, Fahy BN, Ramsamooj R, et al. Incidence, mechanism and prognostic value of activated AKT in pancreas cancer. Br J Cancer. 2003; 89:2110–5.

57. Yamamoto S, Tomita Y, Hoshida Y, et al. Prognostic significance of activated Akt expression in pancreatic ductal adenocarcinoma. Clin Cancer Res. 2004; 10:2846–50.

58. Guryanova OA, Wu Q, Cheng L, et al. Nonreceptor tyrosine kinase BMX maintains self-renewal and tumorigenic potential of glioblastoma stem cells by activating STAT3. Cancer Cell. 2011;19:498–511.

59. Nikoletopoulou V, Lickert H, Frade JM, et al. Neurotrophin receptors TrkA and TrkC cause neuronal death whereas TrkB does not. Nature. 2010;467:59–63.

60. Mathews LA, Cabarcas SM, Hurt EM, et al. Increased expression of DNA repair genes in invasive human pancreatic cancer cells. Pancreas. 2011; 40:730–9.

61. Williams SA, Anderson WC, Santaguida MT, et al. Patient-derived xenografts, the cancer stem cell paradigm, and cancer pathobiology in the 21st century. Lab Investig. 2013;93:970–82.

62. Adikrisna R, Tanaka S, Muramatsu S, et al. Identification of pancreatic cancer stem cells and selective toxicity of chemotherapeutic agents. Gastroenterology. 2012;143:234–45 e7.

63. Mathews Griner LA, Zhang X, Guha R, et al. Large-scale pharmacological profiling of 3D tumor models of cancer cells. Cell Death Dis. 2016;7:e2492.

A novel feedback loop between high MALAT-1 and low miR-200c-3p promotes cell migration and invasion in pancreatic ductal adenocarcinoma and is predictive of poor prognosis

Meng Zhuo[1†], Cuncun Yuan[2†], Ting Han[1†], Jiujie Cui[1], Feng Jiao[1*] and Liwei Wang[1*]

Abstract

Background: It was demonstrated that long non-coding RNAs occupied an important position in tumor pathogenesis and progression. We have previously found that the metastasis-associated lung adenocarcinoma transcript 1 (MALAT-1) promotes cell proliferation and metastases in pancreatic ductal adenocarcinoma (PDAC). The present study was aimed to discuss the underlying mechanisms.

Methods: Bioinformatics method was used to identify the miRNA target of MALAT-1. Expressions of relative genes were assessed by quantitative real-time PCR and western blotting, respectively. Sulforhodamine B assay and Transwell assay were employed to detect cell proliferation, migration and invasion, respectively. Moreover, RNA immunoprecipitation was performed to determine whether RNA-induced silencing complex contained MALAT-1 and its potential binding miRNA. Luciferase assays was used to confirm potential binding site.

Results: Bioinformatics search predicted that miR-200c-3p was a direct target of MALAT-1. Further, we found a reciprocal suppression between MALAT-1 and miR-200c-3p expression. In terms of mechanisms, high MALAT-1 and low miR-200c-3p may form a novel feedback loop. On the one hand, MALAT-1 functioned as a competing endogenous RNA to suppress miR-200c-3p expression, leading to upregulation of ZEB1 expression. On the other hand, miR-200c-3p inhibited the level of MALAT-1 expression was in a way similar to miRNA-mediated downregulation of target genes. Clinical data further indicated that MALAT-1 and ZEB1 expression was negatively correlated with miR-200c-3p transcript level of PDAC tissues. There was a positive correlation between MALAT-1 and ZEB1 level. MALAT-1 (high)/miR-200c-3p (low) correlated with shorter overall survival of PDAC patients. Multivariate analysis revealed that both MALAT-1 and miR-200c-3p levels were independent prognostic factors.

Conclusion: Our findings firstly revealed a novel feedback loop between high MALAT-1 and low miR-200c-3p. Targeting the feedback loop between high MALAT-1 and low miR-200c-3p will be a therapeutic strategy for PDAC.

Keywords: Pancreatic ductal adenocarcinoma, Metastasis-associated lung adenocarcinoma transcript 1, miR-200c-3p, ZEB1, Feedback loop

* Correspondence: jiao_f@yeah.net; liweiwang@shsmu.edu.cn
†Meng Zhuo, Cuncun Yuan and Ting Han contributed equally to this work.
[1]Department of Oncology, Renji Hospital, School of Medicine, Shanghai Jiaotong University, 160 Pujian Road, Shanghai 200127, China
Full list of author information is available at the end of the article

Background

Pancreatic ductal adenocarcinoma (PDAC) is considered to be one of the most lethal tumor worldwide [1] and will become the second leading cause of tumor-associated mortality in the USA by 2030 [2]. In spite of rapid progress in understanding PDAC tumorigenesis at the molecular level and therapeutic approaches, the prognosis of PDAC remains poor, with a 5-year survival rate less than 5% [3]. PDAC is insensitive to chemotherapy and radiotherapy, meaning the identification of novel therapeutic targets is imperative.

Non-coding RNAs (ncRNAs) are not transcribed and translated into coding-proteins, including micro-RNAs (miRNAs) and long non-coding RNAs (lncRNAs) [4]. LncRNAs have attracted increasing attention in recent years due to important biological effects in carcinogenesis and progression [5, 6]. In recent years, a large number of lncRNAs, such as MALAT-1, HOTAIR, H19 and PVT1 appear to play important roles in PDAC development, as it regulates cell growth, progression and chemo-resistance, etc. [7]. We have previously found that the MALAT-1 promotes tumor growth and metastases in PDAC [8, 9]. However, the underlying molecular mechanisms still need to be further clarified.

Recently interaction research between lncRNAs and miRNAs is attracting an increasing amount of attention [10]. In this study, we revealed a reciprocal suppression between MALAT-1 and miR-200c-3p expression in PDAC, and performed underlying mechanisms analysis.

Methods

Ethics statement

The present study was approved and supervised by the Ethics Committee of the Renji Hospital, School of Medicine, Shanghai Jiaotong University. Written informed consent was obtained from all subjects.

Patients and samples

Sixty-five paraffin embedded samples were collected from the Surgery Department, Renji Hospital, School of Medicine, Shanghai Jiaotong University from January 2009 to December 2012, and were histopathologically confirmed and staged in accordance with the Union for International Cancer Control. The follow-up data was ended in December, 2017.

Cell culture

Human pancreatic ductal cells (HPDE) and PDAC cell lines SW1990, CAPAN-1, HS-766 T, CFPAC-1, BxPC-3, AsPC-1 and PANC-1 were all obtained from Chinese Academy of Sciences Cell Bank (Shanghai, China). SW1990 cell was cultured in L-15 medium supplemented with 10% fetal bovine serum (FBS, all purchased from Gibco, Grand Island, NY, USA), and grown in

room temperature air. The other cells were cultured in RPMI 1640 supplemented with 10% FBS (all purchased from Gibco, Grand Island, NY, USA), grown at 37 °C in 5% CO_2 saturated humidity.

RNA extraction and reverse transcription quantitative real-time polymerase chain reaction (RT-qPCR)

The miRNeasy FFPE Kit (QIAGEN, Hilden, Germany) kit and miniBEST universal RNA extraction kit (Takara Bio, Dalian, China) was used to extract total RNA from tissue samples and cultured cells, respectively. Reverse transcription and RT-qPCR kits were employed to examine MALAT-1 and miR-200c-3p level. RT-qPCR reactions were performed by the ViiATM 7 system (Applied Biosystems Inc. Foster City, CA, USA). The primers used in the reaction for MALAT-1, miR-200c-3p, ZEB1, GAPDH and U6 were purchased from Tiangen (Tiangen, Beijing, China). GAPDH and U6 were detected as the endogenous control to normalize the expression levels of the different genes. Comparative threshold cycle (Ct) ($2^{-\Delta\Delta Ct}$) method was selected to calculate relative expression.

Cell proliferation assay

Cell proliferation was measured via the sulforhodamine B assay. Cells were seeded in 96-well plates and transfected with miR-200c-3p nc, miR-200c-3p inhibitor, or mimics and cultured for 24, 48, 72, and 96 h. Using microtiter plate reader (VERSMax), optical density (OD) values were measured at 560 nm.

Cell migration and invasion assays

Invasion assays were conducted 24 h after transfection. Briefly, 1×10^5 cells in serum-free media were seeded into the upper chamber of an insert (8.0 μm, Millipore, Billerica, MA, USA) that was coated with Matrigel (BD Biosciences, Franklin Lakes, NJ, USA) [9]. Then, 10% FBS-containing medium was placed in the lower chambers of the insert. After incubation for 24 h, the invaded cells were fixed and stained using 0.1% crystal violet staining solution. Finally, the cells were counted by a microscope at a magnification of × 200 in five randomly selected fields. Migration assays were similar to the above-mentioned assay but no Matrigel was used.

RNA binding protein immunoprecipitation (RIP)

RIP assay was performed by the Magna RIP™RNA-Binding Protein Immunoprecipitation Kit (Millipore, Billerica, MA, USA). Cells were lysed in RIP Lysis Buffer. MiR-200c-3p and MALAT-1 were immunoprecipitated with AGO2 antibodies. The complexes that bound on the magnetic beads were immobilized and unbound materials were washed off. Then, miR-200c-3p and MALAT-1 were extracted and analyzed by RT-qPCR.

Luciferase assays

Firstly, 293 T cells were seeded in 24-well plates and transfected with 50 nM miR-200c-3p mimics or miR-200c-3p nc respectively. Secondly, after 24 h transfection, the above 293 T cells were then transfected with 100 ng luciferase reporter vectors that contained either wild-type (MALAT-1-wt) or mutant types (MALAT-1-mut) (both were designed and structured from Obio Technology, Shanghai, Corp. Ltd). The Renilla luciferase reference plasmid was included in each transfection system as an internal control to normalize the transfection efficiency. Finally, at 48 h after transfection, the Dual-Luciferase Reporter Assay using an illuminometers (Promega Corporation, Madison, WI) was performed according to the manufacturer's protocol.

Western blot analysis

Western blot analysis was conducted as previously described [11]. The primary antibodies were as follows: anti-AGO2 (1:1000), anti-ZEB1 (1:1000, Cell Signaling Technology, Beverly, MA, USA), and anti-β-Actin (1:2500, Santa Cruz Biotechnology, Santa Cruz, CA, USA).

Plasmid construction and transfection

Recombinant plasmid pcDNA3.0/ZEB1, miR-200c mimic, miR-200c inhibitor, siRNA against MALAT-1, and negative controls were all obtained or constructed from GenePharma (Shanghai, China). The detail sequences were under Additional file 1. Lipofectamine 2000 (Invitrogen, USA) was used as transfections agents.

Statistical analyses

Data were presented as the mean ± SE. All statistical analyses were conducted by SPSS statistical software 17.0 (SPSS Inc., Chicago, IL, USA). For comparison between two groups, we used two-tailed Student's t test. Multiple group comparisons were calculated with one-way ANOVA analysis. Least-significant difference (LSD) was used for post hoc test. χ2 tests or Fisher's exact methods was used to detect correlation between MALAT-1 level or miR-200c-3p and clinical characteristics, as appropriate. The correlation between MALAT-1, miR-200c-3p and ZEB1 expression was analyzed using Pearson Correlation. Kaplan-Meier method was used to estimate overall survival (OS). Univariate and multivariate COX regression analysis was performed. $P < 0.05$ was considered to indicate a statistically significant difference.

Results

Elevated level of MALAT-1 inhibits miR-200c-3p expression in PDAC

To investigate the interaction among potential miRNAs and MALAT-1, we used the Starbase v2.0 (starbase.sysu.edu.cn LncRNA.php) to search for miRNAs that complementarily base-pair with MALAT-1. Twenty miRNAs were predicted to bind to MALAT-1 (see Additional file 2). We further validated 20 miRNAs expression after knockdown of MALAT-1 in CFPAC-1 and AsPC-1 cell lines, which showed relative high level of MALAT-1 (Fig. 1a and b). Initial profiling identified three miRNAs (miR-200c-3p, miR-92b-3p, and miR-181c-5p) that exhibited > 2-fold-change compared with the control (Fig. 1c and d; $P < 0.05$). Next, miR-200c-3p was chosen for the study because it showed the greatest fold-change in response to the MALAT-1 knockdown.

Anti-miR-200c-3p restores MALAT-1-siRNA function

Subsequently, to study the biological function of miR-200c-3p on PDAC, we transfected AsPC-1 and CFPAC-1 cells with miR-200c-3p nc, inhibitors, or mimics (Fig. 2a; $P < 0.05$). Sulforhodamine B assay showed that there were no differences of cell proliferation ability in different groups, including miR-200c-3p nc, inhibitors, or mimics group (Fig. 2b; $P < 0.05$). Transwell assay revealed that miR-200c-3p mimics transfection decreased the number of migrating cells in comparisons with that of miR-200c-3p nc, while transfection of miR-200c-3p inhibitor increased the number of migrating cells (Fig. 2c; $P < 0.05$). Taken together, miR-200c-3p suppressed cell migration and invasion in PDAC, but not cell proliferation.

Our previous studies have revealed that MALAT-1 promotes tumor growth and metastases in PDAC [8, 9]. To further examine if the effects of MALAT-1 on cell migration and invasion were partially mediated by miR-200c-3p, we co-transfected CFPAC-1 and AsPC-1 cells with MALAT-1 siRNA and miR-200c-3p inhibitor. The results revealed that knockdown of MALAT-1 suppressed cell migration and invasion, whereas miR-200c-3p inhibition partially reversed decreased invasiveness (Fig. 3a and b; $P < 0.05$). These findings were also confirmed in PANC-1 and CAPAN-1 cell lines (see Additional file 3; $P < 0.05$). Together, the data suggested that miR-200c-3p can partially rescue the loss of MALAT-1-mediated PDAC cell migration and invasion.

MALAT-1 upregulates ZEB1 expression by sponging miR-200c-3p

Among the many targets of miR-200c-3p, we focused on ZEB1 because it encodes a zinc finger and homeodomain transcription factor proteins that function in PDAC metastasis. Firstly, the result verified that the miR-200c-3p inhibitor triggered significant endogenous ZEB1 expression, whereas miR-200c-3p overexpression silenced ZEB1 protein expression (Fig. 4a; $P < 0.05$). Furthermore, cotransfection with MALAT-1 siRNA and miR-200c-3p inhibitor revealed that the miR-200c-3p inhibitor weakened down-regulation of ZEB1 by MALAT-1 knockdown (Fig. 4b; $P < 0.05$). Further study

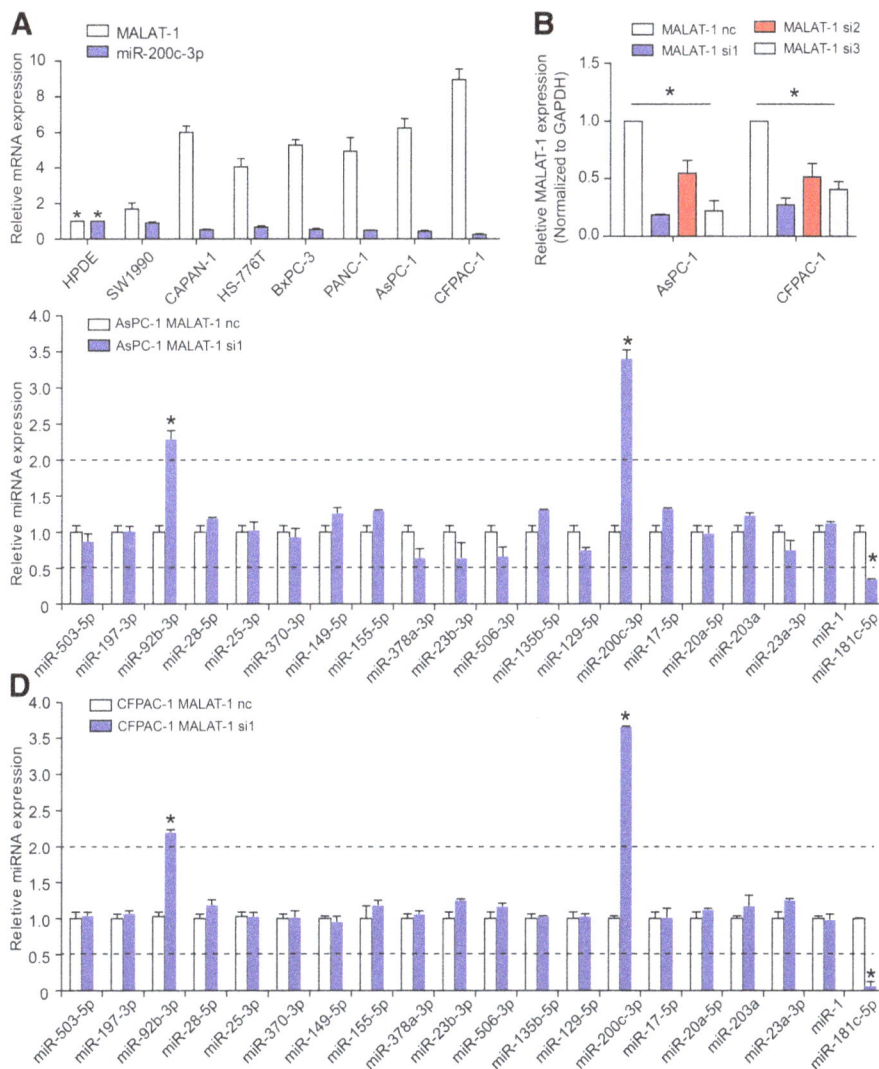

Fig. 1 Elevated level of MALAT-1 inhibits miR-200c-3p expression in PDAC. **a** High level of MALAT-1 and low level of miR-200c-3p were expressed in PDAC cell lines compared to HPDE. **b** RT-qPCR was employ to detect the efficiency of MALAT-1 knockdown in AsPC-1 cell line. **c, d** Twenty miRNAs candidate were chosen to validate in response to knockdown of MALAT-1 in AsPC-1 (**c**) and CFPAC-1 (**d**) cell lines. Initial profiling identified three miRNAs, including miR-200c-3p, miR-92b-3p, and miR-181c-5p, that exhibited > 2-fold-change compared with the control, and miR-200c-3p showed the greatest fold-change in response to the MALAT-1 knockdown

showed that ZEB1 overexpression can rescue the loss of MALAT-1-mediated repression activity in PDAC, including reduced cell migration and invasion (Fig. 5a, b, c and d; $P < 0.05$). This experimental evidence supported that the observed migration/invasion defect in MALAT-1 knockdown or miR200c-3p mimics was in fact mediated via regulation of ZEB1 expression.

MALAT-1 was a target of miR-200c-3p

We then measured MALAT-1 expression levels in response to transfection of miR-200c-3p mimic or inhibitor. The results showed that inhibiting miR-200c-3p up-regulated MALAT-1 levels (Fig. 6a; $P < 0.05$), whereas miR-200c-3p overexpression significantly decreased

MALAT-1 in both cell lines (Fig. 6b; $P < 0.05$). The data above implicated MALALT-1 was also a target of miR-200c-3p.

MALAT-1 and miR-200c-3p are associated with immunoprecipitated AGO2 complex

AGO2 is necessary for miRNA-mediated gene silencing [12]. To investigate whether MALAT-1 expression is controlled by miR-200c-3p, we knocked down AGO2 in AsPC-1 and CFPAC-1 (Fig. 7a; $P < 0.05$). As expected, MALAT-1 expression was increased in AGO2-knockdown cells (Fig. 7b; $P < 0.05$). Also, the stability of miR-200c-3p was significantly impaired in AGO2-knockdown cells

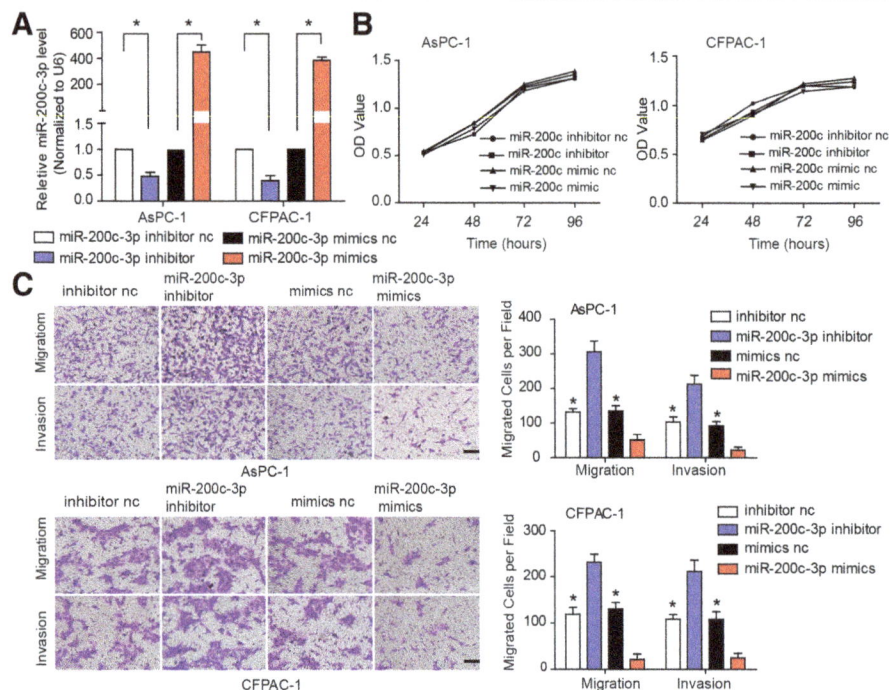

Fig. 2 MiR-200c-3p suppress cell migration and invasion, but not cell proliferation in PDAC. **a** RT-qPCR was employ to detect the transfection efficiency of miR-200c-3p nc, inhibitors, or mimics. **b** Sulforhodamine B assay was used to detect cell proliferation ability in different groups, including miR-200c-3p nc, inhibitors, or mimics group. The cell proliferation ability had no differences **c.** A transwell migration assay to examine the effect of miR-200c-3p on PDAC cell migration and invasion. Transfection of miR-200c-3p mimics reduced the number of migrating cells as compared to that of miR-200c-3p nc, while transfection of miR-200c-3p inhibitor increased the number of migrating cells

(Fig. 7c; $P < 0.05$). These data collectively suggest that miR-200c-3p directly regulates MALAT-1 levels.

To further study the mechanism that underlies the negative regulation of miR-200c-3p by MALAT-1 and to obtain evidence that supports a potential interaction between these two genes, we used Starbase v2.0 to predict the interaction sites between miR-200c-3p and MALAT-1 (Fig. 7d), and cloned the two mutated binding sites to vector, respectively. The mutants were designated as pMALAT-1-mut1 and pMALAT-1-mut2 (Fig. 7d). Then, luciferase assays were performed in 293FT cells that were transfected with pMALAT-1-mut1 or pMALAT-1-mut2. The results showed that luciferase activity decreased in the pMALAT-1 WT group in 293 T-transfected miR-200c-3p mimics compared to control group (Fig. 7e; $P < 0.05$). However, there were no effects on the luciferase reporter activities of pMALAT-1 mut-1 and pMALAT-1 mut-2 (Fig. 7e; $P < 0.05$). Collectively, these results suggested that MALAT-1 was a direct target gene of miR-200c. Further, AGO2 RIP assay showed that transfection with miR-200c-3p mimics enriched MALAT-1 and miR-200c-3p in AGO2 immunoprecipitated from AsPC-1 (Fig. 7f; $P < 0.05$) and CFPAC-1 (Fig. 7g; $P < 0.05$) cell extracts. Collectively, these results were consistent with the hypothesis that MALAT-1 stability is AGO2-dependent and is regulated by miR-200c-3p in PDAC.

MALAT-1 expression is negatively associated with miR-200c-3p in PDAC tissues

We further evaluated the correlation between MALAT-1 and miR-200c-3p expression and the clinicopathological characteristics. The median value was used as cut-off to divide MALAT-1 or miR-200c-3p expression into low level group ($n = 33$) and high level group ($n = 32$). As shown in Additional file 4, MALAT-1 expression is strongly correlated to lymph node metastasis ($P = 0.007$) and clinical stage ($P = 0.007$). And miR-200c-3p expression was negatively correlated with gender ($P = 0.011$), lymph node metastasis ($P = 0.017$), and clinical stage ($P = 0.017$). Bivariate correlation analysis showed that expression of MALAT-1 and ZEB1 was negatively correlated with miR-200c-3p transcript level of PDAC tissues (Fig. 8a; $P < 0.05$). There was a positive correlation between MALAT-1 and ZEB1 level (Fig. 8a; $P < 0.05$). And this phenomenon was consistent at different clinical stages (Fig. 8b and c; $P < 0.05$).

Association between MALAT-1 and miR-200c-3p expression and prognosis in PDAC patients

Kaplan-Meier analysis showed that patients with PDAC tumors expressing high MALAT-1 levels had significantly lower OS than those expressing low MALAT-1

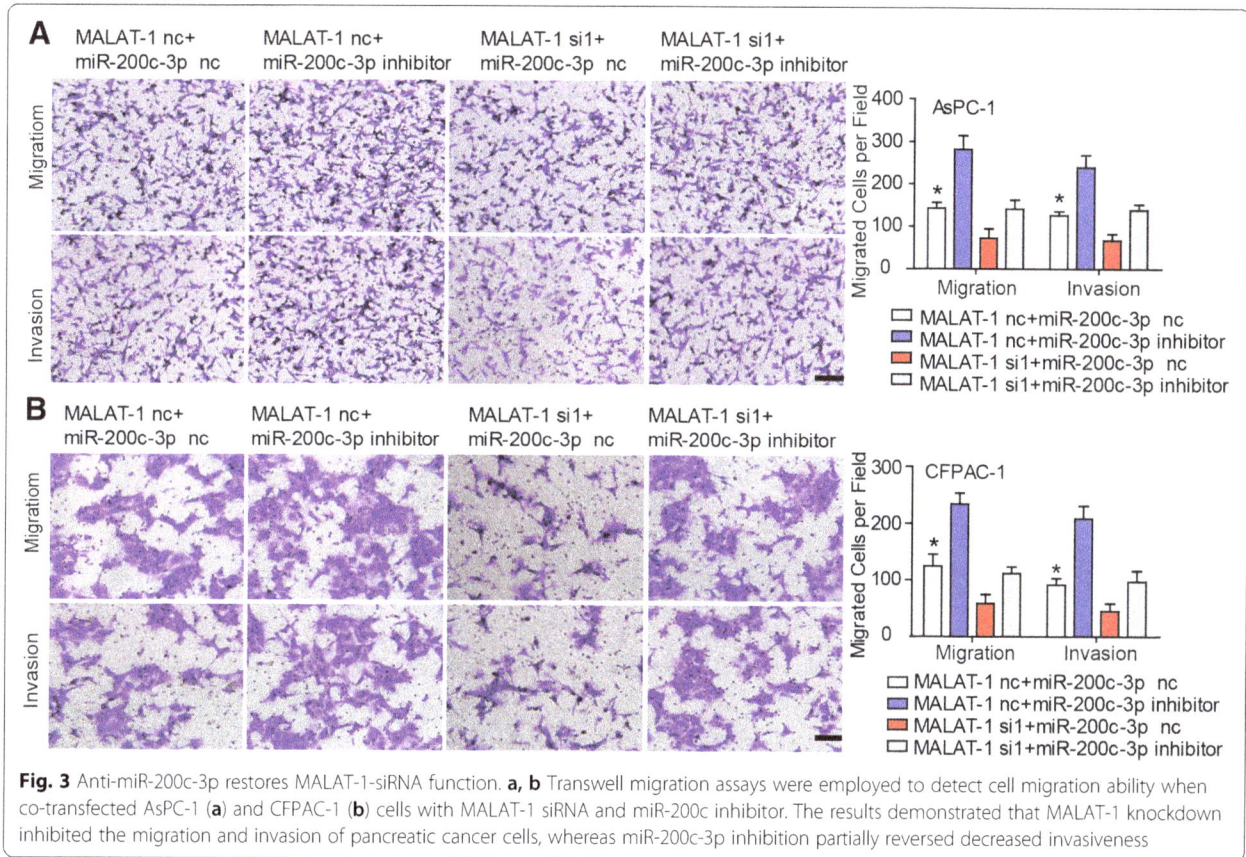

Fig. 3 Anti-miR-200c-3p restores MALAT-1-siRNA function. **a, b** Transwell migration assays were employed to detect cell migration ability when co-transfected AsPC-1 (**a**) and CFPAC-1 (**b**) cells with MALAT-1 siRNA and miR-200c inhibitor. The results demonstrated that MALAT-1 knockdown inhibited the migration and invasion of pancreatic cancer cells, whereas miR-200c-3p inhibition partially reversed decreased invasiveness

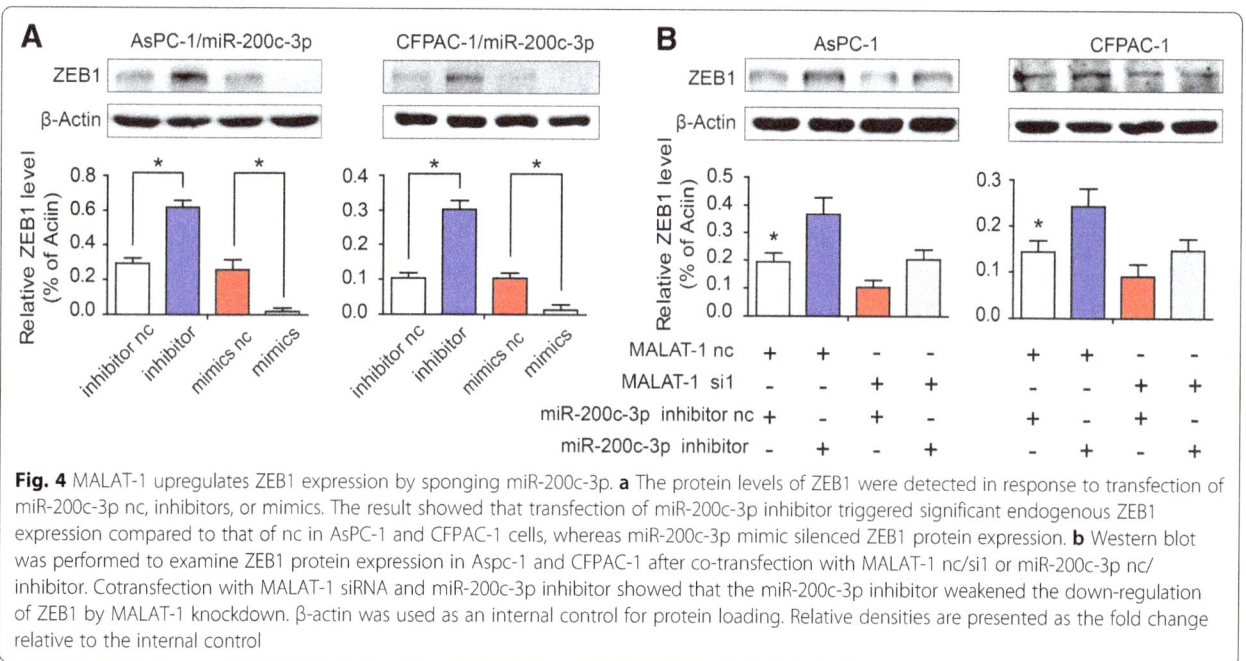

Fig. 4 MALAT-1 upregulates ZEB1 expression by sponging miR-200c-3p. **a** The protein levels of ZEB1 were detected in response to transfection of miR-200c-3p nc, inhibitors, or mimics. The result showed that transfection of miR-200c-3p inhibitor triggered significant endogenous ZEB1 expression compared to that of nc in AsPC-1 and CFPAC-1 cells, whereas miR-200c-3p mimic silenced ZEB1 protein expression. **b** Western blot was performed to examine ZEB1 protein expression in Aspc-1 and CFPAC-1 after co-transfection with MALAT-1 nc/si1 or miR-200c-3p nc/inhibitor. Cotransfection with MALAT-1 siRNA and miR-200c-3p inhibitor showed that the miR-200c-3p inhibitor weakened the down-regulation of ZEB1 by MALAT-1 knockdown. β-actin was used as an internal control for protein loading. Relative densities are presented as the fold change relative to the internal control

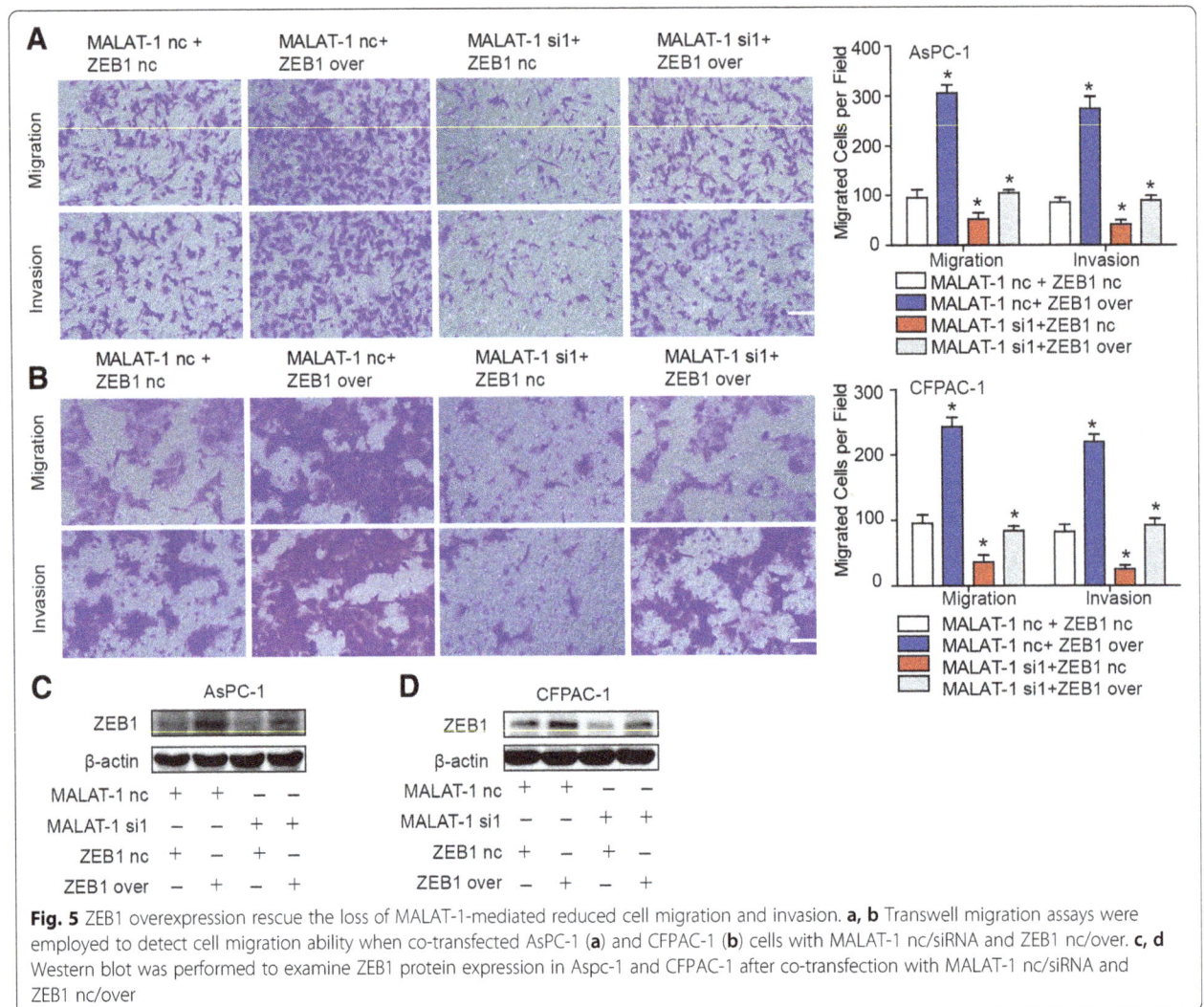

Fig. 5 ZEB1 overexpression rescue the loss of MALAT-1-mediated reduced cell migration and invasion. **a, b** Transwell migration assays were employed to detect cell migration ability when co-transfected AsPC-1 (**a**) and CFPAC-1 (**b**) cells with MALAT-1 nc/siRNA and ZEB1 nc/over. **c, d** Western blot was performed to examine ZEB1 protein expression in Aspc-1 and CFPAC-1 after co-transfection with MALAT-1 nc/siRNA and ZEB1 nc/over

(Fig. 9a; $P < 0.001$), whereas that patients expressing high miR-200c-3p levels had significantly higher OS than those expressing low miR-200c-3p (Fig. 9b; $P < 0.001$). To further investigate the correlation of OS with MALAT-1 and miR-200c-3p expression, the results showed that MALAT-1 (high)/ miR-200c-3p (low) associated with shorter OS of PDAC patients (Fig. 9c; $P < 0.001$).

Using univariate analysis, in addition to clinical stage, both MALAT-1 ($P < 0.001$) and miR-200c-3p ($P < 0.001$) levels were closely associated with OS (see Additional file 5). Multivariate analysis revealed that both MALAT-1 ($P < 0.001$) and miR-200c-3p ($P < 0.001$) level was an independent prognostic factor for PDAC patients (see Additional file 5).

Discussion

Gathering evidence demonstrated that lncRNAs occupies an important position in cancer pathogenesis [4, 13]. Previously, we have outlined the functional lncRNAs in PDAC, such as MALAT-1, HOTAIR, H19 and HULC, and decipher possible mechanisms of lncRNAs [7]. MALAT-1, one of the first lncRNAs, was demonstrated to be associated with lung cancer [14]. Also, MALAT-1 has been linked to several other human tumor entities [15, 16]. In our previous studies, we have found that the MALAT-1 served as oncogenic lncRNA participating in PDAC cell growth and progression [8, 9]. However, the underlying molecular mechanisms are far from being fully elucidated.

Amounting studies indicate that MALAT-1 could exert functions by targeting miRNAs. Han X et al. [17] found that MALAT-1 modulated Srf through miR-133 and discovered a novel correlation among MALAT-1, miR-133, and Srf in myoblast differentiation. Lei R et al. [18] revealed that high level of MALAT-1 promoted cell growth by targeting miR-506 in ovarian cancer. In our study, we found that MALAT-1 knockdown decreased the expression of miR-200c-3p in PDAC. On the other

A novel feedback loop between high MALAT-1 and low miR-200c-3p promotes cell migration and invasion...

185

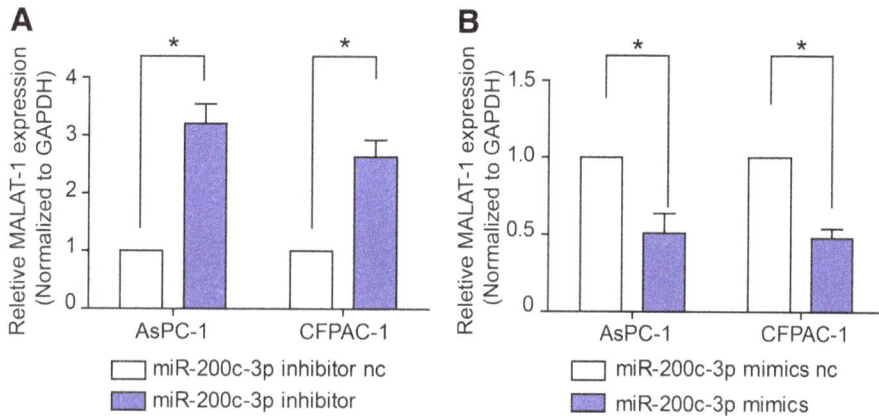

Fig. 6 MALAT-1 was a target of miR-200c-3p. **a, b** RT-qPCR was used to measure MALAT-1 expression levels in response to transfection of miR-200c-3p nc, mimic or inhibitor. The results showed that inhibiting miR-200c-3p up-regulated MALAT-1 levels (**a**), whereas miR-200c-3p overexpression significantly decreased MALAT-1 in both cell lines (**b**)

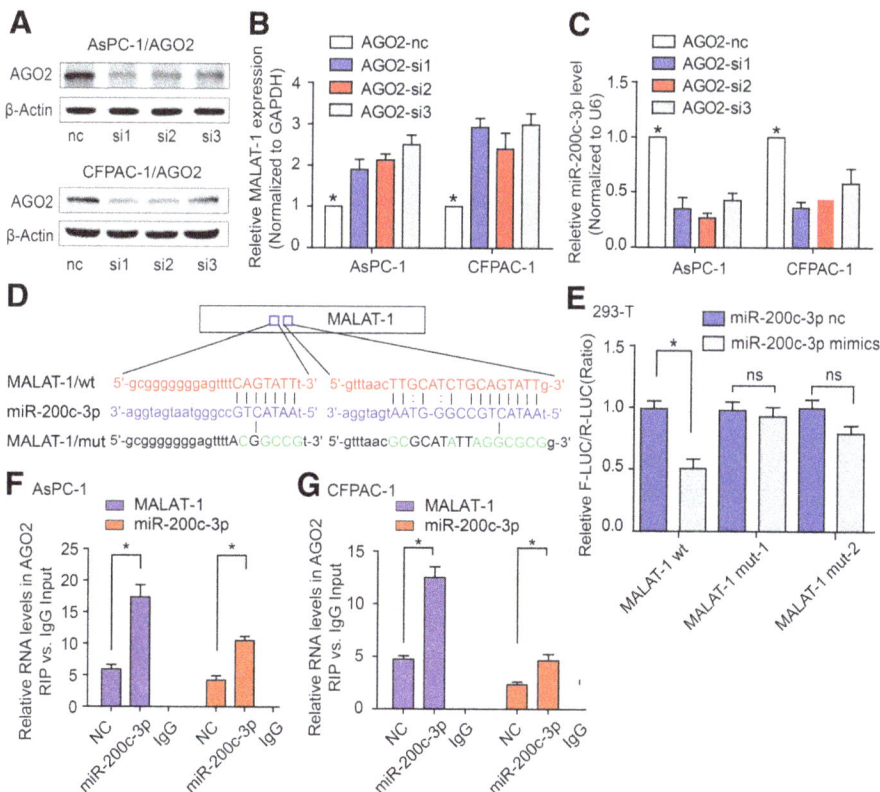

Fig. 7 MALAT-1 and miR-200c-3p are associated with the immunoprecipitated AGO2 complex. **a** Western blot was employed to detect AGO2 expression after AGO2 knockdown in AsPC-1 and CFPAC-1 cells. **b, c** RT-qPCR was use to examine MALAT-1 (**b**) and miR-200c-3p (**c**) level in response to knockdown of AGO2 in AsPC-1 and CFPAC-1, respectively. **d** Binding sites for miR-200c-3p in MALAT-1, as predicted by Starbase v2.0. The parts in the column imply the possible binding sites in MALAT. **e** Seed matches from MALAT-1 wt or its mutants (MALAT-1-mut-1 and MALAT-1-mut-2) that were devoid of specific miR-200c-3p-binding sites were mutagenized and transfected into 293 T cells together with 50 nM of miR-200c-3p mimics or nc. MiR-200-3p mimics significantly decreased luciferase activity only in the MALAT-1-wt construct. **f, g** RIP with monoclonal anti-Ago2 and IgG from AsPC-1 (**f**) and CFPAC-1 (**g**) cell extracts transfected with nc or miR-200c-3p mimics. Levels of MALAT-1 and miR-200c-3p were measured by RT-qPCR

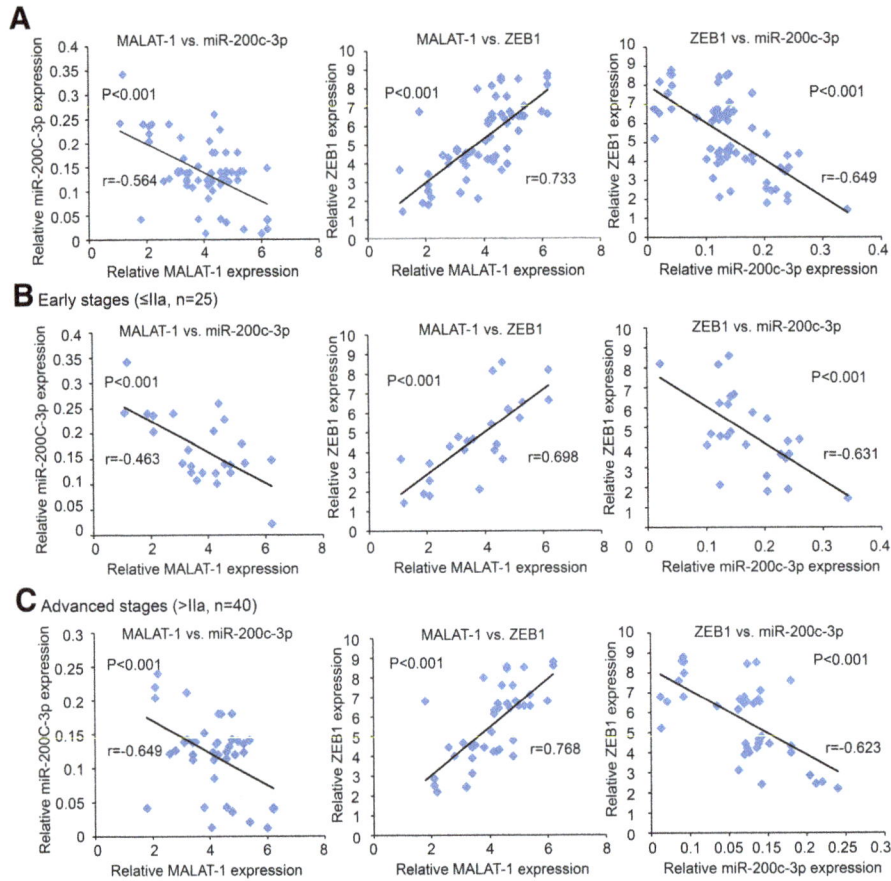

Fig. 8 Correlation between MALAT-1, miR-200c-3p and ZEB1 expression in PDAC patients. **a** Pearson correlation analysis showed that expression of MALAT-1 and ZEB1 was negatively correlated with miR-200c-3p transcript level. And there was a positive correlation between MALAT-1 and ZEB1 level. **b, c** The phenomenon of correlation between MALAT-1, miR-200c-3p and ZEB1 were consistent at different clinical stages, including early (≤ IIa, **b**) and advanced stage (> IIa, **c**)

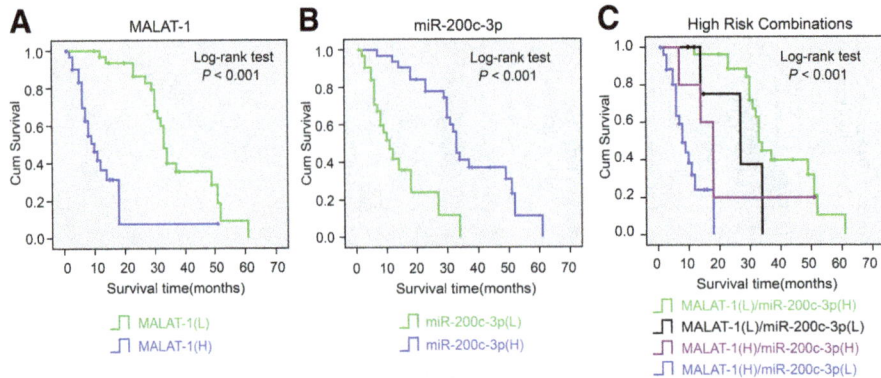

Fig. 9 Association between MALAT-1 and miR-200c-3p expression and prognosis in PDAC patients. **a** The log-rank test showed that patients with PDAC tumors expressing high MALAT-1 levels had significantly lower OS than those expressing low MALAT-1. **b** The patients expressing high miR-200c-3p levels had significantly higher OS than those expressing low miR-200c-3p. **c** The log-rank test showed that MALAT-1 (high)/ miR-200c-3p (low) correlated with shorter OS of PDAC patients compare to that of other groups, including MALAT-1 (low)/miR-200c-3p (low), MALAT-1 (low)/ miR-200c-3p (high) and MALAT-1 (high)/ miR-200c-3p (high)

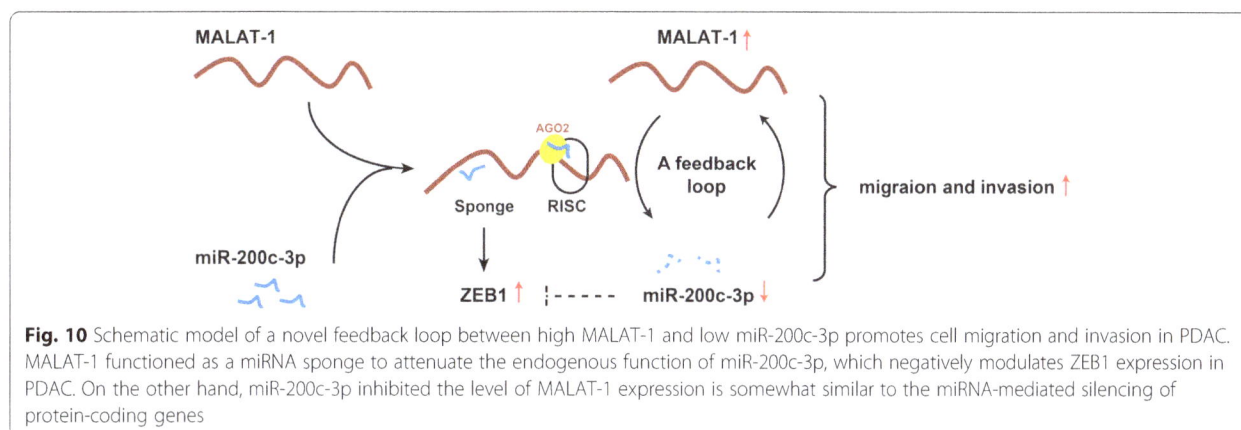

Fig. 10 Schematic model of a novel feedback loop between high MALAT-1 and low miR-200c-3p promotes cell migration and invasion in PDAC. MALAT-1 functioned as a miRNA sponge to attenuate the endogenous function of miR-200c-3p, which negatively modulates ZEB1 expression in PDAC. On the other hand, miR-200c-3p inhibited the level of MALAT-1 expression is somewhat similar to the miRNA-mediated silencing of protein-coding genes

hand, miR-200c-3p mimic decreased the level of MALAT-1, while miR-200c-3p inhibitor upregulated MALAT-1 level. A luciferase assays further confirmed that MALAT-1 was a direct target of miR-200c-3p in PDAC.

Subsequently, we discussed the mechanism of such a feedback loop. It was found that MALAT-1 and miR-200c-3p bind to the same RNA-induced silencing complex. Based on the fact that lncRNAs act as ceRNA to bind specific miRNAs and regulate their function [19, 20]. We supposed that MALAT-1 may inhibit miR-200c-3p expression in such way in PDAC. It was found that MALAT-1 could upregulate ZEB1 expression, which was a target of miR-200c-3p. Together, the above results further confirm our hypothesis. For another, miRNAs regulate protein-coding gene expression at transcriptional level through binding to the 3'-untranslated regions [21, 22]. Leucci E et al. [23] found that miR-9 targeted the AGO2-mediated deregulation of MALAT-1 in the nucleus. Wang X et al. [24] showed that posttranscriptional inhibitory mechanism of MALAT-1 by miR-101 and miR-217 suppressed cell proliferation, migration, and invasion in esophageal squamous cell carcinoma. We proposed that the way that miR-200c-3p inhibited the level of MALAT-1 expression is in a way similar to miRNA-mediated silencing of protein-coding genes. Our data were consistent with recent report in ovarian cancer [12]. Hirata H et al. [25] found that MALAT-1 promoted aggressive phenotype by interacts with miR-205 and EZH2 in renal cell carcinoma. Our previous study had demonstrated that MALAT-1 could recruit EZH2 to the E-cadherin promoter, where it repressed E-cadherin expression, leading to cell migration and invasion in PDAC [26]. In this study, we revealed reciprocal suppression between MALAT-1 and miR-200c-3p expression and clarify the underlying mechanism.

Finally, we found that MALAT-1 and ZEB1 was negatively correlated with miR-200c-3p transcript level of PDAC tissues. And there was a positive correlation between MALAT-1 and ZEB1 level. Survival analysis reveals that both MALAT-1 and miR-200c-3p levels are independent prognostic factors. MALAT-1 (high)/ miR-200c-3p (low) correlated with shorter OS for PDAC patients. Interestingly, Li Q et al. [27] showed that MALAT-1 levels were lower in most endometrioid endometrial carcinoma tissues than in normal tissues, while miR-200c-3p levels were higher. Therefore, different expression model of MALAT-1 and miR-200c-3p in human tumor entities needs further mechanism researches.

Conclusion

In summary, our findings firstly revealed a novel feedback loop between high MALAT-1 and low miR-200c-3p (Fig. 10). MALAT-1 could function as a miRNA sponge to attenuate miR-200c-3p function, leading to ZEB1 upregulation in PDAC. On the other hand, miR-200c-3p inhibited the level of MALAT-1 expression in a way similar to miRNA-mediated silencing of target genes. Targeting the feedback loop between high MALAT-1 and low miR-200c-3p will be a novel therapeutic strategy for PDAC.

Additional files

Additional file 1: The primer sequences of miR-200c mimic, miR-200c inhibitor, siRNA against MALAT-1, and their respective negative controls.

Additional file 2: Initial profiling of miRNAs that have base-pairing with MALAT-1 in response to knockdown of MALAT-1.

Additional file 3: Anti-miR-200c-3p restores MALAT-1-siRNA function in PANC-1 and CAPAN-1 cells. a, b. Transwell migration assays were employed to detect cell migration ability when co-transfected PANC-1 (a) and CAPAN-1 (b) cells with MALAT-1 siRNA and miR-200c inhibitor.

Additional file 4: Correlation between the clinicopathologic characteristics and MALAT-1 and miR-200c-3p expression in PDAC (n = 65).

> **Additional file 5:** Summary of univariate and multivariate COX regression analysis of OS duration in all PDAC patients ($n = 65$).

Abbreviations

FBS: Fetal bovine serum; HPDE: Human pancreatic ductal cells; lncRNAs: Long non-coding RNAs; LSD: Least-significant difference; MALAT-1: Metastasis-associated lung adenocarcinoma transcript 1; miRNAs: Micro-RNAs; ncRNAs: Non-coding RNAs; OD: Optical density; OS: Overall survival; PDAC: Pancreatic ductal adenocarcinoma; RIP: RNA binding protein immunoprecipitation; RT-qPCR: Reverse transcription quantitative real-time polymerase chain reaction

Acknowledgements

We sincerely appreciate the patients who participated in this study.

Funding

This study was supported by the National Natural Science Foundation of China (grant nos. 81502017 for Feng Jiao, 81502018 for Jiujie Cui and 81572315 for Liwei Wang). The funding bodies had no role in study design, data collection and analysis, decision to publish, or preparation of the manuscript.

Authors' contributions

MZ and FJ carried out the cellular and histological studies, the statistical analysis, and drafted the manuscript. CY collected tumor tissues and followed up patients. TH and JC helped perform the cellular and histological studies. FJ and LW participated in designing the study. All authors read and approved the final manuscript.

Competing interests

The authors declare that they have no competing interests.

Author details

[1]Department of Oncology, Renji Hospital, School of Medicine, Shanghai Jiaotong University, 160 Pujian Road, Shanghai 200127, China. [2]Department of Pathology, Eye Ear Nose and Throat Hospital, Fudan University, 83 Fenyang Road, Shanghai 200031, China.

References

1. Siegel RL, Miller KD, Jemal A. Cancer statistics, 2017. CA Cancer J Clin. 2017;67:7–30.
2. Rahib L, Smith BD, Aizenberg R, Rosenzweig AB, Fleshman JM, Matrisian LM. Projecting cancer incidence and deaths to 2030: the unexpected burden of thyroid, liver, and pancreas cancers in the United States. Cancer Res. 2014; 74:2913–21.
3. Kamisawa T, Wood LD, Itoi T, Takaori K. Pancreatic cancer. Lancet. 2016; 388:73–85.
4. Khurana E, Fu Y, Chakravarty D, Demichelis F, Rubin MA, Gerstein M. Role of non-coding sequence variants in cancer. Nat Rev Genet. 2016;17:93–108.
5. Huarte M. The emerging role of lncRNAs in cancer. Nat Med. 2015;21:1253–61.
6. Schmitt AM, Chang HY. Long noncoding RNAs in Cancer pathways. Cancer Cell. 2016;29:452–63.
7. Han T, Hu H, Zhuo M, Wang L, Cui JJ, Jiao F, et al. Long non-coding RNA: an emerging paradigm of pancreatic Cancer. Curr Mol Med. 2016;16:702–9.
8. Jiao F, Hu H, Han T, Yuan C, Wang L, Jin Z, et al. Long noncoding RNA MALAT-1 enhances stem cell-like phenotypes in pancreatic cancer cells. Int J Mol Sci. 2015;16:6677–93.
9. Jiao F, Hu H, Yuan C, Wang L, Jiang W, Jin Z, et al. Elevated expression level of long noncoding RNA MALAT-1 facilitates cell growth, migration and invasion in pancreatic cancer. Oncol Rep. 2014;32:2485–92.
10. Ragusa M, Barbagallo C, Brex D, Caponnetto A, Cirnigliaro M, Battaglia R, et al. Molecular Crosstalking among noncoding RNAs: a new network layer of genome regulation in Cancer. Int J Genomics. 2017;2017:4723193.
11. Han T, Zhuo M, Hu H, Jiao F, Wang LW. Synergistic effects of the combination of 5-AzaCdR and suberoylanilide hydroxamic acid on the anticancer property of pancreatic cancer. Oncol Rep. 2018;39:264–70.
12. Pa M, Naizaer G, Seyiti A, Kuerbang G. Long noncoding RNA MALAT1 functions as a sponge of MiR-200c in ovarian Cancer. Oncol Res. 2017. [Epub ahead of print].
13. Anastasiadou E, Jacob LS, Slack FJ. Non-coding RNA networks in cancer. Nat Rev Cancer. 2018;18:5–18.
14. Ji P, Diederichs S, Wang W, Boing S, Metzger R, Schneider PM, et al. MALAT-1, a novel noncoding RNA, and thymosin beta4 predict metastasis and survival in early-stage non-small cell lung cancer. Oncogene. 2003;22:8031–41.
15. Gutschner T, Hammerle M, Diederichs S. MALAT1 -- a paradigm for long noncoding RNA function in cancer. J Mol Med (Berl). 2013;91:791–801.
16. Wu Y, Huang C, Meng X, Li J. Long noncoding RNA MALAT1: insights into its biogenesis and implications in human disease. Curr Pharm Des. 2015;21: 5017–28.
17. Han X, Yang F, Cao H, Liang Z. Malat1 regulates serum response factor through miR-133 as a competing endogenous RNA in myogenesis. FASEB J. 2015;29:3054–64.
18. Lei R, Xue M, Zhang L, Lin Z. Long noncoding RNA MALAT1-regulated microRNA 506 modulates ovarian cancer growth by targeting iASPP. Onco Targets Ther. 2017;10:35–46.
19. Tay Y, Rinn J, Pandolfi PP. The multilayered complexity of ceRNA crosstalk and competition. Nature. 2014;505:344–52.
20. Salmena L, Poliseno L, Tay Y, Kats L, Pandolfi PP. A ceRNA hypothesis: the Rosetta stone of a hidden RNA language? Cell. 2011;146:353–8.
21. Vannini I, Fanini F, Fabbri M. Emerging roles of microRNAs in cancer. Curr Opin Genet Dev. 2018;48:128–33.
22. Wang Y, Wang L, Chen C, Chu X. New insights into the regulatory role of microRNA in tumor angiogenesis and clinical implications. Mol Cancer. 2018;17:22.
23. Leucci E, Patella F, Waage J, Holmstrom K, Lindow M, Porse B, et al. microRNA-9 targets the long non-coding RNA MALAT1 for degradation in the nucleus. Sci Rep. 2013;3:2535.
24. Wang X, Li M, Wang Z, Han S, Tang X, Ge Y, et al. Silencing of long noncoding RNA MALAT1 by miR-101 and miR-217 inhibits proliferation, migration, and invasion of esophageal squamous cell carcinoma cells. J Biol Chem. 2015;290:3925–35.
25. Hirata H, Hinoda Y, Shahryari V, Deng G, Nakajima K, Tabatabai ZL, et al. Long noncoding RNA MALAT1 promotes aggressive renal cell carcinoma through Ezh2 and interacts with miR-205. Cancer Res. 2015;75:1322–31.
26. Han T, Jiao F, Hu H, Yuan C, Wang L, Jin ZL, et al. EZH2 promotes cell migration and invasion but not alters cell proliferation by suppressing E-cadherin, partly through association with MALAT-1 in pancreatic cancer. Oncotarget. 2016;7:11194–207.
27. Li Q, Zhang C, Chen R, Xiong H, Qiu F, Liu S, et al. Disrupting MALAT1/miR-200c sponge decreases invasion and migration in endometrioid endometrial carcinoma. Cancer Lett. 2016;383:28–40.

Meta-analysis on resected pancreatic cancer: a comparison between adjuvant treatments and gemcitabine alone

Hua Chen, Ruizhi He, Xiuhui Shi, Min Zhou, Chunle Zhao, Hang Zhang[*] and Renyi Qin[*]

Abstract

Background: Pancreatic cancer is a highly malignant tumor with a poor prognosis. Chemotherapy such as gemcitabine is still an important treatment. Gemcitabine (Gem) may prolong survival time and delay the development of recurrent disease after complete resection of pancreatic cancer. Currently, some control studies have been performed between certain drugs and gemcitabine monotherapy after pancreatic cancer surgery, but the outcomes were uncertain. Here, we implemented meta-analysis to compare the efficacy between adjuvant treatments and gemcitabine monotherapy in patients with resected pancreatic cancer.

Methods: PubMed, Embase and the Central Registry of Controlled Trials of the Cochrane Library searches were undertaken to identify randomized controlled trials (RCTs). Date of search ranged from January 1997 to December 2017. The meta-analysis included six RCTs. The major endpoints involved overall survival (OS), disease-free survival/progress free survival/relapse-free survival (DFS/PFS/RFS) and grade 3–4 toxicity.

Results: Pooled meta-analytic estimates were derived using random-effects model. Subgroup analysis used fixed-effects model. The outcome showed that there was no difference in OS (hazard ratio (HR), 0.87; 95% CI, 0.70–1.07; $P = 0.19$) and DFS (HR, 0.85; 95% CI, 0.71–1.02; $P = 0.08$) between the adjuvant treatments group (fluorouracil +folinic acid, S-1, gemcitabine+capecitabine, gemcitabine+erlotinib and gemcitabine+uracil/tegafur) and Gem monotherapy group. However, the subgroup analysis showed that only S-1 chemotherapy, which is an oral fluoropyrimidine agent containing tegafur, gimeracil and oteracil, was significant in OS (HR, 0.59; 95% CI, 0.46–0. 74; $P < 0.0001$) and DFS (HR, 0.63; 95% CI, 0.52–0.75; $P < 0.00001$) compared with Gem alone. Toxicity analysis showed there was an increased incidence of grade 3/4 diarrhea (risk ratio (RR), 5.11; 95%CI, 3.24–8.05; $P < 0.00001$) and decreased incidence of grade 3/4 leucopenia (RR, 0.55; 95%CI, 0.31–0.98; $P = 0.04$), thrombocytopenia (RR, 0.61; 95%CI, 0.39–0.97; $P = 0.04$) in adjuvant treatments group. Neutropenia (RR, 0.69; 95%CI, 0.36–1.29; $P = 0.24$) and fatigue (RR, 1.29; 95%CI, 0.95–1.77; $P = 0.11$) for patients between the two groups were not significantly different.

Conclusions: In our meta-analysis, a significant survival benefit is only observed in the S-1 regimen, but the results are yet to be determined. Optimal cytotoxicity or targeted drug regimens need further validation in clinical trials in the future.

Keywords: Pancreatic cancer, Gemcitabine, Chemotherapy, Meta-analysis

* Correspondence: 172356995@qq.com; ryqin@tjh.tjmu.edu.cn
Department of Biliary-Pancreatic Surgery, Affiliated Tongji Hospital, Tongji Medical College, Huazhong University of Science and Technology, Wuhan 430030, China

Background

In contrast to the steady increase in survival observed for most cancer types, advances have been slow for pancreatic cancers. More than one-half of cases are diagnosed at a distant stage, for which the 5-year survival rates is 3% [1]. Only a small percentage of patients, approximately 10–15%, have a chance of surgical resection [2–4]. However, the postoperative recurrence rate is high, with approximately 75–92% of patients relapsed [5, 6]. Masato et al. [7] reported that 80% local retroperitoneal recurrence, 66% hepatic metastasis, 53% peritoneal dissemination, 47% lymph node recurrence was discovered in postmortem examinations and 87% recurrence, 53% hepatic metastases in antemortem studies. The median survival after resection of pancreatic cancer remains in the range of 11–20 months and is associated with a 5-year survival rate of 7–25% [8, 9]. More radical resection procedures or extensive lymphadenectomy have not improved the course of disease [8]. Accordingly, adjuvant therapy appears to be very important in order to reduce recurrence and prolong survival after surgery.

The main adjuvant therapy after resection of pancreatic adenocarcinoma included chemotherapy and chemoradiation. Chemoradiation (moderate dose radiation with fluorouracil) has been the standard practice in the U.S. since the study (GITSG 9173) was conducted by the Gastrointestinal Tumor Study Group [10]. The results of some studies also support the survival benefit of chemoradiotherapy for patients with resected pancreatic cancer [11, 12]. But other researches have reached the opposite conclusion [13, 14]. The European Study Group for Pancreatic Cancer (ESPAC-1) took on a head-to-head comparison trial and found a lower median survival for chemoradiation,(15.9 months versus 17.9 months for patients who did not receive chemoradiation) and the median time to recurrence was 10.7 months among patients who received chemoradiotherapy and 15.2 months among those who did not receive chemoradiotherapy [15]. This resulted in far less use of adjuvant chemoradiation in Europe [16]. Chemotherapy mainly includes gemcitabine, fluorouracil, FOLFIRINOX (oxaliplatin, irinotecan, fluorouracil, and leucovorin), and gemcitabine in combination with other drugs. At present, most pancreatologists believe that FOLFIRINOX is superior to gemcitabine. But gemcitabine is still an important chemotherapy drug. Previous clinical trials have demonstrated that postoperative chemotherapy with gemcitabine may prolong survival time and significantly delay the development of recurrent disease after complete resection of pancreatic cancer [5, 17]. Furthermore, some control studies have also been performed between certain drugs and gemcitabine monotherapy after pancreatic cancer surgery, but the outcomes were uncertain. Here, we performed a systematic review and quantitative meta-analysis to assess the role of adjuvant treatments compared with gemcitabine alone after macroscopically complete resection of pancreatic cancer.

Methods

Literature search

We retrieved literature with PubMed, Embase and the Central Registry of Controlled Trials of the Cochrane Library and selected studies presented between January 1997, at the time of gemcitabine treatment introduction, and December 2017. The search was performed using the following terms: "pancreatic cancer", "gemcitabine", "chemotherapy" and "randomized controlled trial".

Inclusion and exclusion criteria

Trials were included in this meta-analysis if they met the following criteria: (1) Patients were required to have histologically proved pancreatic exocrine cancer. In each trial, patients underwent surgery with curative intent (R0 or R1 resection, negative or positive nodal status.R0 resection was defined as no tumor within 1 mm of margin); (2) The treatment group received adjuvant treatments with or without Gem, and the control group received Gem alone; (3) Data contained overall survival (OS) and hazard ratio(HR), disease-free survival / progress free survival / relapse-free survival (DFS/PFS/RFS) and hazard ratio(HR), grade 3–4 toxicity, or OS and DFS curves; (4) This analysis only included RCTs which should be prospective, properly randomized.

Trials were excluded if they met any of the following criteria: (1) Patients received chemotherapy, radiotherapy and other antitumor therapy prior to the study entry. (2) Not RCTs such as case reports, reviews and conference reports; (3) duplicate publications.

Data collection and analysis

Two investigators (Min Zhou, Chunle Zhao) independently evaluated the abstracts identified from the database. If one of the investigators concluded an abstract was eligible, the full manuscript was retrieved and reviewed in detail by both investigators. If full text of a study could not be obtained, it would be abandoned because of no detailed data to conduct statistical analysis. If the same study appeared on different publications, the one with the latest data was chosen. Methodologic quality of the trials was assessed using Jadad scale [18]. The following information was extracted from each trial: the author, year of publication, number of patients, chemotherapy regimen, OS, DFS/PFS/RFS, grade 3–4 haematological, non-haematological, performance status, etc. Toxicity profiles were reported according to the WHO's criteria or National Cancer Institute Common Terminology Criteria for Adverse Events (version 3.0).

Statistical analysis

The primary endpoint was OS after randomization. The other end points were DFS/PFS/RFS and adverse effects. All variables were defined as dichotomous data. We standardized the therapeutic results by obtaining the HR between the adjuvant treatments group and the Gem group. When HR was not reported we estimated it from summary statistics with the method described by Tierney and colleagues [19]. Adverse effects were assessed by RR. Publication bias was investigated by visual inspection of funnel plots. Cochrane's Q-test and I^2 statistics were used to assess heterogeneity. For the survival outcome sensitivity analysis was performed to assess the impact of studies with higher risk for bias. A two-tailed p value of less than 0.05 was considered statistically significant. All analyses were performed strictly with RevMan software (version 5.3, Cochrane).

Results

Trial flow of trials selection

The flow chart of this study is shown in Fig. 1. Of the nine trials, three trials are excluded because one reported by Tempero et al. [20] is ongoing trial, the other two by Sinn et al. [21] and Yoshitomi et al. [22] can not obtained detailed data. Both investigators finally agreed to include 6 RCTs in the meta-analysis.

Characteristics of included trials

These randomized controlled studies are summarized in Additional files 1, 2 and 3. All trials qualities were considered high, with a score of 3 in Jadad scale. Of the six trials, two were randomized phase II trials [23, 24] and the others were randomized phase III trials [25–28]. This meta-analysis evaluated 2787 patients in six randomized trials, of whom 1387 patients were included into the Gem alone arm and 1400 patients into other adjuvant treatments arm. In all six trials, gemcitabine was given 1000 mg/m^2 once a week for 3 of every 4 weeks. OS and HR with 95% CI, DFS/PFS/RFS and HR with 95% CI were recorded in most of the trials. Grade 3–4 toxicity was recorded in all trials.

Baseline characteristics of the individual trials including gender, performance status (ECOG performance status 0 or Karnofsky performance status (KPS) 60–100%), stage IV of Tumor, pathological resection margin and lymph nodes are indicated in Additional file 1. The distribution of baseline patient characteristics within the respective six trials was found to be homogeneous.

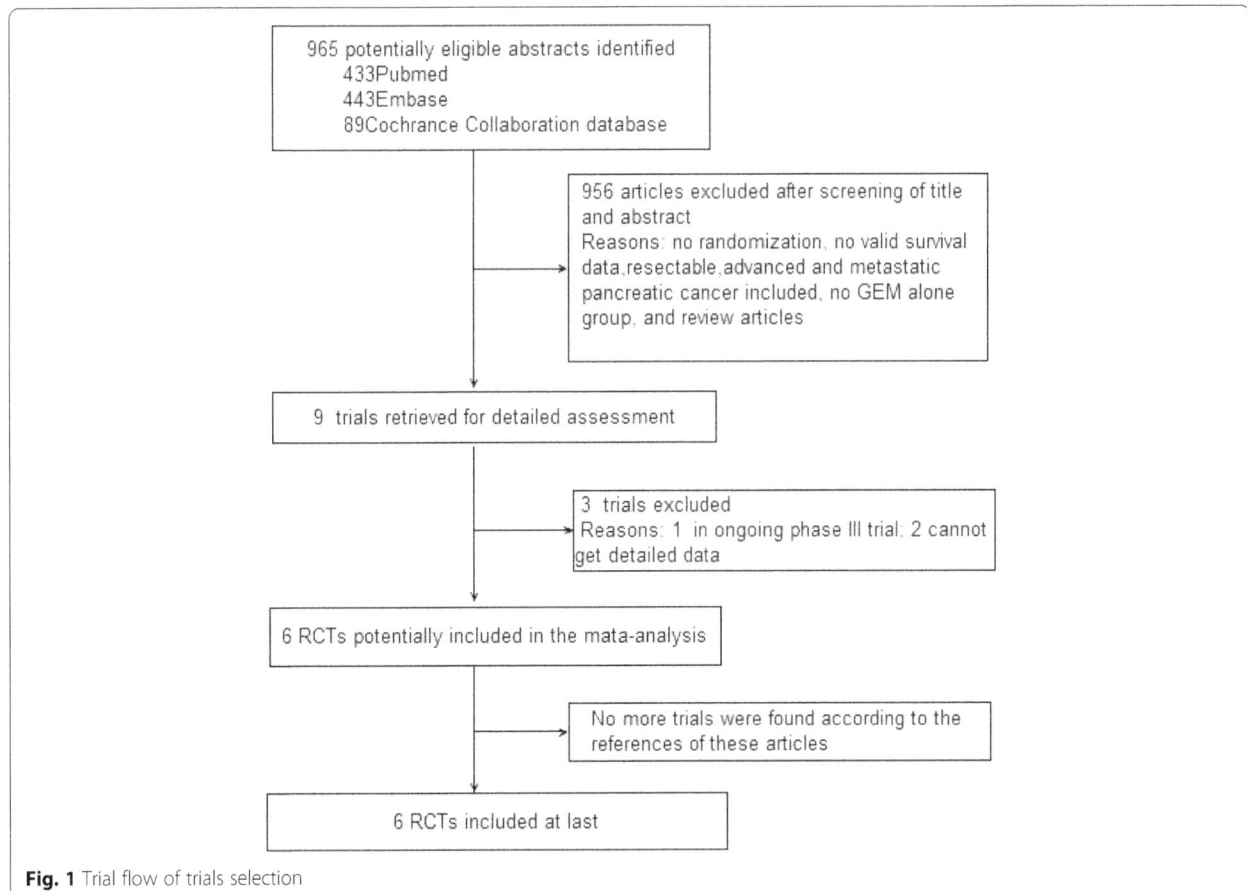

Fig. 1 Trial flow of trials selection

However, patients recruited into the study in CONKO-005 were provided with R0 resection.

Overall survival and sensitivity analysis

The overall survival of six trials are summarized in Additional file 2. The result of the test for heterogeneity of the therapeutic effect was significant ($P = 0.0006$; $I^2 = 77\%$). Therefore, we selected random effect model. There was not significant in HRs of OS for the adjuvant treatments arm compared with Gem alone arm (HR, 0.87; 95% CI, 0.70–1.07; $P = 0.19$). A sensitivity analysis was performed by excluding JASPAC 01 as it show a best survival benefit ($p < 0.0001$) in the adjuvant treatments group and was therefore considered as an outlier. The meta-analysis of the five remaining studies confirmed no difference in OS between the two arms (HR, 0.96; 95% CI, 0.88–1.06; $P = 0.44$).

Disease-free survival and sensitivity analysis

The disease-free survival of six trials are summarized in Additional file 2. The result of the test for heterogeneity of the therapeutic effect was significant ($P = 0.0007$; $I^2 = 77\%$). The outcome of random effect model was not significant in HR of DFS for the adjuvant treatments compared with Gem alone (HR, 0.85; 95% CI, 0.71–1.02; $P = 0.08$). The meta-analysis of the five remaining studies (excluding JASPAC 01) also confirmed no difference in DFS between the two arms (HR, 0.92; 95% CI, 0.80–1.06; $P = 0.25$).

Subgroup analysis

According to the adjuvant treatments protocol, we divided the trial into three groups such as group1: Fluorouracil +folinic acid (FU + FA) treatment, group 2: S-1 (an oral fluoropyrimidine) treatments and group 3: Gem combined treatments.

Figure 2 shows the subgroup analyses of HR of OS. The heterogeneity of subgroup was not significant, which was showed in group 2 ($P = 0.58$; $I^2 = 0\%$) and group3 ($P = 0.19$; $I^2 = 39\%$). So we used fixed effect mode. There was not significant in HR of OS for Gem combined treatments group (HR, 0.89; 95% CI, 0.78–1.02; $P = 0.09$) and FU + FA group (HR, 1.06; 95% CI, 0.93–1.22; $P = 0.39$). But for the S-1 group, it was significant (HR, 0.59; 95% CI, 0.46–0.74; $P < 0.0001$).

Figure 3 shows the subgroup analyses of HR of DFS. The heterogeneity of subgroup was not significant, which was showed group 2 ($P = 0.57$; $I^2 = 0\%$) and group 3 ($P = 0.41$; $I^2 = 0\%$). There was not significant in HR of DFS for Gem combined treatments group compared with Gem alone (HR, 0.92; 95% CI, 0.82–1.05; $P = 0.21$) and for FU + FA group (HR, 1.04; 95% CI, 0.91–1.19; $P = 0.57$). But for S-1 group, it was significant (HR, 0.63; 95% CI, 0.52–0.75; $P < 0.00001$).

Toxic effects of chemotherapy

Six trials reported the incidence of grade 3/4 leucopenia and thrombocytopenia [23–28], five trials reported the incidence of grade 3/4 neutropenia [23, 25–28] and four trials reported the incidence of grade 3/4 anaemia [23, 24, 26, 27]. Five trials reported the incidence of grade 3/4 diarrhea [23, 25–28] and four trials reported the incidence of grade 3/4 fatigue and nausea [25–28].

Grade 3–4 toxicity of subgroup was calculated using method for dichotomous data (RR, 95% CI),

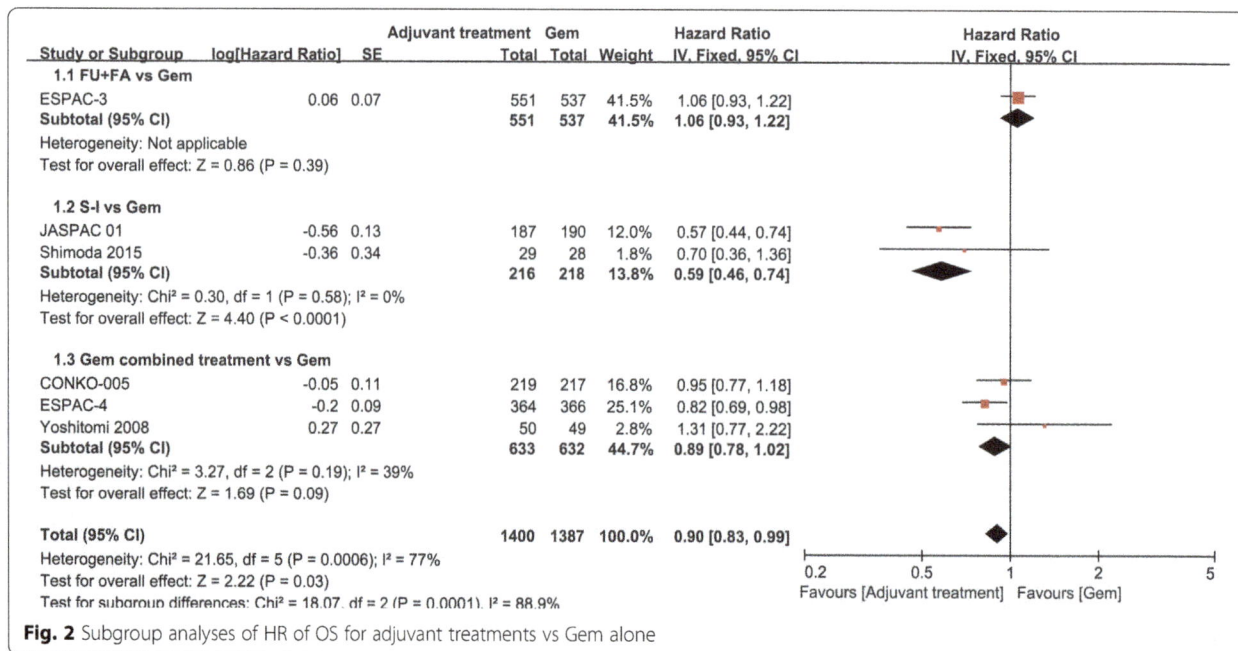

Study or Subgroup	log[Hazard Ratio]	SE	Adjuvant treatment Total	Gem Total	Weight	Hazard Ratio IV, Fixed, 95% CI
1.1 FU+FA vs Gem						
ESPAC-3	0.06	0.07	551	537	41.5%	1.06 [0.93, 1.22]
Subtotal (95% CI)			551	537	41.5%	1.06 [0.93, 1.22]
Heterogeneity: Not applicable						
Test for overall effect: Z = 0.86 (P = 0.39)						
1.2 S-I vs Gem						
JASPAC 01	-0.56	0.13	187	190	12.0%	0.57 [0.44, 0.74]
Shimoda 2015	-0.36	0.34	29	28	1.8%	0.70 [0.36, 1.36]
Subtotal (95% CI)			216	218	13.8%	0.59 [0.46, 0.74]
Heterogeneity: Chi² = 0.30, df = 1 (P = 0.58); I² = 0%						
Test for overall effect: Z = 4.40 (P < 0.0001)						
1.3 Gem combined treatment vs Gem						
CONKO-005	-0.05	0.11	219	217	16.8%	0.95 [0.77, 1.18]
ESPAC-4	-0.2	0.09	364	366	25.1%	0.82 [0.69, 0.98]
Yoshitomi 2008	0.27	0.27	50	49	2.8%	1.31 [0.77, 2.22]
Subtotal (95% CI)			633	632	44.7%	0.89 [0.78, 1.02]
Heterogeneity: Chi² = 3.27, df = 2 (P = 0.19); I² = 39%						
Test for overall effect: Z = 1.69 (P = 0.09)						
Total (95% CI)			1400	1387	100.0%	0.90 [0.83, 0.99]
Heterogeneity: Chi² = 21.65, df = 5 (P = 0.0006); I² = 77%						
Test for overall effect: Z = 2.22 (P = 0.03)						
Test for subgroup differences: Chi² = 18.07, df = 2 (P = 0.0001), I² = 88.9%						

Fig. 2 Subgroup analyses of HR of OS for adjuvant treatments vs Gem alone

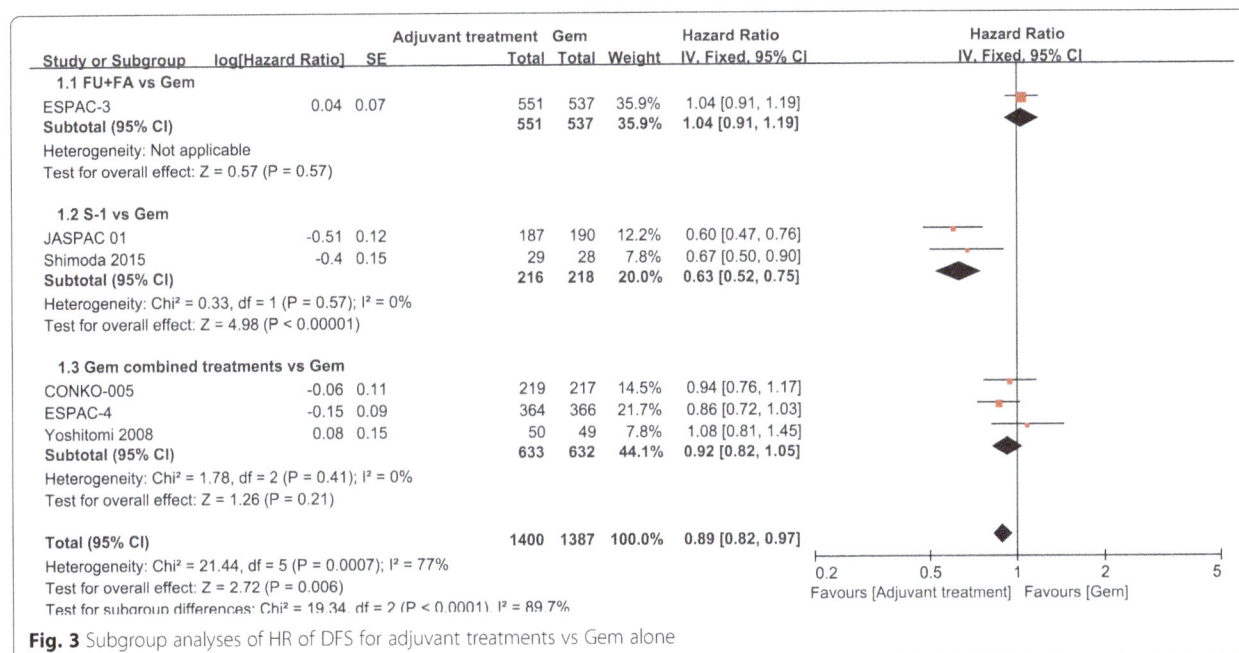

Study or Subgroup	log[Hazard Ratio]	SE	Adjuvant treatment Total	Gem Total	Weight	Hazard Ratio IV, Fixed, 95% CI	Hazard Ratio IV, Fixed, 95% CI
1.1 FU+FA vs Gem							
ESPAC-3	0.04	0.07	551	537	35.9%	1.04 [0.91, 1.19]	
Subtotal (95% CI)			551	537	35.9%	1.04 [0.91, 1.19]	
Heterogeneity: Not applicable							
Test for overall effect: Z = 0.57 (P = 0.57)							
1.2 S-1 vs Gem							
JASPAC 01	-0.51	0.12	187	190	12.2%	0.60 [0.47, 0.76]	
Shimoda 2015	-0.4	0.15	29	28	7.8%	0.67 [0.50, 0.90]	
Subtotal (95% CI)			216	218	20.0%	0.63 [0.52, 0.75]	
Heterogeneity: Chi² = 0.33, df = 1 (P = 0.57); I² = 0%							
Test for overall effect: Z = 4.98 (P < 0.00001)							
1.3 Gem combined treatments vs Gem							
CONKO-005	-0.06	0.11	219	217	14.5%	0.94 [0.76, 1.17]	
ESPAC-4	-0.15	0.09	364	366	21.7%	0.86 [0.72, 1.03]	
Yoshitomi 2008	0.08	0.15	50	49	7.8%	1.08 [0.81, 1.45]	
Subtotal (95% CI)			633	632	44.1%	0.92 [0.82, 1.05]	
Heterogeneity: Chi² = 1.78, df = 2 (P = 0.41); I² = 0%							
Test for overall effect: Z = 1.26 (P = 0.21)							
Total (95% CI)			1400	1387	100.0%	0.89 [0.82, 0.97]	
Heterogeneity: Chi² = 21.44, df = 5 (P = 0.0007); I² = 77%							
Test for overall effect: Z = 2.72 (P = 0.006)							
Test for subgroup differences: Chi² = 19.34, df = 2 (P < 0.0001), I² = 89.7%							

0.2   0.5   1   2   5
Favours [Adjuvant treatment]   Favours [Gem]

Fig. 3 Subgroup analyses of HR of DFS for adjuvant treatments vs Gem alone

(Additional file 3). The pooled results of the meta-analysis revealed an increased incidence of grade 3/4 diarrhea (RR, 5.11; 95%CI, 3.24–8.05; $P < 0.00001$) and decreased incidence of grade 3/4 leucopenia (RR, 0.55; 95%CI, 0.31–0.98; $P = 0.04$), thrombocytopenia (RR, 0.61; 95%CI, 0.39–0.97; $P = 0.04$) in adjuvant treatments group. Neutropenia (RR, 0.69; 95%CI, 0.36–1.29; $P = 0.24$) and fatigue (RR, 1.29; 95%CI, 0.95–1.77; $P = 0.11$) for patients between the two groups was not significantly different.

Assessment for publication bias
Additional files 4 and 5 represent funnel plots that test for publication bias. Funnel plots for OS (Additional file 4) and DFS (Additional file 5) supported the lack of evidence for publication bias.

Discussion
For pancreatic cancer treatment, surgery is preferred for best survival [4, 29]. However, the prognosis of the patient remains poor even after curative surgery owing to the high recurrence rate. Since 1996, gemcitabine has become the cornerstone for the treatment of pancreatic cancer. Burris et al. [30] further demonstrated that gemcitabine had a modest survival advantage over treatment with 5-FU in patients with advanced pancreatic cancer. The median survival duration of patients treated with gemcitabine was 5.65 months, compared with 4.41 months for patients treated with 5-FU. The CONKO-001 trial [31] also showed that the median DFS was 13.4 months in the gemcitabine-treated group and 6.7 months in the observation group after radical pancreatic cancer resection (HR, 0.55; 95%CI, 0.44–0.69; $P < 0.001$). Patients randomized to

adjuvant gemcitabine therapy had longer OS than those randomized to observation alone (HR, 0.76; 95%CI, 0.61–0.95; $P = 0.01$), with 5-year OS of 20.7% vs 10.4%, respectively, and 10-year OS of 12.2% vs 7.7%. Furthermore, some clinical trials have aimed at assessing the potential superiority of adjuvant chemotherapy over single-agent gemcitabine in resected pancreatic cancer, but the results were not determinate.

In this study, we evaluated six randomized controlled trials comparing adjuvant treatments with gemcitabine monotherapy in first-line treatment of patients undergoing pancreatectomy. Our pooled analysis revealed the overall clinical efficacy of adjuvant chemotherapy was not superior to that of gemcitabine monotherapy in OS (HR, 0.87; 95% CI, 0.70–1.07; $P = 0.19$) and DFS (HR, 0.85; 95% CI, 0.71–1.02; $P = 0.08$). The incidence of adverse events in adjuvant treatments group were increased in grade 3/4 diarrhea and decreased in grade 3/4 leucopenia, thrombocytopenia compared with gemcitabine alone. Although our analysis did not show that adjuvant therapy was superior to gemcitabine monotherapy for resected pancreatic cancer, further stratification analysis was needed given the large heterogeneity of the pooled results.

We next analyzed the clinical efficacy of FU + FA regimen, S-1 regimen and Gem combined regimen respectively, and found that only patients receiving S-1 treatment had a benefit compared with patients receiving gemcitabine alone.

Toxicity of subgroup in S-1 regimen showed the lower incidence of leucopenia, thrombocytopenia, neutropenia and higher diarrhea. Pooled analysis of subgroup analysis showed that S-1 chemotherapy had a significant OS benefit (HR, 0.59; 95% CI, 0.46–0.74; $P < 0.0001$) and DFS benefit (HR, 0.63; 95% CI, 0.52–0.75; $P < 0.00001$). But it should be pointed out that this was only included the results of two trials ($n = 434$). Most patients in the JASPAC 01 [27] study had stage II disease, whereas the majority in another study had stages III and IV [23]. The JASPAC 01 study was only enrolled with patients of Asians. At the same dose, Asians had lower toxic reaction to S-1 than Europeans due to different metabolism. Furthermore, the CAP-002 study [22] also reported that S-1and Gem+S-1(GS) provided similar efficacy to Gem as the adjuvant chemotherapy for resected pancreatic cancer. Two year DFS rate was 24.2%, 28.1% and 34.4% in Gem, S-1 and GS, respectively and the median OS was 21 m in Gem, 26 m in S-1 and 27.9 m in GS.

The ESPAC-1 trial reported that fluorouracil plus folinic acid regimen could improve OS after pancreatic cancer resection, increasing the estimated 2 year and 5 year survival to 40% and 21% compared with 30% and 8.0% for surgery alone [15]. However, the ESPAC-3 [28] trial showed no difference in OS and PFS between the study groups (median OS and 2-year survival rate, 23.0 months and 48.1% in the FU + FA group vs 23.6 months and 49.1% in the Gem group, respectively; $P = 0.39$. median PFS and 2-year survival rate, 14.1 months and 30.7% in the FU + FA group vs 14.3 months and 29.6% in the Gem group, respectively; $P = 0.53$). The outcome of univariate analysis of the ESPAC-3 trial revealed that tumor grade, tumor size, nodal status, resection margin, postoperative CA19–9 levels, performance status, and smoking were independent prognostic factors of OS. But resection margin status was not significant on multivariate analysis, confirming the results of the ESPAC-1 trial that increasingly differentiated tumors, tumor size, and lymph-node status were associated with prognosis. Toxicity analysis of the ESPAC-3 trial showed the lower incidence of leucopenia, thrombocytopenia and higher diarrhea in FU + FA group.

Our subgroup analysis showed that Gem combined therapy did not had a significant OS benefit (HR, 0.89; 95% CI, 0.78–1.02; $P = 0.09$) and DFS benefit (HR, 0.92; 95% CI, 0.82–1.05; $P = 0.21$). It had higher incidence of diarrhea in gemcitabine-based combination therapy group, but leucopenia, thrombocytopenia and neutropenia were no difference between the three groups. In the ESPAC-3 trial [28], the outcome demonstrated that gemcitabine was not superior to fluorouracil plus folinic acid in overall survival for patients with completely resected pancreatic cancer and suggested further comparison of the effects between gemcitabine combined with fluorouracil and folinic acid and gemcitabine monotherapy. Afterward, gemcitabine plus capecitabine (ESPAC-4) [26] trial showed a increase in overall survival, with an estimated 5 year OS of 28.8% (22.9–35.2) compared with 16.3% (10.2–23.7) with Gem and found that prognosis was relationship with postoperative CA19–9 concentrations and pathological margin. However, gemcitabine plus uracil/tegafur had no benefit compared with GEM alone for patients with resected pancreatic cancer. 1-year DFS rate was 50.0% in GU group and 49.0% in the Gem group. Median survival time was 21.2 months and 29.8 months, respectively [24]. Moreover, there were no significant differences in DFS and OS rates between N1, N2 and R0, R1 patients. Although gemcitabine plus erlotinib (GemErlo) had demonstrated a mild survival advantage for advanced pancreatic cancer [32, 33], it did not improve median DFS (GemErlo 11.4 months; Gem 11.4 months) or median overall survival (GemErlo 24.5 months; Gem 26.5 months) in patients with R0 resections in CONKO-005 trial [25]. Similarly, the combination therapy of Gem with sorafenib for 12 months can not improve DFS or OS for R1 resected pancreatic cancer patients in the CONKO-006 trial [21].

At present, some trials demonstrated that the oxaliplatin, irinotecan, fluorouracil, and leucovorin (FOLFIRINOX) and the combination chemotherapy of gemcitabine and nab-paclitaxel regimens had effect on metastatic pancreatic ductal adenocarcinoma (PDAC) [34–36]. Compared with gemcitabine, FOLFIRINOX and nab-paclitaxel plus gemcitabine showed survival advantage [34, 36]. Now, gemcitabine and nab-paclitaxel regimen is being investigated in ongoing phaseIII trial for its efficacy in the adjuvant setting (APACT [NCT01964430: Nab-Paclitaxel and Gemcitabine vs Gemcitabine Alone as Adjuvant Therapy for Patients With Resected Pancreatic Cancer]) [20].

The limitations of this study was the fact that the medicines tested in the trials were different, including chemotherapy drug and molecular targeted drug, which was used alone or in combination. Another limitation was the small number of trials that be included in the study because there were not many of these researches. The third limitation was relatively small number patients of some trials, although the total number of patients included in the meta- analysis was conspicuous.

Conclusion

In our meta-analysis, a significant survival benefit is only observed in the S-1 regimen, but the results are yet to be determined. Optimal cytotoxicity or targeted drug regimens need further validation in clinical trials in the future. Here, we think that a controlled trial of gemcitabine in combined with S-1 versus FOLFIRINOX or some of the other gents may be a viable option.

Additional files

Additional file 1: Table S1. Characteristics of randomized controlled trials.

Additional file 2: Table S2. Survival results from randomized trials (adjuvant treatments vs Gem alone).

> **Additional file 3: Table S3.** The incidence of grade 3/4 adverse events (adjuvant treatments vs Gem alone).
>
> **Additional file 4: Figure S1.** Funnel plot for OS for adjuvant treatments vs Gem alone. The outcome supported the lack of evidence for publication bias.
>
> **Additional file 5: Figure S2.** Funnel plot for DFS for adjuvant treatments vs Gem alone. The outcome supported the lack of evidence for publication bias.

Abbreviations

Cap: Capecitabine; CI: Confidence interval; DFS: Disease-free survival; Erlo: Erlotinib; FA: Folinic acid; FU: 5-Fluorouracil; Gem: Gemcitabine; GemErlo: Gemcitabine+erlotinib; GU: Gemcitabine+uracil/tegafur; HR: Hazard ratio; KPS: Karnofsky performance status; NA: Data not available; OS: Overall survival; PFS: Progress free survival; RCTs: Randomized controlled trials; RFS: Relapse-free survival; RR: Risk ratio; UFT: Uracil/tegafur

Acknowledgements
Not applicable.

Funding
No.

Availability of data and materials
Not applicable.

Authors' contributions
HC and RH conducted electronic database searches. MZ and CZ independently inspected all candidate articles and conducted study selection. HC, RH and XS conducted data extraction. HC and HZ performed the statistical analysis. HC drafted the manuscript. RQ conceived of the study together with HZ, participated in its design and coordination. All authors read and approved the final manuscript.

Consent for publication
Not applicable.

Competing interests
The authors declare that they have no competing interests.

References
1. Siegel RL, Miller KD, Jemal A. Cancer statistics, 2018. CA Cancer J Clin. 2018; 68:7–30.
2. Beger HG, Rau B, Gansauge F, Poch B, Link KH. Treatment of pancreatic cancer: challenge of the facts. World J Surg. 2003;27:1075–84.
3. Cress RD, Yin D, Clarke L, Bold R, Holly EA. Survival among patients with adenocarcinoma of the pancreas: a population-based study (United States). Cancer Causes Control. 2006;17:403–9.
4. Sener SF, Fremgen A, Menck HR, Winchester DP. Pancreatic cancer: a report of treatment and survival trends for 100,313 patients diagnosed from 1985-1995, using the National Cancer Database. J Am Coll Surg. 1999;189:1–7.
5. Oettle H, Post S, Neuhaus P, Gellert K, Langrehr J, Ridwelski K, Schramm H, Fahlke J, Zuelke C, Burkart C, et al. Adjuvant chemotherapy with gemcitabine vs observation in patients undergoing curative-intent resection of pancreatic cancer: a randomized controlled trial. JAMA. 2007;297:267–77.
6. Van den Broeck A, Sergeant G, Ectors N, Van Steenbergen W, Aerts R, Topal B. Patterns of recurrence after curative resection of pancreatic ductal adenocarcinoma. Eur J Surg Oncol. 2009;35:600–4.
7. Kayahara M, Nagakawa T, Ueno K, Ohta T, Takeda T, Miyazaki I. An evaluation of radical resection for pancreatic cancer based on the mode of recurrence as determined by autopsy and diagnostic imaging. Cancer. 1993; 72:2118–23.
8. Alexakis N, Halloran C, Raraty M, Ghaneh P, Sutton R, Neoptolemos JP. Current standards of surgery for pancreatic cancer. Br J Surg. 2004;91: 1410–27.
9. Brunner TB, Grabenbauer GG, Meyer T, Golcher H, Sauer R, Hohenberger W. Primary resection versus neoadjuvant chemoradiation followed by resection for locally resectable or potentially resectable pancreatic carcinoma without distant metastasis. A multi-centre prospectively randomised phase II-study of the Interdisciplinary Working Group Gastrointestinal Tumours (AIO, ARO, and CAO). BMC Cancer. 2007;7:41.
10. Kalser MH, Ellenberg SS. Pancreatic cancer. Adjuvant combined radiation and chemotherapy following curative resection. Arch Surg. 1985;120: 899–903.
11. Regine WF, Winter KA, Abrams RA, Safran H, Hoffman JP, Konski A, Benson AB, Macdonald JS, Kudrimoti MR, Fromm ML, et al. Fluorouracil vs gemcitabine chemotherapy before and after fluorouracil-based chemoradiation following resection of pancreatic adenocarcinoma: a randomized controlled trial. JAMA. 2008;299:1019–26.
12. Yeo CJ, Abrams RA, Grochow LB, Sohn TA, Ord SE, Hruban RH, Zahurak ML, Dooley WC, Coleman J, Sauter PK, et al. Pancreaticoduodenectomy for pancreatic adenocarcinoma: postoperative adjuvant chemoradiation improves survival. A prospective, single-institution experience. Ann Surg. 1997;225:621–33 discussion 633-626.
13. Neoptolemos JP, Dunn JA, Stocken DD, Almond J, Link K, Beger H, Bassi C, Falconi M, Pederzoli P, Dervenis C, et al. Adjuvant chemoradiotherapy and chemotherapy in resectable pancreatic cancer: a randomised controlled trial. Lancet. 2001;358:1576–85.
14. Smeenk HG, van Eijck CH, Hop WC, Erdmann J, Tran KC, Debois M, van Cutsem E, van Dekken H, Klinkenbijl JH, Jeekel J. Long-term survival and metastatic pattern of pancreatic and periampullary cancer after adjuvant chemoradiation or observation: long-term results of EORTC trial 40891. Ann Surg. 2007;246:734–40.
15. Neoptolemos JP, Stocken DD, Friess H, Bassi C, Dunn JA, Hickey H, Beger H, Fernandez-Cruz L, Dervenis C, Lacaine F, et al. A randomized trial of chemoradiotherapy and chemotherapy after resection of pancreatic cancer. N Engl J Med. 2004;350:1200–10.
16. Twombly R. Adjuvant chemoradiation for pancreatic cancer: few good data, much debate. J Natl Cancer Inst. 2008;100:1670–1.
17. Ueno H, Kosuge T, Matsuyama Y, Yamamoto J, Nakao A, Egawa S, Doi R, Monden M, Hatori T, Tanaka M, et al. A randomised phase III trial comparing gemcitabine with surgery-only in patients with resected pancreatic cancer: Japanese study Group of Adjuvant Therapy for pancreatic Cancer. Br J Cancer. 2009;101:908–15.
18. Jadad AR, Moore RA, Carroll D, Jenkinson C, Reynolds DJ, Gavaghan DJ, McQuay HJ. Assessing the quality of reports of randomized clinical trials: is blinding necessary? Control Clin Trials. 1996;17:1–12.
19. Tierney JF, Stewart LA, Ghersi D, Burdett S, Sydes MR. Practical methods for incorporating summary time-to-event data into meta-analysis. Trials. 2007;8:16.
20. Tempero MA, Cardin DB, Biankin A, Goldstein D, Moore M, O'Reilly EM, Philip PA, Riess H, Macarulla T, Yung L, et al. nab-paclitaxel (nab-P) plus gemcitabine (Gem) vs Gem alone as adjuvant treatment for resected pancreatic cancer (PC) in a phase III trial (APACT). J Clin Oncol. 2015;33:TPS4153.
21. Sinn M, Liersch T, Gellert K, Riess H, Stübs P, Waldschmidt DT, Pelzer U, Stieler J, Striefler JK, Bahra M, et al. LBA18CONKO-006: A randomized double-blinded phase IIB-study of adjuvant therapy with gemcitabine + sorafenib/placebo for patients with R1-resection of pancreatic cancer. Ann Oncol. 2014;25:mdu438 418-mdu438.418.
22. Yoshitomi H, Shimizu H, Yoshidome H, Ohtsuka M, Kato A, Furukawa K, Takayashiki T, Kuboki S, Okamura D, Suzuki D, et al. A randomized phase II trial of adjuvant chemotherapy with S-1 versus S-1 and gemcitabine (GS) versus gemcitabine alone (GEM) in patients with resected pancreatic cancer (CAP-002 study). J Clin Oncol. 2013;31:4056.
23. Shimoda M, Kubota K, Shimizu T, Katoh M. Randomized clinical trial of adjuvant chemotherapy with S-1 versus gemcitabine after pancreatic cancer resection. Br J Surg. 2015;102:746–54.
24. Yoshitomi H, Togawa A, Kimura F, Ito H, Shimizu H, Yoshidome H, Otsuka M, Kato A, Nozawa S, Furukawa K, et al. A randomized phase II trial of adjuvant

chemotherapy with uracil/tegafur and gemcitabine versus gemcitabine alone in patients with resected pancreatic cancer. Cancer. 2008;113:2448–56.

25. Sinn M, Bahra M, Liersch T, Gellert K, Messmann H, Bechstein W, Waldschmidt D, Jacobasch L, Wilhelm M, Rau BM, et al. CONKO-005: adjuvant chemotherapy with gemcitabine plus erlotinib versus gemcitabine alone in patients after R0 resection of pancreatic cancer: a multicenter randomized phase III trial. J Clin Oncol. 2017;35:3330–7.

26. Neoptolemos JP, Palmer DH, Ghaneh P, Psarelli EE, Valle JW, Halloran CM, Faluyi O, O'Reilly DA, Cunningham D, Wadsley J, et al. Comparison of adjuvant gemcitabine and capecitabine with gemcitabine monotherapy in patients with resected pancreatic cancer (ESPAC-4): a multicentre, open-label, randomised, phase 3 trial. Lancet. 2017;389:1011–24.

27. Uesaka K, Boku N, Fukutomi A, Okamura Y, Konishi M, Matsumoto I, Kaneoka Y, Shimizu Y, Nakamori S, Sakamoto H, et al. Adjuvant chemotherapy of S-1 versus gemcitabine for resected pancreatic cancer: a phase 3, open-label, randomised, non-inferiority trial (JASPAC 01). Lancet. 2016;388:248–57.

28. Neoptolemos JP, Stocken DD, Bassi C, Ghaneh P, Cunningham D, Goldstein D, Padbury R, Moore MJ, Gallinger S, Mariette C, et al. Adjuvant chemotherapy with fluorouracil plus folinic acid vs gemcitabine following pancreatic cancer resection: a randomized controlled trial. JAMA. 2010;304:1073–81.

29. Imamura M, Doi R, Imaizumi T, Funakoshi A, Wakasugi H, Sunamura M, Ogata Y, Hishinuma S, Asano T, Aikou T, et al. A randomized multicenter trial comparing resection and radiochemotherapy for resectable locally invasive pancreatic cancer. Surgery. 2004;136:1003–11.

30. Burris HA 3rd, Moore MJ, Andersen J, Green MR, Rothenberg ML, Modiano MR, Cripps MC, Portenoy RK, Storniolo AM, Tarassoff P, et al. Improvements in survival and clinical benefit with gemcitabine as first-line therapy for patients with advanced pancreas cancer: a randomized trial. J Clin Oncol. 1997;15:2403–13.

31. Oettle H, Neuhaus P, Hochhaus A, Hartmann JT, Gellert K, Ridwelski K, Niedergethmann M, Zulke C, Fahlke J, Arning MB, et al. Adjuvant chemotherapy with gemcitabine and long-term outcomes among patients with resected pancreatic cancer: the CONKO-001 randomized trial. JAMA. 2013;310:1473–81.

32. Gresham GK, Wells GA, Gill S, Cameron C, Jonker DJ. Chemotherapy regimens for advanced pancreatic cancer: a systematic review and network meta-analysis. BMC Cancer. 2014;14:471.

33. Moore MJ, Goldstein D, Hamm J, Figer A, Hecht JR, Gallinger S, Au HJ, Murawa P, Walde D, Wolff RA, et al. Erlotinib plus gemcitabine compared with gemcitabine alone in patients with advanced pancreatic cancer: a phase III trial of the National Cancer Institute of Canada Clinical Trials Group. J Clin Oncol. 2007;25:1960–6.

34. Conroy T, Desseigne F, Ychou M, Bouche O, Guimbaud R, Becouarn Y, Adenis A, Raoul JL, Gourgou-Bourgade S, de la Fouchardiere C, et al. FOLFIRINOX versus gemcitabine for metastatic pancreatic cancer. N Engl J Med. 2011;364:1817–25.

35. Von Hoff DD, Ramanathan RK, Borad MJ, Laheru DA, Smith LS, Wood TE, Korn RL, Desai N, Trieu V, Iglesias JL, et al. Gemcitabine plus nab-paclitaxel is an active regimen in patients with advanced pancreatic cancer: a phase I/II trial. J Clin Oncol. 2011;29:4548–54.

36. Von Hoff DD, Ervin T, Arena FP, Chiorean EG, Infante J, Moore M, Seay T, Tjulandin SA, Ma WW, Saleh MN, et al. Increased survival in pancreatic cancer with nab-paclitaxel plus gemcitabine. N Engl J Med. 2013;369: 1691–703.

Permissions

All chapters in this book were first published in CANCER, by BioMed Central; hereby published with permission under the Creative Commons Attribution License or equivalent. Every chapter published in this book has been scrutinized by our experts. Their significance has been extensively debated. The topics covered herein carry significant findings which will fuel the growth of the discipline. They may even be implemented as practical applications or may be referred to as a beginning point for another development.

The contributors of this book come from diverse backgrounds, making this book a truly international effort. This book will bring forth new frontiers with its revolutionizing research information and detailed analysis of the nascent developments around the world.

We would like to thank all the contributing authors for lending their expertise to make the book truly unique. They have played a crucial role in the development of this book. Without their invaluable contributions this book wouldn't have been possible. They have made vital efforts to compile up to date information on the varied aspects of this subject to make this book a valuable addition to the collection of many professionals and students.

This book was conceptualized with the vision of imparting up-to-date information and advanced data in this field. To ensure the same, a matchless editorial board was set up. Every individual on the board went through rigorous rounds of assessment to prove their worth. After which they invested a large part of their time researching and compiling the most relevant data for our readers.

The editorial board has been involved in producing this book since its inception. They have spent rigorous hours researching and exploring the diverse topics which have resulted in the successful publishing of this book. They have passed on their knowledge of decades through this book. To expedite this challenging task, the publisher supported the team at every step. A small team of assistant editors was also appointed to further simplify the editing procedure and attain best results for the readers.

Apart from the editorial board, the designing team has also invested a significant amount of their time in understanding the subject and creating the most relevant covers. They scrutinized every image to scout for the most suitable representation of the subject and create an appropriate cover for the book.

The publishing team has been an ardent support to the editorial, designing and production team. Their endless efforts to recruit the best for this project, has resulted in the accomplishment of this book. They are a veteran in the field of academics and their pool of knowledge is as vast as their experience in printing. Their expertise and guidance has proved useful at every step. Their uncompromising quality standards have made this book an exceptional effort. Their encouragement from time to time has been an inspiration for everyone.

The publisher and the editorial board hope that this book will prove to be a valuable piece of knowledge for researchers, students, practitioners and scholars across the globe.

List of Contributors

Hirofumi Harima, Seiji Kaino, Taro Takami, Shuhei Shinoda, Koichi Fujisawa, Naoki Yamamoto and Isao Sakaida
Department of Gastroenterology and Hepatology, Yamaguchi University Graduate School of Medicine, 1-1-1 Minami-Kogushi, Ube, Yamaguchi 755-8505, Japan

Takahiro Yamasaki
Department of Oncology and Laboratory Medicine, Yamaguchi University Graduate School of Medicine, 1-1-1 Minami-Kogushi, Ube, Yamaguchi 755-8505, Japan

Toshihiko Matsumoto
Department of Gastroenterology and Hepatology, Yamaguchi University Graduate School of Medicine, 1-1-1 Minami-Kogushi, Ube, Yamaguchi 755-8505, Japan
Department of Oncology and Laboratory Medicine, Yamaguchi University Graduate School of Medicine, 1-1-1 Minami-Kogushi, Ube, Yamaguchi 755-8505, Japan

Kanishka Chakraborty, Janet Lightner, Keely Hilton and Koyamangalath Krishnan
Division of Hematology-Oncology, Department of Internal Medicine, James H. Quillen College of Medicine, East Tennessee State University, Johnson City, TN 37614, USA

Victoria E. Palau
Division of Hematology-Oncology, Department of Internal Medicine, James H. Quillen College of Medicine, East Tennessee State University, Johnson City, TN 37614, USA
Department of Pharmaceutical Sciences, Gatton College of Pharmacy, East Tennessee State University, Johnson City, TN 37614, USA

Daniel Wann
Department of Internal Medicine, Beth Israel Deaconess Medical Center, Harvard Medical School, Boston, MA 02215, USA

Marianne Brannon and William Stone
Department of Pediatrics, James H. Quillen College of Medicine, East Tennessee State University, Johnson City, TN 37614, USA

Jacek Hajda and Monika Lehmann
Coordination Centre for Clinical Trials, University Hospital Heidelberg, Marsilius-Arkaden, Tower West, Im Neuenheimer Feld 130.3, 69120 Heidelberg, Germany

Ottheinz Krebs, Michael Dahm and Bernard Huber
Oryx GmbH and Co KG, Marktplatz 1, 85598 Baldham, Germany

Meinhard Kieser
Institute of Medical Biometry and Informatics, University Hospital Heidelberg, Marsilius-Arkaden, Tower West, Im Neuenheimer Feld 130.3, 69120 Heidelberg, Germany

Karsten Geletneky
Department of Neurosurgery, Klinikum Darmstadt, Grafenstraße 9, 64283 Darmstadt, Germany

Dirk Jäger, Christine E. Engeland, Christoph Springfeld and Guy Ungerechts
Department of Medical Oncology, National Center for Tumor Diseases (NCT), Im Neuenheimer Feld 460, 69120 Heidelberg, Germany

Tilman Schöning
Central Pharmacy, University Hospital Heidelberg, Im Neuenheimer Feld 670, 69120 Heidelberg, Germany

Oliver Sedlaczek
Department of Radiology, German Cancer Research Center, Im Neuenheimer Feld 280, 69120 Heidelberg, Germany

Albrecht Stenzinger
Department of Pathology, University Hospital Heidelberg, Im Neuenheimer Feld 224, 69120 Heidelberg, Germany

Niels Halama
Tissue Imaging and Analysis Center (TIGA), University Heidelberg – BioQuant, Im Neuenheimer Feld 267, 69120 Heidelberg, Germany

Volker Daniel
Institute of Immunology, Transplantation Immunology, University Hospital Heidelberg, Im Neuenheimer Feld 305, 69120 Heidelberg, Germany

Barbara Leuchs, Assia Angelova and Jean Rommelaere
Department of Applied Tumor Virology, German Cancer Research Center, Im Neuenheimer Feld 242, 69120 Heidelberg, Germany

Takuma Goto, Mikihiro Fujiya, Hiroaki Konishi, Junpei Sasajima, Shugo Fujibayashi, Akihiro Hayashi, Tatsuya Utsumi, Hiroki Sato, Takuya Iwama, Masami Ijiri, Aki Sakatani, Kazuyuki Tanaka, Yoshiki Nomura, Nobuhiro Ueno, Shin Kashima, Kentaro Moriichi, Yusuke Mizukami and Toshikatsu Okumura
Division of Gastroenterology and Hematology/Oncology, Department of Medicine, Asahikawa Medical University, 2-1 Midorigaoka-higashi, Asahikawa, Hokkaido 078-8510, Japan

Yutaka Kohgo
Department of Gastroenterology, International University of Health and Welfare Hospital, Nasushiobara, Japan

Shu-ta Wu, Kajal R. Grover, Bailey C. Allen, Ru Zhou, Mahboubeh Yazdanifar and Pinku Mukherjee
Department of Biological Sciences, University of North Carolina at Charlotte, Charlotte, NC 28223, USA

Anthony J. Fowler, Corey B. Garmon, Adam B. Fessler, Joshua D. Ogle and Craig A. Ogle
Department of Chemistry, University of North Carolina at Charlotte, Charlotte, NC 28223, USA

Chandra D. Williams
Department of Animal Laboratory Resources, University of North Carolina at Charlotte, Charlotte, NC 28223, USA

Berta Laquente
Institut Català d'Oncologia-IDIBELL (Institut d'Investigació Biomèdica de Bellvitge), Barcelona, Spain

Jose Lopez-Martin
University Hospital and Research Institute, Madrid, Spain

Donald Richards
US Oncology Research, Tyler, USA

Gerald Illerhaus
Hematology, Onkology, and Palliative Care, Klinikum Stuttgart, Stuttgart, Germany

David Z. Chang
Virginia Oncology Associates, Eastern Virginia Medical School, US Oncology Research, Hampton, VA, USA

George Kim
21st Century Oncology, University of Florida Health Oncology, Jacksonville, USA

Philip Stella
St. Joseph Mercy Hospital, Ypsilanti, MI, USA

Dirk Richel
Academic Medical Center, Amsterdam, Netherlands

Cezary Szcylik
Department of Oncology, Military Institute of Medicine, Warsaw, Poland

Stefano Cascinu
Department of Oncology and Hematology, Universitá di Modena e Reggio Emilia, Policlinico di Modena, Modena, Italy

G. L. Frassineti
Department of Oncology, Istituto Scientifico Romagnolo per lo Studio e la Cura dei Tumori (IRST) IRCCS, Meldola, Italy

Tudor Ciuleanu
Institute of Oncology Ion Chiricuta, University of Medicine and Pharmacy Iuliu Hatieganu, Cluj Napoca, Romania

Karla Hurt, Scott Hynes, Ji Lin and Aimee Bence Lin
Eli Lilly and Company, Indianapolis, IN, USA

Daniel Von Hoff
Translational Genomics Research Institute (TGen) and HonorHealth Research Institute, Phoenix, AZ, USA

Emiliano Calvo
START Madrid-CIOCC, Centro Integral Oncológico Clara Campal, Medical Oncology Division, Hospital Universitario Madrid Norte Sanchinarro, Calle Oña, 10, 28050 Madrid, Spain

Danielle C. Glassman, Randze L. Palmaira, Christina M. Covington, Avni M. Desai, Geoffrey Y. Ku, Jia Li, James J. Harding, Anna M. Varghese and Eileen M. O'Reilly
David M. Rubenstein Center for Pancreatic Cancer Research, Memorial Sloan Kettering Cancer Center, Weil Cornell Medical College, New York, NY, USA

Kenneth H. Yu
David M. Rubenstein Center for Pancreatic Cancer Research, Memorial Sloan Kettering Cancer Center, Weil Cornell Medical College, New York, NY, USA Gastrointestinal Oncology Service, Memorial Sloan Kettering Cancer Center, 300 East 66th Street, New York, NY 10065, USA

Feng Wang, Lijuan Hu, Yunfei Liu, Rui Cui and Wencong Tian
The Institute of Integrative Medicine for Acute Abdominal Diseases, Nankai Hospital, No. 6, Changjiang Road, Nankai, Tianjin 300100, China

Hongyi Liu
The Post-doctoral Working Station, Tianjin Medical University, Tianjin 300070, China

Yijie Duan
The Institute of Integrative Medicine for Acute Abdominal Diseases, Nankai Hospital, No. 6, Changjiang Road, Nankai, Tianjin 300100, China
The Centre of Disease Control, Dagang, Tianjin 300270, China

Anas M. Saad
Faculty of Medicine, Damascus University, Damascus, Syria

Tarek Turk
Faculty of Medicine, Damascus University, Damascus, Syria

Muneer J. Al-Husseini
Faculty of Medicine, Ain Shams University, Cairo, Egypt

Omar Abdel-Rahman
Clinical Oncology Department, Faculty of Medicine, Ain Shams University, Lofty Elsayed Street, Cairo 11566, Egypt
Department of Oncology, University of Calgary and Tom Baker Cancer Center, Calgary, Alberta, Canada

Mohammad Al-Kandari
Division of Anatomical Pathology, Vancouver General Hospital, Vancouver, British Columbia, Canada

Basile Tessier-Cloutier
Division of Anatomical Pathology, Vancouver General Hospital, Vancouver, British Columbia, Canada
Department of Pathology and Laboratory Medicine, University of British Columbia, Vancouver, British Columbia, Canada

Dongxia Gao
Division of Medical Oncology, University of British Columbia, Vancouver, British Columbia, Canada

David F. Schaeffer
Division of Anatomical Pathology, Vancouver General Hospital, Vancouver, British Columbia, Canada
Department of Pathology and Laboratory Medicine, University of British Columbia, Vancouver, British Columbia, Canada

Genetic Pathology Evaluation Centre, University of British Columbia, Vancouver, British Columbia, Canada
Pancreas Centre BC, Vancouver, British Columbia, Canada

Katy Milne
Deeley Research Centre, British Columbia Cancer Agency, Victoria, British Columbia, Canada

Brad H. Nelson
Deeley Research Centre, British Columbia Cancer Agency, Victoria, British Columbia, Canada
Department of Biochemistry and Microbiology, University of Victoria, Victoria, British Columbia, Canada

Steve E. Kalloger
Department of Pathology and Laboratory Medicine, University of British Columbia, Vancouver, British Columbia, Canada
Pancreas Centre BC, Vancouver, British Columbia, Canada
Division of Medical Oncology, British Columbia Cancer Agency, Vancouver, British Columbia, Canada
Department of Anatomical Pathology, Abbotosford Regional Hospital and Cancer Centre, Abbotsford, British Columbia, Canada

Daniel J. Renouf
Division of Medical Oncology, University of British Columbia, Vancouver, British Columbia, Canada
Pancreas Centre BC, Vancouver, British Columbia, Canada
Division of Medical Oncology, British Columbia Cancer Agency, Vancouver, British Columbia, Canada

Brandon S. Sheffield
Department of Anatomical Pathology, Abbotosford Regional Hospital and Cancer Centre, Abbotsford, British Columbia, Canada

Daniel L. P. Holyoake, Emmanouil Fokas and Maria A. Hawkins
CRUK/MRC Oxford Institute for Radiation Oncology, Department of Oncology, University of Oxford, Old Road Campus Research Building, Roosevelt Drive, Oxford OX3 7DQ, UK

Elizabeth Ward
Oncology Clinical Trials Office, Department of Oncology, University of Oxford, Old Road Campus Research Building, Roosevelt Drive, Oxford OX3 7DQ, UK

Derek Grose and David McIntosh
The Beatson West of Scotland Cancer Centre, 1053 Great Western Rd, Glasgow G12 0YN, UK

David Sebag-Montefiore
The University of Leeds, Cancer Research UK Leeds Centre, 14 Leeds Institute of Cancer and Pathology, Cancer Genetics Building, St James's University Hospital, 15 Beckett Street, Leeds, West Yorkshire LS9 7TF, UK
Leeds Cancer Centre, Leeds Teaching Hospitals NHS Trust, Bexley Wing, Beckett Street, Leeds LS9 7TF, UK

Ganesh Radhakrishna
Leeds Cancer Centre, Leeds Teaching Hospitals NHS Trust, Bexley Wing, Beckett Street, Leeds LS9 7TF, UK

Neel Patel and Michael Silva
Oxford University Hospitals NHS Foundation Trust, Old Road, Headington, Oxford OX3 7LE, UK

Somnath Mukherjee
CRUK/MRC Oxford Institute for Radiation Oncology, Department of Oncology, University of Oxford, Old Road Campus Research Building, Roosevelt Drive, Oxford OX3 7DQ, UK
Oxford University Hospitals NHS Foundation Trust, Old Road, Headington, Oxford OX3 7LE, UK

Victoria Y. Strauss and Lang'o Odondi
Centre for Statistics in Medicine, Nuffield Department of Orthopaedics, Rheumatology and Musculoskeletal Sciences, University of Oxford, Botnar Research Centre, Windmill Road, Oxford OX3 7LD, UK

Alan Melcher
The Institute of Cancer Research, Chester Beatty Laboratories, 237, Fulham Rd, London SW3 6JB, UK

Jan-Paul Gundlach, Charlotte Hauser, Thomas Becker and Jan-Hendrik Egberts
Department of General Surgery, Visceral, Thoracic, Transplantation and Pediatric Surgery, University Hospital Schleswig-Holstein (UKSH), Campus Kiel, Arnold-Heller Str. 3, Haus 18, 24105 Kiel, Germany

Franka Maria Schlegel, Christian Röder and Holger Kalthoff
Institute for Experimental Cancer Research, University of Kiel, Arnold-Heller Str. 3 (Haus 17), D-24105 Kiel, Germany

Christine Böger and Christoph Röcken
Department of Pathology, University Hospital Schleswig-Holstein (UKSH), Campus Kiel, Arnold-Heller Str. 3, Haus 14, 24105 Kiel, Germany

Anna Trauzold
Department of General Surgery, Visceral, Thoracic, Transplantation and Pediatric Surgery, University Hospital Schleswig-Holstein (UKSH), Campus Kiel, Arnold-Heller Str. 3, Haus 18, 24105 Kiel, Germany

Institute for Experimental Cancer Research, University of Kiel, Arnold-Heller Str. 3 (Haus 17), D-24105 Kiel, Germany

I. Otte and J. Vollmann
Institute for Medical Ethics and History of Medicine, Ruhr University Bochum, Markstr. 258a, D-44795 Bochum, Germany

S. Salloch
Institute for Ethics and History of Medicine, University Medicine Greifswald, Ellernholzstr. 1-2, D-17487 Greifswald, Germany

A. Reinacher-Schick
Department for Hematology, Oncology and Palliative Care, St. Josef-Hospital, Ruhr-University Bochum, Gudrunstr. 56, D-44791 Bochum, Germany

Akira Yamauchi, Masumi Itadani, Kayoko Kobiki and Futoshi Kuribayashi
Department of Biochemistry, Kawasaki Medical School, 577 Matsushima, Kurashiki, Okayama 701-0192, Japan

Masahiro Yamamura, Naoko Okada and Yoshiyuki Yamaguchi
Department of Clinical Oncology, Kawasaki Medical School, Okayama, Japan

Naoki Katase
Department of Molecular and Developmental Biology, Kawasaki Medical School, Okayama, Japan

Masafumi Nakamura
Department of Surgery and Oncology, Graduate School of Medical Sciences, Kyushu University, Fukuoka, Japan

Yoshiki Hirooka
Department of Endoscopy, Nagoya University Hospital, 65 Tsuruma-cho, Showa-ku, Nagoya 466-8550, Japan

Hideki Kasuya, Itzel B. Villalobos, Yoshinori Naoe and Toru Ichinose
Cancer Immune Therapy Research Center, Nagoya University Graduate School of Medicine, Nagoya, Japan

Takuya Ishikawa, Hiroki Kawashima, Eizaburo Ohno and Hidemi Goto
Department of Gastroenterology, Nagoya University Graduate School of Medicine, Nagoya, Japan

Nobuto Koyama and Maki Tanaka
Takara Bio Inc., Otsu, Japan

Yasuhiro Kodera
Department of Surgery II, Nagoya University Graduate School of Medicine, Nagoya, Japan

Tristan Lerbs and Martin Schneider
Department of General, Visceral and Transplantation Surgery, Im Neuenheimer Feld 110, 69120 Heidelberg, Germany

Savita Bisht, Peter Brossart and Georg Feldmann
Department of Internal Medicine 3, Center of Integrated Oncology (CIO) Cologne-Bonn, University Hospital of Bonn, Bonn, Germany

Sebastian Schölch, Mathieu Pecqueux, Thilo Welsch, Christoph Reissfelder, Nuh N. Rahbari, Johannes Fritzmann and Jürgen Weitz
Department of Gastrointestinal, Thoracic and Vascular Surgery, Medizinische Fakultät Carl Gustav Carus, Technische Universität Dresden, Fetscherstr. 74, 01307 Dresden, Germany

Glen Kristiansen
Department of Pathology, Center of Integrated Oncology Cologne-Bonn, University Hospital of Bonn, Bonn, Germany

Bianca T. Hofmann
Department of General, Visceral and Thoracic Surgery, University Medical Center Hamburg-Eppendorf, Martinistrasse 52, 20246 Hamburg, Germany

Christoph Kahlert
Department of General, Visceral and Transplantation Surgery, Im Neuenheimer Feld 110, 69120 Heidelberg, Germany
Department of Gastrointestinal, Thoracic and Vascular Surgery, Medizinische Fakultät Carl Gustav Carus, Technische Universität Dresden, Fetscherstr. 74, 01307 Dresden, Germany

Dandan Li and Udo Rudloff
Rare Tumor Initiative, Cancer for Cancer Research, National Cancer Institute, Building 10, Room 2B-38E, Bethesda, MD, USA

John E. Mullinax
Sarcoma Department, Moffitt Cancer Center, Tampa, FL, USA

Taylor Aiken
Thoracic and GI Oncology Branch, Center for Cancer Research, National Cancer Institute, Bethesda, MD, USA
Department of Surgery, University of Wisconsin School of Medicine and Public Health, Madison, WI, USA

Hongwu Xin
Laboratory of Oncology, Center for Molecular Medicine and Department of Molecular Biology and Biochemistry, School of Basic Medicine, Yangtze University, Jingzhou, Hubei, China

Gordon Wiegand
Flow Cytometry Core, Hollings Cancer Center, Medical University of South Carolina, Charleston, SC, USA

Andrew Anderson
Gilead Sciences, Foster City, CA, USA

Snorri Thorgeirsson
Laboratory of Experimental Carcinogenesis, Center for Cancer Research, National Cancer Institute, NIH, Bethesda, USA

Itzhak Avital
St. Peter's Hospital, Rutgers University, Robert Wood Johnson School of Medicine, New Brunswick, NJ, USA

Meng Zhuo, Ting Han, Jiujie Cui, Feng Jiao and Liwei Wang
Department of Oncology, Renji Hospital, School of Medicine, Shanghai Jiaotong University, 160 Pujian Road, Shanghai 200127, China

Cuncun Yuan
Department of Pathology, Eye Ear Nose and Throat Hospital, Fudan University, 83 Fenyang Road, Shanghai 200031, China

Hua Chen, Ruizhi He, Xiuhui Shi, Min Zhou, Chunle Zhao, Hang Zhang and Renyi Qin
Department of Biliary-Pancreatic Surgery, Affiliated Tongji Hospital, Tongji Medical College, Huazhong University of Science and Technology, Wuhan 430030, China

Index

A

Acetonitrile, 13-14, 49, 56

Acid Sphingomyelinase, 11-12, 23-24

Antiproliferative Activity, 1-2, 4-5, 7-8, 10

C

Cancer Cachexia, 78-80, 86, 88-89

Cancer Cell Migration, 134-135, 139, 141, 143

Caveolin,, 11

Cellular Proliferation, 2, 4, 9, 12, 43

Ceramide Distribution, 11

Ceramide Synthesis, 11-12, 14-17, 20-22

Ceramide Transport, 11-12, 17-18, 24

Chemoradiation, 116, 190, 195

Chemoresistance, 44, 155, 163, 172-176

Chemotaxis, 134, 136-139, 142-144

Chemotherapeutic Drug, 46-47

Clinical Oncology, 144

Clinical Protocol, 26

Confocal Microscopy, 13, 46

Cytokine, 78, 80, 83, 88

D

De Novo Pathway, 11-12, 14, 16, 22

Death Receptor, 13, 23-24, 118-119, 126-127

Deferasirox, 1-3, 8, 10

Deferoxamine, 1-2, 10

Dihydroceramide, 11-13, 16

Dihydroceramide Desaturase, 11

Diphenyltetrazolium Bromide, 46, 50

Dose-limiting Toxicity, 115, 145, 148

E

Epithelial-mesenchymal Transition, 1, 9, 144, 154, 161-162, 175

Exosome,, 35

F

Fluorescein Diacetate, 46, 48-52, 54, 56

Fluoropyrimidine Agent, 189

Fluorouracil, 2, 34, 47, 56, 65, 68-69, 76-77, 96, 116, 150, 152, 189-190, 192, 194-196

G

Gastrinoma, 91

Gemcitabine, 10, 26-27, 29-31, 34, 43-45, 47, 57, 59-61, 63-70, 73, 75-77, 100, 114-117, 128, 130-133, 145-148, 150-153, 163, 165-173, 175-176, 189-191, 193-196

I

Immunhistology, 118

Immuno-oncology, 101

Immunofluorescence, 11-13, 19-22, 165

Intraductal Papillary Mucinous Neoplasm, 35-36, 44

Iron Chelator, 1-2, 5, 7, 10

L

Lactate Dehydrogenase, 8

Leukemia, 7, 10, 16, 24

Lipid Transport, 11

Lung Adenocarcinoma, 101, 144, 178, 188

M

Membrane Lipid, 11, 24, 169

Membrane Sphingomyelin, 16, 24

Metastasis, 9-10, 12, 23, 25, 27-30, 33-34, 43-44, 47, 57, 76, 87, 105, 118-119, 121, 123, 126-127, 134-135, 143, 146, 154, 156-157, 161-164, 176, 178, 180, 182, 188, 190, 195

Metastatic Pancreatic Cancer, 10, 25, 34, 59-60, 63, 65-66, 76-77, 150, 152-153, 176, 196

N

Nab-paclitaxel, 10, 26, 29, 34, 47, 57, 60, 65-66, 68-69, 76-77, 150, 152-153, 176, 194-196

Nanoliposomal Irinotecan, 68, 76

Neuronal Tissue, 31

Neutropenia, 59, 63, 65, 74, 147, 189, 192-194

Nuclear Localization, 118, 120-121, 126

O

Oncolytic Virotherapy, 26

Oncolytic Virus, 34, 145-146, 152

Optimal Cytotoxicity, 189, 194

Orthotopic Tumor Model, 50

P

Paclitaxel, 2, 10, 26, 29, 34, 46-49, 56-58, 60, 65-66, 68-69, 76-77, 132, 150, 152-153, 176, 194-196

Pancreatic Cancer, 1-12, 14-18, 20-21, 23, 25-28, 31-36, 44, 56-57, 59-60, 63, 65-68, 75-81, 83, 87-92, 96-97, 99-102, 106, 126-127, 143-146, 158, 170, 172-173, 183, 193-196

Pancreatic Carcinoma, 10, 34, 88, 100, 109, 126, 128, 152-153, 174, 195

Pancreatic Ductal Adenocarcinoma, 26, 44-46, 56-58, 69, 76-77, 101-102, 108-109, 113, 118-119, 126, 130, 155-156, 161-162, 175-179, 188

Parvovirus, 26

Pharmacokinetic, 30, 61, 64, 69, 73

Phosphorylation, 10, 20, 22, 24, 79, 134, 136-138, 141-143, 171, 176
Poly Lactic-co-glycolic Acid, 46-47
Propidium Iodide, 1, 3, 167, 175

S
Somatostatinoma, 91
Sphingomyelin, 11-18, 20-22, 24
Sphingosine, 12-13, 23-24, 144
Stereotactic Body Radiation Therapy, 110-111, 115, 117

T
Tetrazolium, 1-2
Thrombocytopenia, 59, 63-64, 147, 189, 192-194

Tocotrienol, 11-12, 23
Tumor Marker, 27, 35, 151
Tyrosine Kinase, 14, 143, 163, 173, 175, 177

W
Warburg Effect, 78-80, 83, 86-87

X
Xenografted Tumor, 9

www.ingramcontent.com/pod-product-compliance
Lightning Source LLC
Chambersburg PA
CBHW080659200326

41458CB00013B/4910